Fundamentals of Endocrinology

Fundamentals of Endocrinology

W. Roy Slaunwhite, Jr.
State University of New York
Buffalo, New York

MARCEL DEKKER, INC.   New York and Basel

Library of Congress Cataloging-in-Publication Data

Slaunwhite, W. Roy
   Fundamentals of endocrinology / by W. Roy Slaunwhite, Jr.
      p.   cm.
   Includes bibliographies and index.
   ISBN 0-8247-7714-X
   1. Endocrinology.   I. Title.
   [DNLM: 1. Endocrine Glands–physiology.   2. Hormones–physiology.
WK 102 S6302f]
QP187.S473 1988
612'.4--dc19
DNLM/DLC
for Library of Congress   87-30574
                                                                            CIP

MARCEL DEKKER, INC.
270 Madison Avenue, New York, New York 10016

Current printing (last digit):
10 9 8 7 6 5 4 3 2 1

PRINTED IN THE UNITED STATES OF AMERICA

To Maria Slaunwhite
for her support
during the prolonged gestation
of this book

Foreword

In the remote 1950s, when Roy Slaunwhite and I were young, there flowed from Buffalo, where he and Avery Sandberg worked together in biochemistry, what seemed to the envious rest of us junior endocrinologists an endless stream of sharply focused, superbly executed, clearly presented studies on every facet of the metabolism of steroid hormones. Trained in part by the great Leo T. Samuels of the University of Utah, Slaunwhite and Sandberg displayed impressive technical expertise; the application of it was at once practical and theoretically valid. Their studies on the disposition in the human body of corticosteroids and androgens, on the role of the enterohepatic circulation in what might be called the detoxification of estrogens, and on many other topics of wide application still stand as landmarks in the field, not likely to be supplanted or surpassed.

That body of superior work has uniquely qualified the author to write a book like this. So have his thirty years of teaching medical students, medical technologists, and pre- and postdoctoral fellows in biochemistry and endocrinology at the State University of New York. What is peculiarly his own is his capacity, manifested notably in this volume, to write about a complex subject simply and clearly. That is not to say that he oversimplifies at the expense of the intricate truth. Slaunwhite's book is no primer for children. He is wise enough to recognize that endocrinology is a subject broad and deep, based on hard chemical data but delicate, nevertheless; wide-ranging but not embracing the cosmos. He senses its limits and knows his own. Endocrinology (indeed, each individual patient with an endocrine disorder) forms a complicated mosaic. Professor Slaunwhite knows, and his book demonstrates, that you cannot force simplicity upon a subject intrinsically complicated and one wherein.many questions remain unanswered.

The organization of this text is original and at the same time masterly. It is no longer possible to present endocrine science in the conventional textbook-of-medicine manner, with chapters neatly arranged to correspond with the little clusters of cells traditionally regarded as "the" endocrine glands: pituitary, thyroid, parathyroids, adrenal cortex and medulla, endocrine pancreas, ovary, and testis. Most textbooks of endocrinology still follow a modified version of this old scheme. Professor Slaunwhite holds a wider view, taking into account modern concepts of what a hormone is and a much expanded idea of the definition of a gland, including, among many other organs and tissues, the placenta, the lung, and—perhaps the biggest and most elaborate gland of all—the gut. He leaves out nothing important: Neither the brain nor the hypothalamus nor the ubiquitous prostaglandins are omitted. Hormone receptors and genetic factors are properly emphasized. Best of all, for either the new or the seasoned student of endocrinology, the materials are arranged along functional lines. The author has brought off the impossible: an approach that is novel but that is based upon classical biological and chemical data.

This book is a readable, indeed a compelling, account of a rapidly moving area of science, a narrative that does not pretentiously try to freeze highly mutable information into definitive stone. We have here a useful and trustworthy guide for the novice, and an imaginative and stimulating treatise for the experienced endocrinologist, young or old.

Nicholas P. Christy, M.D.
Professor of Medicine
Health Science Center at Brooklyn, SUNY, and
Chief of Staff
Brooklyn VAMC, New York

Preface

One does not lightly undertake writing a text, even an introductory one. The precipitating event in my case was the need to write extensive handouts for dental and medical school classes because existing texts slighted burgeoning and exciting discoveries in the biochemical aspects of endocrinology. Graduate classes were even more severely handicapped.

Next came the need to "organize" the presentation of a large amount of material. I had always "followed the pack" as it were, using an organ approach, but I decided to break with tradition and organize each chapter about a biological function. Although this requires discussing the thyroid in two chapters and the adrenal cortex in three, it does allow a holistic treatment of broad areas, which I have found satisfying.

The most difficult issue with which I still constantly struggle is the matter of detail. Where does one draw the line, so to speak? Several principles guide me. I wanted a readable, stimulating text for beginners, not a sophisticated reference for experts. The beginners must, however, have a basic background in biology, chemistry, and perhaps one semester of biochemistry, although this last requirement could be abridged by a capable and willing instructor. Hence, this book should be suitable for upperclassmen, graduate, or professional students.

Each chapter summarizes the biological aspects of the subject so that the student can place the modern biochemistry and physiology in the overall context of the body's ecology. Selected clinical aspects are included to illustrate the practical applications of endocrinology in humans. These sections are always found at the end of each chapter and may be readily omitted at the discretion of the instructor.

To maintain intellectual vigor, relevant critical techniques and experiments are inserted so that an impression of a dynamic, expanding discipline is transmitted. Open-ended questions are posed, which instructors and students may pursue if they so wish. And finally, bibliographies at the end of each chapter may be used to delve deeper into intriguing topics.

Before closing, I must acknowledge my indebtedness to my students, who criticized early drafts, and to several colleagues who offered many helpful suggestions: Kent Crickard, Chester Deluca, Margaret MacGillivray, Robert Pedersen, Stephen Spaulding, Judith Van Liew, and Julian Walters.

W. Roy Slaunwhite, Jr.

Introduction

In one sense, endocrinology is timeless, but in another it is modern, in the vanguard of the biomedical sciences. Ancient writings including the Bible mention eunuchs, and it has been known for some time that castration produces a pliable and docile animal, as well as one incapable of reproduction. Greek and Egyptian physicians knew the basic symptoms of diabetes mellitus. Although they had no instruments or scientific technology, they used their senses to the fullest. They observed that the urine of certain individuals attracted flies and was sweet. These individuals ate and drank a great deal, but perversely grew thinner and weaker until they died. Presumably, they were looking at what we call Type I diabetes (see Chapter 9). (Due to their shorter life span and different lifestyles, it is unlikely that Type II diabetes occurred often among the ancients.)

The science of endocrinology, the study of the endocrine glands or those glands that secrete their products into the vascular compartment, started in the late nineteenth century with the demonstration that a lipid testicular extract painted on the comb of a capon or injected would reverse the effects of castration, restoring the typical male plumage. It would be many decades before the active principle in that lipid extract would be identified as testosterone (see Chapter 8), but the technique of excising a gland or tissue, noting the panoply of effects produced, administering an extract of the organ or tissue excised, and noting the disappearance of the syndrome became the basis of endocrinology. Often one aspect of the syndrome was especially sensitive and easy to quantitate, and one had a bioassay to use in the purification of the active principle.

In the first half of the twentieth century, pioneers in endocrinology removed glands and isolated in pure form the active substances. Some glands turned out to be very complex. The adrenal was found grossly and histologically to be two tissues: The inner medulla was neural in origin while the outer cortex, derived from mesoderm, made three different types of steroid hormones. Similarly, the pituitary or hypophysis contained in many species, but not man, three lobes, one of which, the neurohypophysis or posterior pituitary, was an extension of the brain. It was found to contain two related hormones. The adenohypophysis or anterior pituitary was the most complex, secreting no fewer than six hormones!

These were indeed exciting years, as one hormone after another was identified, isolated, and characterized. The excitement was not in identifying another substance, for many other natural compounds were characterized during this period; rather it was the realization that these hormones were special. In spite of their small, indeed, often minute, concentrations, they had dramatic effects on the body. Moreover, some of the syndromes produced in animals bore a remarkable resemblance to certain pathological conditions in humans. Perhaps, mankind was on the verge of explaining some inexplicable human disease states! Alas, it was not to be that easy. While medicine gained some valuable tools, science had progressed only one step toward a molecular explanation of endocrine disease.

During the second half of the twentieth century, while isolation of new hormones continued in full swing, many scientists turned their attention to the mechanisms of action of hormones. After several dead ends had been explored, Sutherland discovered a cytosolic cyclic nucleotide, cyclic adenosine monophosphate (cAMP). What a lodestone this was to be! During the following years, it provided an answer to a conundrum that had frustrated endocrinologists: How were cells able to respond to hormones so large and so hydrophilic that they could not readily pass through plasma cell membranes? Could it be that the membrane might contain transducing molecules that could respond to a specific hormone, the primary signal, with the production of an intracellular "second messenger"? The answer is, of course, yes, and cAMP was the first of a series of intracellular messengers to be discovered.

Since hormones are transported in the blood, every cell (except possibly those behind the blood-brain barrier) is exposed to dozens of hormones, yet each cell type responds to only a small number. This demands that the exofacial side of the plasma membrane contain substances with a very high affinity for a specific hormone. We call this class of substances receptors. The ability to detect and quantitate receptors depended on the development of a new technique called radioimmunoassay. Historically, Yalow developed this technique for the measurement of hormones in plasma, but its properties of sensitivity and specificity ideally suited it to the measurement of receptors also. With the marriage of these two discoveries, investigators rapidly demonstrated that many hormones utilized cAMP-dependent protein kinases to propagate the hormonal message. Significantly, some hormones did not work this way, and other second messengers were discovered (see Chapter 1). The intracellular messengers for some hormones, most notably insulin, have not yet been discovered.

The last major breakthrough in endocrinology has been the application of techniques of molecular biology that are more powerful and easier to use, in general, than those of polypeptide biochemistry. In an

Table Nobel Prizes Awarded for the Study of Hormones

Year	Name	Subject
1909	Theodor Kocher	Study of the thyroid
1923	Frederic Banting	Isolation of insulin
	John J. R. Macleod	
1939	Adolf Butenandt (declined)	Chemistry of sex hormones
1947	Bernado A. Houssay	Study of the pituitary
1950	Philip S. Hench	Study of adrenocortical hormones
	Edward C. Kendall	
	Tadeus Reichstein	
1955	Vincent duVigneaud	Isolation of oxytocin and vasopressin
1958	Frederick Sanger	Technique of polypeptide sequencing; application to insulin
1966	Charles B. Huggins	Hormonal treatment of prostatic cancer
1971	Earl W. Sutherland, Jr.	Discovery of cAMP
1977	Roslyn Yalow	Radioimmunoassay
	Roger C. L. Guillemin	Isolation of hypothalamic hormones
	Andrew V. Schally	
1982	Sune Bergstrom	Isolation and biochemistry of prostaglandins
	Bengt Samuelsson	
	John R. Vane	
1984	Robert Merrifield	Automated synthesis of peptide hormones and enzymes

Source: From *Information Please Almanac,* 1985, Houghton Mifflin Co., Boston, pp 637–643.

amazingly short time (<10 years), the genes for a number of receptors as well as prohormones have been isolated and sequenced. Not too surprisingly, the nucleotide sequences of some oncogenes producing abnormal growth show some similarity to those of receptors for growth factors regulating normal growth. We are getting closer to answering some basic questions concerning cancer.

As you can see, endocrinology is an exciting area, and it will surely remain at the forefront of medical science for some decades to come. It is also a demanding discipline, for it is a truly interdisciplinary science, imposing additional burdens on the novice, but I hope that you will find it, as I have, rewarding.

I am a stranger to you, and why should you trust my enthusiasm? Let me give a more general perspective. Each year since 1901, a group of august authorities gathers to award Nobel Prizes in chemistry and in medicine and physiology. This is an exceedingly difficult task, for there are many outstanding scientists working in many different areas. No one knows the details of their deliberations, but their annual announcements form a pattern. It is not sufficient to be outstanding in your field: The field itself is important. In the table notice how frequently the Nobel Prize has been awarded to those working in endocrinology!

W. Roy Slaunwhite, Jr.

Contents

Foreword (*Nicholas P. Christy, M.D.*)   *v*
Preface   *vii*
Introduction   *ix*

1   Endocrinology: A Perspective   1
2   Hormones: An Overview   47
3   Nutrition and Regulatory
    Polypeptides of the
    Gastrointestinal Tract   67
4   Growth   99
5   Thyroid Hormones   129
6   Salt and Water Metabolism   155
7   Metabolism of Calcium and
    Phosphorus   195
8   Reproduction   223
9   Fuel Metabolism   315
    Appendixes   395

    Index   *403*

1

Endocrinology: A Perspective

Definition of a Hormone   2
The Chemical Nature of Hormones   3
Some Properties of Hormones   3
    Prohormones and preprohormones   4
    Secretion   7
    Transport   8
    Negative feedback   8
    Diurnal rhythm   10
    Episodic secretion   10
    Biological amplification   10
    Receptor-mediated hormone action   11
Paracrine and Neurocrine Hormones   23
Cholesterol and Steroidogenesis   24
Techniques   27
    Ablation–replacement   27
    Saturation analysis   27
    Monoclonal antibodies   30
Clinical Aspects   31
    Definitions   31
    Hypofunction and hyperfunction   32
    The role of genes   33
    Techniques   36
    Serum or plasma versus urine sampling   36
    Treatment   37
Summary   37
Supplemental Bibliography   41

Endocrinology as an entity is about 100 years old and as a science about 70 years of age. The attractiveness of endocrinology as a science is its multidisciplinary approach to understanding endocrine syndromes. The integration of knowledge from physiology, histology, biochemistry, pathology, pharmacology, biophysics, and medicine appeals to those who resist narrow compartmentalization. Endocrinology is dynamic and constantly changing. This text tries to inculcate the basic information upon which all changes will be built while exposing you to new hypotheses, some of which must inevitably fall to the onslaught of new data. With these challenges, let us begin!

The most frightening aspect of a new, technical area is the "jargon" that necessarily accompanies it. Although there is no way to escape it, there is no dictum that it must all be learned at once. So, relax! Each term will be explained again in later chapters. At the moment, try to ignore the trees and see the forest. There are principles which, once grasped, enable one to assimilate details more readily.

DEFINITION OF A HORMONE

It used to be easy to define a hormone: it was the product of secretion, as opposed to excretion, from an endocrine gland. With the recent introduction of the concepts of paracrine and neurocrine hormones, demarcations have become fuzzy and attempts to classify and categorize have led to frustration. So, let me first simplify by limiting our discussion to the classic endocrine hormones. After all, the overwhelming bulk of the endocrine literature is concerned with them. Later, I will return to the newer concepts.

Hormones are chemicals that
1. Are *secreted* in minute amounts directly into the blood stream (through the extracellular fluid), classically from "ductless" glands. (We must recognize, however, that there are bits of endocrine tissue scattered throughout exocrine organs, such as the pancreas, gut, and kidney; they do, however, obey the principle of secretion.)
2. Are *transported* by the vascular system, some of them tightly bound to specific plasma proteins.
3. Act at *remote* loci (in cellular terms) on *specific* target cells producing a *specific* effect. (Note that one hormone may have multiple targets and several actions.)
4. Act, together with the neural system, as physiologic regulators of the metabolism of the whole body and, either in a positive or negative sense, physiologic integrators of metabolism, usually in concert with one or more other hormones.

It is the complexity of this last aspect that is most fascinating to investigators and dismaying to students.

THE CHEMICAL NATURE OF HORMONES

Hormones are mostly polypeptides that cover the gamut in size from a tripeptide to subunit proteins having a molecular mass of about 30,000 daltons (30 kDa). Some are also glycopeptides. The primary structure of most of the known hormones has been established, and sequence homology among some suggests their relatedness and allows us to group them into "families." A few have been extensively investigated. For example, x-ray crystallographic structures are available for several forms of insulin. Also, analogues of many of the smaller hormones have been synthesized, and some of them have interesting properties.

A few hormones are derivates of tyrosine, e.g., dopamine, epinephrine, norepinephrine, thyroxine, and triiodothyronine.

Another small group consists of the steroids. These are produced by the adrenal cortex, gonads, corpus luteum, and the fetoplacental unit. They may be broadly classified as glucocorticosteroids and mineralocorticosteroids, progestins, androgens, and estrogens. In addition, a modified steroid formed in the kidney regulates calcium absorption from the intestine.

SOME PROPERTIES OF HORMONES

Classically, hormones have been isolated from endocrine tissue by following the bioactivity associated with that tissue through a process of extraction and fractionation. Insulin, the second polypeptide hormone to be isolated by this procedure (1921), is important, not only in endocrinology, but in protein chemistry. Initially, scientists believed that the primary structure (amino acid sequence) of insulin, like that of ribonuclease, contained all the information needed for formation of the correct secondary and tertiary structure. The failure of reduced insulin to regain appreciable bioactivity upon gentle oxidation with air meant, however, that there had to be a larger precursor form of insulin. Indeed, with the advent of radioimmunoassay (RIA), larger, inactive forms of many polypeptide hormones were detected in human plasma. The techniques of gene expression then provided incontrovertible evidence that some polypeptide hormones exist initially as larger precursors called prohormones.

There is no consensus on the nomenclature of a "classic," active hormone. I use the term "mature" because it denotes a time-related process and shun the term "native" because of the implication that the precursor forms are not native.

Prohormones and Preprohormones

This facet of endocrinology is still unfolding, and judgment must be reserved on the classifications that I present. Based largely on the translation of appropriate mRNAs in cell-free systems and on the sequencing of corresponding DNAs (or cDNAs), one can discern presently three classes of precursor hormones (Table 1.1). The common feature to all, however, is the presence of a signal sequence of variable length (19 to 29 amino acids). In accord with Blobel's initial observations, about two-thirds of these are hydrophobic residues, possibly to aid in penetration of the phospholipid membrane of the endoplasmic reticulum. The COOH-terminal residue of the signal sequence is frequently glycine or alanine, but it may also be serine, threonine, or proline; all, however, are small. This preliminary or leader sequence is commonly denoted simply as *pre-* followed by the name of the hormone, e.g., preproinsulin.

In one group of hormones removal of the leader sequence immediately produces the mature hormone. Prolactin, somatotropin (or growth hormone), and chorionic somatomammotropin are illustrative of this group. These three hormones also comprise a "family" having extensive sequence homology (see Chap. 4). Thus, this group may not represent a class, but merely a family.

Another group represented by insulin and parathyroid hormones yields a prohormone upon removal of the signal sequence. Remember that this is an extremely rapid process. Current concepts visualize removal of the signal sequence from the NH_2-terminus of the prohormone as it enters the cisternae of the endoplasmic reticulum, perhaps even before synthesis has been completed on the polysomes. The residual prohormone then travels down the cisternae to the Golgi apparatus where it is packaged into secretory granules for storage. If the stimulus for secretion is not too great, another small peptide is clipped off, leaving the mature hormone ready for secretion. Large, and especially prolonged, stimuli promote the secretion of a mixture of hormone and prohormone.

Table 1.1 Prohormones and Preprohormones

Hormone	Species	Pro sequence No. amino acids	Pre sequence No. amino acids	Amino acid −1[a]
Insulin	Rat	33	23	Ala
PTH	Bovine	6	25	Gly
Prosomatostatin	Porcine, piscine	79	26	Gly
PRL	Human, rat, bovine	None	28, 29	Pro, Thr
STH	Human, rat	None	26	Ala, Ala
CS	Human	None	26	Ala
Glucagon	Piscine (angler)	32	19	Ser
Proopiomelanocortin	Bovine, murine	NA	26	Gly
Proenkephalin	Bovine	NA	—	—
Propressophysin	Rat	NA	—	—

NA, not applicable.

[a]The numbering in prohormones and preprohormones starts at +1 at the amino terminal end of the prohormone; pre-sequences are numbered *negatively* starting at the carboxyl terminus with −1 and increasing consecutive negative numbers as one progresses to the amino terminus of the preprohormone.

Structurally, the *pro* sequence may be located either NH$_2$-terminally or internally. It is usually separated from the mature hormone by a basic dipeptide—Lys-Lys, Lys-Arg, or Arg-Arg. Proinsulin, for example, consists of a single polypeptide chain with the pro sequence located internally. The intact prohormone correctly positions three disulfide bonds required for the biological activity of mature insulin. Prohormones have weak to no biological activity.

A third class may be called the multihormone gene products. Translation of a single gene produces a large polypeptide containing more than one hormone molecule separated from each other by the customary basic dipeptide. Cleavage of the basic dipeptides produces equimolar quantities of the relevant hormones. Proopiomelanocortin, proenkephalin, propressophysin, and proglucagon are examples of this class. (Piscine proglucagon is slightly different from the other three in that it contains two glucagon-related sequences arranged in tandem, and the propressophysin gene codes for a hormone and its carrier protein.)

The liberation of active, mature hormone from the prohormone requires a highly specific, trypsin-type peptidase. Glandular kallikreins (EC 3.4.28.8) are members of a closely related subfamily of serine proteases that may do this. For many years, tissue kallikreins have been known to act on kininogen to liberate kinins, e.g., lysylbradykinin, a vasoactive decapeptide. The recent isolation and sequencing of rat pancreatic kallikrein mRNA has allowed the prediction of its amino acid sequence. The predicted preprozymogen of 265 amino acids (29,227 daltons) includes a secretary prepeptide of 17 amino acids and an activation peptide of 11 amino acids. The amino acid sequence of the predicted active form has extensive homology with kallikreins from other exocrine tissues from both rat and pig, as well as with the γ-subunit of mouse nerve growth factor (see Chap. 4), epidermal growth factor-binding protein (see Chap. 4), and rat tonin, indicating their derivation from a common gene. These proteases have high specificity with a general, but not absolute, preference for residues that bear positively charged side chains and a strong bias for arginine over lysine. It remains to be demonstrated (by hybridization, for example) that kallikreins are also present in endocrine tissue.

Some hormones require the entire, intact structure of the mature hormone for biological activity, and relatively minor modifications, such as methylation, acylation, or oxidation/reduction of a sulfur, may drastically curtail activity. In a few, biological activity resides in a small fragment of the polypeptide sequence, which may be located at either the NH_2- or COOH-terminus of the peptide. When a small polypeptide does contain substantial bioactivity, total synthesis of the peptide obviates the commercial need for isolation or for synthesis through recombinant DNA techniques—an important economic advantage.

Amidation of the COOH-terminal group is frequently essential for biological activity. Hydrolysis of this one group may markedly or totally abolish bioactivity.

Secretion

Polypeptide and adrenergic hormone discharge (exocytosis or emiocytosis) from secretory granules is an active, energy-dependent (ATP) process in which the granular membrane fuses with the cellular plasma membrane, followed by rupture of the membrane at the point of contact. Cyclic AMP is involved in most, if not all, cases. Exocytosis is strongly influenced by calcium. Colchicine, a microtubular poison, inhibits secretion, thereby presenting circumstantial evidence that microtubules may also be involved.

Initiation of secretion is dependent upon a specific stimulus—an ion, a metabolite, or another hormone—which is a property of the particular hormone being discussed. A weak to moderate stimulus releases active hormone, whereas a strong or prolonged stimulus may cause the release of some prohormone as well. Frequently strong stimuli produce a biphasic response—a brief (5–10 min) surge of excretion followed by a slowly increasing wave of secretion. The latter, but not the former, is sensitive to protein synthesis inhibitors.

Steroid hormones are not stored, and thyroid hormones are stored in a different manner. In each group, however, we have an example of a prohormone. Thyroxine, the principal secretory product of the thyroid, is the precursor of the more active hormone, 3,3′,5-triiodothyronine (T_3). Similarly, testosterone from the testes is converted to the more active dihydrotestosterone in certain target tissues.

Transport

A characteristic of endocrine organs is their high degree of vascularity; there is a capillary running by essentially every endocrine cell. This is logical because hormones depend upon the vascular system for transport. Most hormones are transported either in a free form or lossely bound to plasma proteins principally albumin. Thyroid and steroid hormones are two exceptions. These hormones bind to specific β-globulins having very high association constants(10^7 to 10^{10} M^{-1}) so that there is very little that is left free or unbound (0.03–10%, depending upon the specific system). The bound hormone is *physiologically inactive* (with some reservations) and *metabolically inert*. Only the tiny unbound amount is small enough to diffuse into cells. The binding process is, however, reversible and the equilibrium,

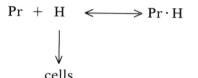

as shown, is pulled to the left as hormone leaves the vascular system. The bound hormone forms a readily available pool that serves as a cushion, or buffer, during the time an endocrine gland is shut off (see Episodic Secretion, below).

Negative Feedback

If hormones regulate the entire economy of the body, what then regulates the regulators? At this point, endocrinology becomes truly complex. The principle, however, is quite straightforward. The nervous systems and the endocrine systems acting in concert through a system of checks and balances regulate each other, i.e., each system is finely tuned through a network of positive-feedforward signals and negative-feedback signals (Fig. 1.1). *No system is independent*; each is interconnected with several others.

The analogy with electronics is a good one. In a public address system, an amplifier without adequate feedback is apt to oscillate or "squeal." An endocrine system that loses its regulation (becomes autonomous) produces a disease (endocrinopathy) that may be life-threatening.

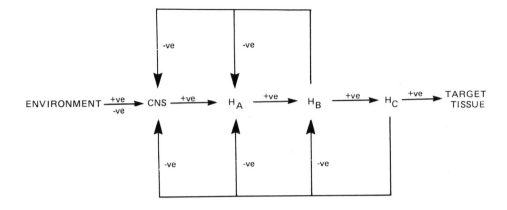

Figure 1.1 A schematic representation of a hypothetical endocrine system with positive-feedforward and negative-feedback signals: H_A, H_B, and H_C represent different hormones. Although this scheme is applicable to the hypothalamoadenohypophyseal-target endocrine organ system, it is not restricted to it, nor is it implied that there are equal responses at the different levels to the same feedback signal: +ve, positive; −ve, negative.

Some correlates are worth mentioning. The system just described produces in each of us a condition called *homeostasis*, a constancy of our internal environments in the face of varying, and sometimes very hostile, external environments. To accomplish this, the CNS may change the *setpoint* (gain) of the system to compensate for extremes in environment. After all, running a marathon on a hot day is much more taxing than rocking in front of the fireplace on a cool autumn evening!

A signal is generated in response to a nonsteady-state condition. That signal must be *short-lived*, otherwise it is in danger of becoming a false signal as the system responds and approaches the steady state. Nerve impulses are by nature virtually instantaneous and are extremely short-lived (milliseconds). Chemical messages (hormones) are circumscribed by the capacity of the vascular system to transport them to their respective target tissues. Hence, half-lives (in plasma) range from about 1 min to an hour. There are a few logical exceptions.

Diurnal Rhythm

We all have within us a biological clock that has defied anatomical localization; presumably it lies somewhere within the CNS. Some candidates are the hippocampus, amygdala, and suprachiasmatic nuclei of the hypothalamus.

Even when most external time clues (clocks, radios, TV, day/night) are removed and the rest are standardized, people maintain a diurnal or circadian rhythm of activity and of the secretion of certain hormones. Initiation of rhythm is sleep-related. For example, working with sleep physiologists, endocrinologists have found that secretion of somatotropin, prolactin, and adrenocorticotropin is initiated at different stages of sleep. Later in the day, secretion is greatly diminished.

Episodic Secretion

For those hormones depending upon events in the CNS and the hypothalamus, episodic (ultradian) secretion is common. Examples are adrenocorticotropin (ACTH), luteotropin (LH), and follicle-stimulating hormone (FSH). With ACTH, episodic secretion is superimposed on circadian rhythm. Between secretory episodes, a gland may be shut off completely.

Biological Amplification

Hormones control nearly all the metabolism that occurs in our bodies, both organic and inorganic, as we shall learn in later chapters. On the other hand, hormones are made in minute amounts, microgram to milligram quantities daily for each hormone. Even though more hormones are being discovered, it is probable that there are only a few dozen taken all together. Therefore, for each category of metabolite, whether it be sodium/potassium or calcium or the energy stores of the body (protein, fat, and carbohydrate), a very small number of hormones in very small amounts controls the disposition of that entire pool of metabolite. Such a process is called biological amplification.

Since the gain or amplification of a regulatory enzymatic step may be 100-fold or less, it is obvious that cascading will be required for a few milligrams of hormone to control kilograms of metabolite. The synthesis/phosphorolysis of glycogen under the control of insulin/epinephrine/glucagon is a typical textbook example. Later, we shall consider others.

Receptor-Mediated Hormone Action

Target tissues recognize and select the appropriate hormone(s) from the delivery wagon (the adjacent capillary bloodstream) by virtue of special, very high affinity (K_d, ca. 10^{-10} M) proteins, called receptors. For most (polypeptidic) hormones, these receptors are located on the external surface of the plasma membrane, thus obviating the need for large and for hydrophilic molecules to pass through this lipid bilayer. Lipophilic hormones, such as thyroid and steroid hormones, diffuse freely through the plasma membrane and interact with internal receptors. These two groups will be discussed separately.

Plasma Cell Membrane Receptors

Function and regulation.   Receptors have two functions. The first function is recognition of a specific hormone by virtue of the highly specific and favorable energetics of interaction or binding. Conversely, most of the other 30 to 40 hormones floating by have absolutely no interaction.

Remember that the elimination of an amide group or the substitution of a D-amino acid for its L-epimer may drastically reduce binding. This is not to say, however, that there cannot be some cross talk. For example, oxytocin and vasopressin differ by only two of nine amino acids, and each expresses some of the biological activity of the other and binds to some extent to the receptor for the other hormone.

The second function is the expression of a characteristic biological activity whether it be glycogenolysis, lipolysis, increased synthesis of thyroid hormones, or urinary excretion of phosphate. In many cases, posttranslational phosphorylation of key enzymes by a kinase is a critical step. In spite of years of searching, as yet, only a few of these key enzymes have been identified. The evidence accumulated indicates, however, that for each kinase activity there must be a corresponding phosphoprotein phosphatase so that termination as well as initiation of hormone action may be rapid (minutes). Naturally, to prevent futile cycling, activation of one enzyme deactivates the other, i.e., if phosphorylation activates a kinase, the same reaction deactivates the phosphoprotein phosphatase.

Regulation of cellular response to a given concentration of hormone may occur by one of two (or perhaps both) mechanisms.

Continued exposure of a tissue, either in vivo or in vitro, to a hormone, especially at high concentrations, leads to its desensitization or refractoriness. Binding studies show that the *number* of receptors has decreased; this is called downregulation. Examination of a limited number of systems reveals that the receptors have been internalized and that they will recycle to the cell surface if the elevated hormonal signal does not persist. Prolonged exposure to high concentrations of hormone will, of course, lead to lysosomal degradation of the internalized receptors.

The second regulatory mechanism uses a decreased sensitivity (K_d) of the receptors without any change in their number. This is accomplished by phosphorylation of the receptors. Although cAMP (see Second messengers, below) is involved, it is not known whether a cAMP-dependent kinase is directly responsible for this reaction.

The responsiveness of tissues to hormones can be modified by pathologic changes or pharmacological treatment; these can not be construed as physiologic regulation.

Structure. Again, little is known. Adrenergic receptors and the receptor for insulin are discussed in Chapter 9, and those for some growth factors in Chapter 4. Some are monomeric, whereas that for insulin, which is tetrameric, is the largest. The sequences of two receptors, those for insulin and epidermal growth factor, both contain a lipophilic section which is interpreted as favoring insertion into the membrane, i.e., a transmembrane receptor. Coincidentally, both possess tyrosine kinase activity. No conclusions should be drawn from such limited observations.

Second messengers. Because hydrophilic hormones do not pass through the plasma cell membrane, there must be a mechanism for transmitting information through the membrane and generating another signal inside the cell. This internal signal is called a *second messenger.*

Four second messengers have now been identified; insulin's second messenger is still unknown. Cyclic AMP, generated from ATP by adenylate cyclase, is the oldest known messenger. Most of the polypeptide hormones, as well as α_1-, β_1- and β_2-adrenergic receptors, act through cAMP.

Transient increases in intracellular calcium ion concentrations may also act as a second messenger. Normally, the cytosolic calcium concentration is quite low (100 to 200 nM) with the bulk of the cellular calcium being stored in the endoplasmic reticulum and mitochondria. An appropriate hormonal–receptor interaction activates phospholipase C, releasing diacylglycerol (DG) and inositol-1,4,5-triphosphate (PI_3) (Fig. 1.2). Both of these substances are second messengers. The PI_3 causes release of calcium from endoplasmic reticulum by an unknown mechanism, producing a transient increase in calcium concentration that is sufficient to activate calmodulin and other enzymes (see next section). In the meantime, diacylglycerol is activating C-kinase. These two branches have different temporal roles; the calmodulin branch mediates the initial phase of the reaction, and the C-kinase branch mediates the sustained phase.

Protein kinases and phosphoprotein phosphatases. The protein kinases catalyze the ATP-dependent phosphorylation of specific substrate proteins, thereby altering their kinetic or structural properties. There are three major groups of protein kinases.

Cyclic AMP-Dependent Protein Kinases. One of the important functions for cAMP is its interaction with cAMP-dependent protein kinase. This tetrameric enzyme has the structure, R_2C_2, with two catalytic and two regulatory subunits. The tetramer is

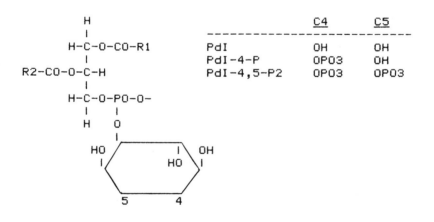

Figure 1.2 Structures of phosphoinositides. The structures of the inositol phosphates (not shown) follow logically from hydrolysis of the glycerol-3-phosphate bond: R1 and R2 are fatty acyl groups. PdI, phosphatidyl inositol; PdI-4-P and PdI-4,5-P_2, the 4-phosphate and 4,5-biphosphate of PdI.

inactive. The binding of cAMP to the regulatory subunits (K_d, 10^{-5} M) releases the active catalytic subunits. These enzymes require both magnesium and calcium for activity.

Calcium–Calmodulin-Dependent Protein Kinase. Preoccupation with adenylate cyclase and cAMP for many years diverted attention from the importance of calcium ions. In about 1976, commencing with the discovery that the α-adrenergic activation of glycolysis and gluconeogenesis in rat liver involves Ca^{2+} rather than cAMP, investigators have sought, found, and characterized a cellular calcium-binding receptor.

The criteria that must be satisfied before a protein may be classified as a Ca^{2+} receptor are as follows:

1. High specific affinity for Ca^{2+}
2. Mandatory binding of Ca^{2+} for expression of its role
3. Regulation of vital intracellular processes common to all eukaryotic cells
4. Ubiquity
5. A highly conserved structure

Calmodulin (CaM), a heat-stable, 17,000-dalton calcium-binding protein, meets all these requirements. It contains four equivalent calcium-binding sites (K_d, 2.4×10^{-6} M) that do not bind magnesium under physiologic conditions. Calcium binding induces a more helical conformation of the protein and exposes a highly lipophilic region that interacts with the enzymes that it activates (demonstrated for phosphodiesterase, myosin light-chain kinase and calcium–magnesium ATPase). So far, 15 enzymes, including several kinases, have been reported to require CaM as a regulatory component (Table 1.2). Calmodulin is ubiquitous, occurring in primitive algae, slime molds, and coelenterates, as well as in more advanced plants and mammals. Its amino acid sequence is relatively invariant from mammals to the sea pansy, differing by no more than seven conservative amino acid substitutions, only one of which (in the sea pansy) occurs in a calcium-binding domain.

The characteristics just discussed imply that intracellular calcium concentrations should vary significantly with various stimuli, and they do. Normally free intracellular calcium concentrations are about 100 nM so the calcium-binding sites on CaM

Table 1.2 Calmodulin-Regulated Enzymes

Cyclic nucleotide phosphodiesterase
Adenylate cyclase
Guanylate cyclase
cGMP protein kinase
Myosin light-chain kinase
Calcium–magnesium ATPase
Phosphorylase kinase
NAD^+ kinase
Phosphoprotein phosphatase
Phospholipase A_2
Tryptophan 5′-monooxygenase
Succinate dehydrogenase
O-Methyltransferase
N-Methyltransferase

Immunocytochemical experiments suggest that CaM is also involved in microtubule polymerization–depolymerization, chromosome movement, axonal transport, synaptic transmission, flagellar and ciliary motility, and the acrosome reaction.
Source: From Means, Tash, and Chafouleas, *Physiol Rev 62*:1–39, 1982; with permission.

are largely unoccupied. When a stimulus increases this concentration to 5 μM, more than one-half (on the average) of the binding sites on CaM would be occupied, thereby converting (some of) the protein to an active form that can, in turn, activate any of the enzymes listed in Table 1.2 that happen to be present.

Calcium–Phospholipid-Dependent Protein Kinase. In 1975 Michell proposed that stimulation of phosphatidylinositol (PdI) metabolism may couple receptor occupancy to generation of an intracellular calcium signal. In the 1980s, both Michell and Berridge modified this hypothesis, suggesting that the initial enzymic reaction stimulated by this class of ligands is the phospholipase C-mediated hydrolysis of phosphatidylinositol-4,5-biphosphate (PdI-4,5-P_2) to yield diacylglycerol (DG) and inositol-1,4,5-triphosphate (IP_3)(see Fig. 1.2 for structures). Berridge further suggested that IP_3 is the intracellular messenger that mediates mobilization of calcium from cellular stores.

The phosphatidylinositides comprise a small (< 10%) fraction of the total cellular phospholipids, but their rapid turnover marks them as important, dynamic constituents of the plasma membrane. Figure 1.3 summarizes the pathways of phosphoinositide metabolism. Because of the cyclic (scavenging) as well as de novo pathways of synthesis, only two compounds are uniquely derived, namely, PdI-4,5-P_2 and IP_3 (from PdI-4-P and PdI-4,5-P_2, respectively). The PdI-4-P and PdI-4,5-P_2 are truly trace lipids, each making up about 2.5% of inositol lipids or 0.25% of total cellular lipids.

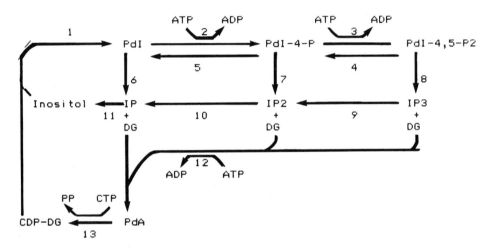

Figure 1.3 Pathways of phosphoinositide metabolism. Enzymes: (1) cytidine disphosphate-diacylglycerol:inositol transferase; (2) phosphatidylinositol kinase; (3) phosphatidylinositol-4-phosphate kinase; (4) phosphatidylinositol-4,5-biphosphate phosphomonoesterase; (5) phosphotidylinositol-4-phosphate phosphomonoesterase; (6) phosphotidylinositol phospholipase C; (7) phosphotidylinositol-4-phosphate phospholipase C; (8) phosphotidylinositol-4,5-biphosphate phospholipase C; (9) inositol-1,4,5-triphosphate phosphatase; (10) inositol-1, 4-biphosphate phosphatase; (11) inositol phosphate phosphatase; (12) diacylglycerol kinase; (13) cytidine diphosphate-diacylglycerol synthetase. Substances: PdI, PdI-4-P, PdI-4,5-P2, see Figure 1.2; IP, IP2, IP3, DG, the hydrolysis products of the phosphatides, i.e., inositol-1-phosphate, inositol-1,4-biphosphate, inositol-1,4,5-triphosphate, diacylglycerol, respectively; CDP-DG, cytidine diphosphodiacylglycerol.

The calcium-activated, phospholipid-dependent protein kinase or protein kinase C (C-kinase) exists in two forms, depending upon its association with membrane phospholipids. In its nonassociated form, it is a relatively poor kinase that is relatively insensitive to activation by calcium. Association with diacylglycerol and phospholipids, particularly phosphatidylserine, produces a highly active protein kinase that is sensitive to changes in the calcium concentration in the micromolar to submicromolar range.

Phosphoprotein Phosphatases. The rapid relaxation of a stimulated cell to its basal level depends upon the transience of each second messenger and on an increase in activity of phosphoprotein phosphatases. These enzymes are less well studied than the protein kinases, but it is known that they are regulated by at least three mechanisms: by phosphorylation of an inhibitor protein, by phosphorylation of the complex of cAMP with the regulatory subunit of cAMP-dependent kinase, or by a calcium–CaM-dependent phosphatase (see Table 1.2). The two phosphorylated products act as inhibitors of phosphoprotein phosphatase (see Chap. 9).

Interactions. Coupling of Receptors to Adenylate Cyclase.   A current view of the mechanism of transfer of information across the membrane to cAMP is summarized in Figure 1.4. Hormonal receptors (R) of varying size and form located on the exofacial side of the cellular plasma membrane confer hormonal specificity. There may be receptors to more than one hormone on a given cell. Adenylate cyclase, lying on the cytoplasmic face of the plasma membrane, is composed of a regulatory and a catalytic subunit. When it is activated, it generates cAMP from ATP. As usual, the destruction of the byproduct of this reaction, inorganic pyrophosphate, by pyrophosphatase makes this reaction irreversible.

Lying within the plasma membrane are two types of regulatory subunits. Because both of these subunits bind guanine nucleotides and magnesium, they are frequently called nucleotide-binding protein or N (also sometimes guanine nucleotide-binding protein or G). Most recently, investigators have shown that these are each heterotrimers having opposing actions. Hormone-receptor complexes that interact with N_s stimulate

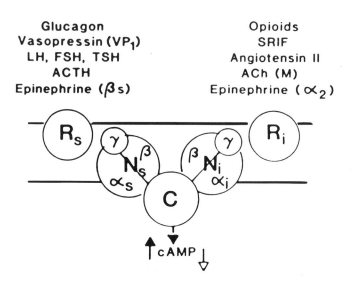

Figure 1.4 Basic constituents of a hormone-sensitive adenylate cyclase system. R_s and R_i are receptors for hormones that have stimulatory and inhibitory effects, respectively. These interact with stimulatory and inhibitory nucleotide-binding proteins (N_s and N_i) which control adenylate cyclase (*Source*: From Birnbaumer et al. 1985, with permission).

activation of adenylate cyclase, whereas those that interact with N_i inhibit activation of this enzyme. The mechanism of regulation of the adenylate cyclase is not known mostly because of an inability to purify it from somatic cells of mammalian origin.

In the meantime, knowledge concerning N_s and N_i has blossomed (Fig. 1.5). Both consist of α, β, and γ-subunits, both bind GTP and its analogues, as well as Mg, both are substrates for the ADP-ribosyltransferase activity of bacterial toxins, and both are GTPases. Both are 4S proteins with molecular mass of about 80 to 100 kDa. Both proteins, upon treatment with Mg and a nonhydrolyzable GTP analogue, undergo subunit dissociation to give α-subunits of N_s or N_i with guanine nucleotide bound to them and a complex of $\beta\gamma$–subunits.

The α_s- and a_i-subunits differ in several ways. Cholera toxin ADP-ribosylates the α_s-subunit, whereas pertussis toxin acts

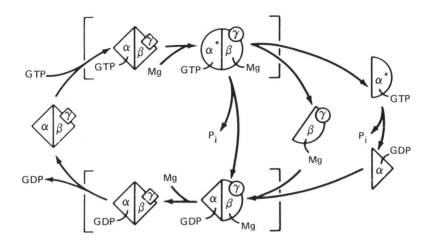

Figure 1.5 Regulatory cycle of N_s and N_i (indistinctly represented as N) as it may occur under the influence of GTP and Mg. The cycle has been divided into four steps: association of GTP with N, activation of N, hydrolysis of GTP and concomitant deactivation of N, and dissociation of GDP. Which form of the N protein hydrolyzes the GTP is not known (*Source*: From Birnbaumer et al. 1985, with permission).

similarly on the α_i-subunit. In most tissues, α_s shows size heterogeneity with a predominating form of 42 kDa and lesser amounts of a 51 to 52-kDa form, whereas there appears to be only one form of α_i, 40 to 41 kD. The β- and γ-subunits of N_s and N_i are very similar, if not identical, with the former having a molecular mass of 35 kDa and the latter about 5 to 8 kDa.

Although Figure 1.5 implies that the regulation of N_s and N_i are similar, this is not quite true. The apparent K_m of N_s for GTP (or its analogues) is about 1 μM so that at the prevailing intracellular concentrations of GTP (ca. 100 μM), N_s is always saturated with guanine nucleotides. The apparent K_m for Mg, which is required for activation of N_s, is 5 to 10 mM. Because the intracellular concentration of Mg is about 0.5 mM, binding of Mg appears to be rate-limiting, a rather odd fact. The subunit N_i differs from N_s in its high affinity for magnesium, hence, N_i is saturated with both guanine nucleotides and magnesium under physiologic conditions. Study of N_i has occurred mostly in membranes of an N_s-deficient *cyc*− mutant of S49 lymphoma cells.

The model shown in Figure 1.5 leaves several questions unanswered. Most important is the question of physiological significance. Reconstitution experiments in liposomes are not the equivalent of natural membranes. The nature of the interaction of the hormone–receptor complex with N_s and N_i is not understood. And while it is known that N_s and N_i react noncompetitively with adenylate cyclase, the mechanism of the interaction, as stated earlier, is not understood.

(A note of caution, however. Models are tools useful in the design of experiments. The reality implied by the model can never be proved, only disproved. After many experiments testing the validity of the model fail to disprove it, the model becomes generally accepted. Sometimes years later, perhaps with the introduction of a new technique, a single experiment may consign the model to the trash heap.)

In summary, the trigger is the hormone–receptor interaction. The receptor may or may not have previously associated with the appropriate nucleotide-binding protein. At any rate, these three must form a ternary complex, HRN. Because the prevailing concentration of GTP is much greater than its K_d for N, HRN is active, and adenylate cyclase is activated. When H dissociates from the HRN complex, the GTPase action of N rapidly terminates adenylate cyclase activity.

(The claim that the affinity of RN for H is less than that of RN-GTP is probably physiologically irrelevant because RN is presumably always saturated with GTP.)

Interrelationships of the Calcium and cAMP Messenger Systems.   It would be a mistake to think of the calcium and cAMP messengers acting in different cell types to regulate specific aspects of cellular function. Rather, these two messengers participate jointly to regulate the intracellular domain (Table 1.3). Yet, their interactions are not stereotyped. In fact, they may be diametrically opposed.

Table 1.3 shows the effects of Ca_4CaM, the calcium–calmodulin complex, on several enzymes involved in the regulation of cAMP concentrations as well as the effect of cAMP on $[Ca^{2+}]$ and the CaM-dependent kinase. Both are involved in the regulation of secretion of aldosterone, cortisol, insulin, and prolactin, as well as the regulation of glycogenolysis. More details will be given in the appropriate chapters.

Table 1.3   Interactions between the Ca^{2+} and cAMP Messenger Systems

---

Biochemical interactions: Ca_4CaM effects on cAMP system
  Ca_4CaM stimulates phosphodiesterase ——⟩↓ cAMP
  Ca_4CaM stimulates adenylate cyclase ——⟩↑ cAMP
  Ca_4CaM stimulates protein kinases and phosphorylates some of the
  same proteins as cAMP-dependent protein kinase
Biochemical interactions: cAMP effects on Ca^{2+} system
  cAMP increases plasma membrane Ca^{2+} influx rate ——⟩↑ $[Ca^{2+}]$
  cAMP increases plasma membrane Ca^{2+} efflux rate ——⟩↓ $[Ca^{2+}]$
  cAMP increases sarcoplasmic/endoplasmic reticulum Ca^{2+} uptake rate
  ——⟩↓ $[Ca^{2+}]$
  cAMP increases sensitivity of Ca_4CaM-regulated protein kinase to Ca^{2+}
  cAMP decreases sensitivity of Ca_4CaM-regulated protein kinase to Ca^{2+}
Cellular interactions
  Coordinate regulation — fly salivary gland, thyroid gland
  Hierachical regulation — secretion of insulin, cortisol, or prolactin,
  neurotransmitter release, nerve cell activity
  Redundant regulation — glycogenolysis, aldosterone secretion
  Sequential action — adrenergic stimulation of cardiac function
  Antagonistic action — platelet activation, smooth muscle contraction
Set-point control by cAMP
  cAMP increases responsiveness to a standard activation of the Ca^{2+}
  messenger system — insulin, aldosterone, prolactin secretion
  cAMP decreases responsiveness to a standard activation of the Ca^{2+}
  messenger system — platelet release, smooth muscle contraction

---

Source: Reprinted by permission *N Engl J Med 314*:1167, 1986, from an article by
H. Rasmussen.

**Relationship of Calcium to the Arachidonic Acid
Cascade.** When a receptor linked to the calcium messenger
system is activated, phospholipase C causes the release of
diacylglycerol (as well as IP_3). Phospholipase A_2, activated by Ca^{2+}
acts on phosphatidylcholine, promoting the release of
arachidonic acid. Through the cyclooxygenase pathway,
arachidonic acid is converted to thromboxanes, prostaglandins,
or leukotrienes (see Chap. 9).

Cytosolic and Nuclear Receptors

Steroid and thyroid hormones, being lipophilic, have no trouble passing through phospholipid membranes by diffusion. In the cytosol, the dogma states, steroid hormones bind to receptor proteins producing a conformational change as a prerequisite for transport into the nucleus. In other words, the cytosolic receptor plays an obligatory role in cellular transport.

Two recent reports are causing a reevaluation of the accepted model. Both reports used monoclonal antibodies to estrophilin, the cytosolic estrogen receptor. Both groups showed, by use of cytochemical techniques, that specific staining was confined to the nuclei of human and animal target tissues. The expected cytosolic staining was not seen. Why?

Our understanding of the initial nuclear events is minuscule. Must the steroid hormone bind to specific strands of chromatin to initiate transcription of genes that will initiate the specific biological response of that target cell? Whether the steroid interacts with a nuclear histone or nonhistone protein is not clear. Or, is the steroid important only for transport of the receptor into the nucleus? Some very recent work indicates that the latter may be true. Von der Ahe and colleagues claim that the receptors for estrogen, progesterone, androgen, and glucocorticoid interact in the promoter region of chicken lysozyme and that the regulatory elements for different hormones may be similar or may share some structural features.

Knowledge concerning the events of transcription and translation is both fragmentary and uneven. The greatest advances are occurring in the area of progesterone action in the avian oviduct and in the cloning of the human estrogen receptor cDNA for the MCF-7 human breast cancer cell line. Progress is also being made with progesterone action in mammalian breast tissue, an extremely complicated target tissue. These advances will be discussed in Chapter 8.

Triiodothyronine (thyroxine is, in most tissues, a prohormone) acts a little differently. There is a cytosolic, high-affinity protein, but interaction with it is *not* a prerequisite for nuclear transport or for the initiation of nuclear events. The role of the cytosolic protein is not clear. It may act as a trap, creating an intracellular pool of hormone.

The time scale for steroid- and thyroid-initiated reactions is much longer than for hormones binding to plasma membrane receptors. With sensitive indicators, usually radioactive isotopes, initial events can be detected in less than an hour. In practical, biological terms, however, responses require many hours or, occasionally, a day or two for full expression.

PARACRINE AND NEUROCRINE HORMONES

It is now evident that some polypeptides do not function as classic hormones, i.e., their serum concentration does not increase concurrently with increased biological response. This group may tentatively be divided into two parts: those having a paracrine function, and those with a neurocrine function.

Paracrine polypeptides act locally by diffusion through adjacent cells or perhaps through extracellular fluid bathing nearby cells. Even though low concentrations of such peptides may be detectable in serum, this fact is viewed as a coincidental "leakage" or "spillage" into the circulatory system. Somatostatin is a prime example of a paracrine polypeptide. The wide distribution of D cells of the gastroenteropancreatic system, their separation from each other, and their high population density all make this hypothesis—and it is nothing more—attractive. (In Chapter 4, however, we shall see somatostatin acting as a conventional hormone.) Prostaglandins are also an excellent example of paracrine substances as most of them act locally.

Neurocrine polypeptides constitute an evergrowing group that is found in both neural tissue and the gut. The small clusters of cells that produce hormones in the gut are derived embryologically from the neural crest, thus, it is not surprising that they produce neurocrine polypeptides. Three of this group were first isolated from brain (thyrotropin-releasing hormone, ovine and porcine hypothalamus; substance P, bovine hypothalamus; enkephalins, porcine brain) and were later detected in the gastrointestinal tract, mostly of laboratory animals. On the other hand, there is a much larger group of gastrointestimal hormones that have been detected either directly or by measurement of hormone-specific receptors in the brain. These include gastrin, cholecystokinin, insulin, motilin, vasoactive intestinal peptide, and neurotensin. In addition, bombesin, originally identified as a component of frog skin, is found in both places. Dual location, however, is not enough to qualify for the label of neurocrine.

Neurocrine cells, without exception I believe, possess amine-handling properties and, therefore, belong to the *a*mine *p*recursor *u*ptake and *d*ecarboxylation (APUD) series. Recently Fujita and Kobayashi have expanded the APUD concept into the paraneuronal cell concept. Paraneurons are neuroepithelium-derived cells having neuronlike properties without actually being nerve cells. Gastroenteropancreatic (GEP) endocrine cells closely resemble certain neurons in their granule structure, in the chemistry and metabolism of secretion, in the mechanisms of stimulus recognition, and in the type of stimulus-secretion coupling. The granules mentioned liberate their contents by exocytosis, in quanta, as do the synaptic vesicles. These granules, it is postulated, may contain more than one secretory product, probably in integer ratios to each other. Thus, granules may contain peptide hormones with their carrier proteins (if appropriate) in addition to amines or even ATP.

Although this hypothesis requires experimental verification, there is supporting evidence in non-GEP, but closely related systems. For example, the neuroendocrine supraoptic nuclei of the hypothalamus synthesize a precursor of arginine vasopressin and its carrier protein, neurophysin. Furthermore, an adrenal medullary protein, containing seven copies of met-enkephalin and one of leu-enkephalin, has been isolated which explains the met-enkephalin/leu-enkephalin ratio. Thus, in these two instances, dual secretory products are made in a finite ratio.

How do neurocrine peptides act? They "seem to regulate local neuronal activity in a hormone-like manner. They facilitate or inhibit neuronal communication by interfering with neuronal excitability or indirectly by influencing the functioning of synaptic mechanisms such as the release of neurotransmitters" (Lovnen and Soudijn, 1979). They act locally over short distances and, compared with biogenic amines, they are relatively long-acting.

CHOLESTEROL AND STEROIDOGENESIS

The structures in Figure 1.6 demonstrate the chemical relatedness of all the steroid hormones to the sterol, cholesterol,

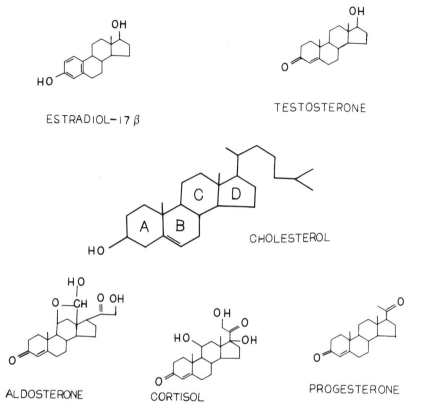

ESTRADIOL–17 β

TESTOSTERONE

CHOLESTEROL

ALDOSTERONE

CORTISOL

PROGESTERONE

Figure 1.6 The structural relationship of steroid hormones to cholesterol, the sterol from which they are all derived.

i.e., they all possess the tetracyclic steroid nucleus, an oxygen at C-3, unsaturation in ring A or B and a hydroxyl or an acetyl group or both at C-17. (In addition, 1,25-dihydroxycholecalciferol, although not a true steroid itself, is derived from the cholesterol precursor, 7-dehydrocholesterol.) Indeed, the pathways of synthesis of all these hormones are well established. The pattern is degradative (Fig. 1.7). Following the initial loss of six carbons from the cholesterol side chain leading to the formation of progestins, glucocorticosteroids, and mineralocorticosteroids, the last two carbons of the side chain are removed for the formation

```
C27 ---------------> C21 ---------------> C19 -------------> C18
```

cholesterol   progesterone   testosterone   estradiol
                         cortisol   dehydroepiandrosterone
                         aldosterone

Figure 1.7   Generalized pattern of steroidogenesis.

of androgens. Finally, the C-19 angular methyl group is lost con-
comitantly with aromatization of ring A in the formation of
estrogens.

What is the source of cholesterol? Early experiments showed
that all steroidogenic tissue (see Table 2.1) can synthesize cholesterol de novo, i.e., from acetylcoenzyme A (acetyl-CoA) through
3-hydroxymethyl-3-methylglutaryl CoA (HMG-CoA), mevalonate,
squalene, and lanosterol. Other experiments, however, showed extensive uptake of plasma cholesterol (labeled) by some of these
tissues. More recently, the identification and partial characterization of the low-density and high-density lipoproteins (LDL and
HDL) and their receptors in certain tissues have led to a more complete understanding of the relationships involved.

First, under normal circumstances, the greater part of
substrate cholesterol in the adrenal, ovary, and placenta (testes
still uncertain) is derived from uptake of lipoprotein cholesterol.
This applies to most, but not all, species.

Second, there are two distinct receptor-mediated pathways.
The LDL pathway, which is most common, is specific for lipoprotein particles containing either apo-B or apo-E (some HDL) in
humans. Uptake occurs by endocytosis followed by lysosomal
degradation. The HDL pathway, which has been convincingly
demonstrated only in rodents, relies on receptor recognition of
apo-E, a major constituent of HDL in the rat. Complete lysosomal
degradation of apolipoprotein may not be necessary.

Third, uptake is hormonally regulated except in the placenta.
Appropriate trophic hormonal stimulation increases the number
of lipoprotein receptors or, in cultured bovine granulosa cells,
receptor affinity, leading to an increase in the rate of internalization of lipoprotein. The availability of maternal LDL is the rate-
limiting step in LDL uptake by the human placenta.

Cellular cholesterol, regardless of the source, is esterified by long-chain fatty acids through their acyl-CoA derivates. In humans, arachidonate is the predominant fatty acid. The cholesteryl esters are deposited in steroidogenic organs as lipid droplets. Trophic hormone (ACTH, LH, or human chorionic gonadotropin; LCG) stimulation produces multiple coordinated changes in cholesterol metabolism. Not only is uptake of cholesterol increased, but the mobilization of cholesterol esters is enhanced by activation of cholesterol esterases, movement of cholesterol into mitochondria is stimulated, and the first and rate-limiting step in steroidogenesis is promoted, namely, side-chain cleavage to produce pregnenolone. All these facets of steroidogenesis are considered in detail in Chapters 8 and 9.

TECHNIQUES

Even though some may feel that a discussion of techniques does not properly belong in an introductory course, there are three that are so basic that I must include them.

Ablation–Replacement

This technique forms the basis of endocrinology. Even though newer techniques have largely supplanted it, it remains, and will always remain, the basic technique. Surgical removal of a gland or tissue, or more recently, neutralization of the putative secretory product of that organ with specific antibodies, produces a symptom or a syndrome (a group of symptoms) that is corrected by administration of an extract of the organ or of a pure substance isolated from that extract. This generalized statement is more precisely presented in Table 1.4. These criteria have become ever more restrictive as hormones of decreasing concentration in the body and of increasing potency are isolated. Criterion B4 (Table 1.4) is especially difficult to meet for the polypeptides, but also especially important because of problems in assuring purity.

Saturation Analysis

This technique, introduced in the late 1950s by Ekins in England for the assay of thyroxine and by Yalow in the United States for

Table 1.4   Hormonal Criteria

A hormone should fulfill all of the following criteria:

A. Physiological criteria
    1. is released from specific site(s) of origin by physiological stimuli
    2. has specific actions on remote specific structures or organs
    3. its effects persist after elimination of all neural connections between the site of origin and the site of action *or* an effect can be shown in vitro

B. Biochemical criteria
    1. chemically identified in extracts of putative source
    2. chemically or immunologically identified in blood
    3. serum concentration is proportional to the physiological stimulus
    4. administration of physiologic amounts of exogenous (preferably synthetic) agent produces actions similar to those of the endogenous one

Source: Modified from Andersson, 1973.

the assay of insulin, has revolutionized clinical chemistry and endocrinology. The basis of the assay is a protein (*Pr*) having a high affinity and low capacity to bind the analyte in question. The protein need not be pure, but it should be the only high-affinity, low-capacity protein present. One must have, on the other hand, pure analyte labeled with a radioisotope(H^*)—iodine-125 or tritium are the most commonly used. The hormone–analyte (*H*) in a standard or in a sample, when mixed with (*Pr*) and (H^*), competes for a limited number of binding sites on (*Pr*).

$$Pr \cdot H \leftrightarrow H + Pr + H^* \leftrightarrow Pr \cdot H^*$$

Thus, an equilibrium between all species is established. The relative concentrations of (*Pr · H*) and (*Pr · H**) depend upon the relative concentrations of (*H*) and (H^*). Then, by the law of mass action, the association constant (K_a) of the reaction may be written

$$K_a = (H)(Pr)/(Pr \cdot H) = (H^*)(Pr)/(Pr \cdot H^*)$$

Rearranging terms,

$$(Pr \cdot H^*)/(H^*) = (Pr \cdot H)/(H)$$

It is obvious that the ratio of protein-bound (b) to unbound (u) radioactive analyte is the same as that of the natural analyte. Also, increasing (H) in the presence of a constant total concentration of binding protein and of radiolabeled analyte decreases the number of binding sites available to (H^*). Upon separation of protein-bound from unbound labeled analyte and measurement of radioactivity, one has all the information needed for an assay. One may plot b/u, b, or $1/b$ on the ordinate, the quantity of standard (H) added on the abscissa and then read the values of (H) in the samples from the standard curve.

Of the four critical determinants of clinical chemistry—sensitivity, specificity, accuracy, and reproducibility—sensitivity is the most crucial. With the availability of highly radioactively labeled ligands (specific activity of more than 50 Ci/mmol), sensitivity (the smallest amount detectable) is an inverse function of the association constant of the binding protein. Typically these lie in the range of 10^8 to 10^{10} M^{-1}.

The sensitivity achieved by saturation analysis is truly spectacular. Calibration curves frequently start from a few picograms, equivalent to a few femtomoles or less depending upon the molecular weight of the analyte. Remember, too, that Avogadro's number is about 6×10^{23} molecules per mole. One may be measuring fewer than 10^8 molecules!

The implications for endocrinology were breathtaking! The restrictions on design of experiments because of large sample sizes of 1–10 ml of serum or plasma were gone. Saturation analysis, using only 10–100 μl of sample, made measurements, or even repeated measurements, on infants or small laboratory animals possible.

Almost as significant were the advances in specificity provided by saturation analysis. This is a characteristic of the binding protein employed, and thus, at this point, one must divide saturation analysis into three broad categories: competitive protein binding assay (CPBA), using endogenous circulating plasma proteins; radioimmunoassay (RIA), using induced antibodies; and radioreceptor assay (RRA), using target tissue protein. The CPBA is now mainly of historical interest, the only wide application being the assay of cortisol (Keane et al., 1975). Because of our ability to tailor antibodies to specific regions of a large molecule (NH$_2$-terminal region, COOH-terminal region, an internal region of a polypeptide, the A/B ring, or the side-chain–D ring region of a steroid), RIA is today the dominant technique. Such sophistication places an additional burden on the analyst, for frequently multiple assays for the same analyte produce *different* values. Which, if any, are accurate?

There is one basic reason for such disparate results. Antibodies, although highly specific, are not *absolutely specific*, and they may also bind related molecules having little or no biological activity. For example, the antibody may recognize a circulating prohormone, or it may recognize an inactive metabolite. One recourse is the use of RRA, a more difficult assay, but one more closely related to biological activity. Indeed, RRA can be viewed as a microbioassay.

Monoclonal Antibodies

A third technique, although new, has already had a large impact. This is the use of monoclonal antibodies (MAbs). On the basis of a technique published by Köhler and Milstein (1975), a myeloma cell line containing the genetic information required to proliferate indefinitely in tissue culture is fused (currently using polyethylene glycol) with lymphocytes from an immunized animal. Each normal B lymphocyte contains the genetic information to produce a single antibody, but it lacks the ability to proliferate as a cell line. Furthermore, the myeloma cells are deficient in hypoxathine–guanine–phosphoribosyl transferase (HPRT), and aminopterin is added to the culture medium. Thus, both the main and the salvage pathways for the synthesis of nucleic acid are blocked; neither the myeloma cells nor the lymphocytes can grow independently, but the fused, hybrid cells can. The lymphocytes contribute the genetic information for formation of HPRT and immunoglobulin, and the myeloma cells contribute the genetic information for cellular proliferation.

Offsetting this principle is the technical difficulty of selecting the hybrid cell producing the required antibody of designated characteristics from among the tens of thousands present. Thus, the major prerequisite for the production of MAbs is the availability of a rapid, sensitive, and accurate screening assay. As you can see, the production of MAbs is still a major undertaking. In many cases, the results are worth the effort. This is particularly true of receptors; MAbs to receptors for estrogen, thyrotropin, adrenergic chemicals, acetylcholine, and transferrin have been produced. Once obtained, these antibodies can be used for receptor purification, receptor radioassays, immunocytochemistry, and immunopathogenic studies. Monoclonal antibodies to soluble antigens are more difficult to make. So far, MAbs to insulin, parathyroid hormone, somatotropin, and substance P have been produced, as well as to partially purified factors, such as mullerian-inhibiting factor and osteoclast-activating factor.

CLINICAL ASPECTS

Definitions

The prefixes shown in Table 1.5 are attached to the names of endocrine organs (hyperthyroid, hypogonad) or of endocrine compounds (hypocortisolemia), although the latter can be quite mouth-filling. Implied in such labels is the definition of normality. Normality in terms of physical measurements is *not*, however, a constant. Age, stature (body mass or surface area), sex, time of day, reproductive status, and nutritional status are just some of the variables that may affect the definition of normality.

The so-called normal values for the concentrations of hormones (or their products) in sera, plasma, urine, etc., which are widely quoted, are usually those for average-sized adult men or nonpregnant women. The neonatologist, pediatrician, obstetrician, and geriatrician may each use different sets of normal values.

More recently, the descriptors "inappropriately low" or "inappropriately high" have been used to describe abnormal responses to tests of endocrine function or of abnormal body fluid concentrations. Even though the meaning is the same, the statement automatically raises the question, "What is 'appropriate'?"

Table 1.5 General Definitions of Function or of Concentration

State	Prefix	Descriptor
Below normal	Hypo-	Inappropriately low
Normal	Eu-	Appropriate
Above normal	Hyper-	Inappropriately high

It also avoids premature labeling of patients, a procedure that might conceivably prejudice their chances of employment or of obtaining life insurance.

True hypofunction or hyperfunction of an endocrine organ or tissue defines an endocrinopathy, a disease state of that organ. The symptons of the syndrome may all be forthrightly expressed; here, the syndrome is said to be frank or classic. Often such cases can be spotted by a trained observer as they walk down the street. More commonly, only a few symptoms are expressed and their expression is frequently more subtle. Obviously, these pose a greater challenge for correct diagnosis.

Certain endocrinopathies may be subdivided on the basis of their etiology into primary, secondary, or tertiary disease. For example, a defect in a hypogonadal patient may be located in the gonads (primary); in the pituitary, a result of hyposecretion of gonadotropins (secondary); or in the hypothalamus, a result of hyposecretion of gonadotropin-releasing hormone (tertiary). Obviously, this increases the complexity of diagnosis. The approach to differential diagnosis differs somewhat with the endocrine system in question and with hypofunction vs. hyperfunction.

Hypofunction and Hyperfunction

At this point, we may profitably ask if there are any generalities concerning hypofunction and hyperfunction. There are three major categories of hypofunction. One is a defective hormone-producing organ, which may arise from either a natural or an iatrogenic origin. Destruction of an organ resulting from bacterial or viral infection or infarction is now believed to be less common that that caused by autoimmune disease. For example, whereas Hashimoto's thyroiditis is a classic example of the latter, other instances have been documented. As our knowledge of immunology improves, this area will become better defined.

Medical intervention may also induce hypofunction. For example, prolonged treatment of certain conditions with pharmacologic amounts of glucocorticoids will suppress ACTH release (by negative feedback) and produce severe adrenal atrophy—a functional hypoadrenocorticism. Hyperthyroidism is often replaced by a permanent hypothyroidism. It is not known, however, whether this reflects the natural course of the disease or is a result of treatment.

A secondary category of hypofunction occurs in congenital enzymatic defects in hormone production. Classic examples are the 21-hydroxylase deficiency in congenital adrenal hyperplasia and congenital hypothyroidism (with an unspecified defect). These, as well as other examples, are fully discussed in the appropriate chapters.

The third category of hypofunction occurs at the target organ level. It has been said that most endocrine disease will turn out to be receptor mediated. Our knowledge and techniques are still too elementary to test this assertion, but it does point to an area that will develop during your professional careers. Already we know that the glucose intolerance of obese people is due to a decreased number of insulin receptors. Other less well known conditions are also due to receptor inadequacy. To date, our knowledge of postreceptor events is fragmentary. As these steps become known, undoubtedly it will become apparent that "idiosyncratic" illnesses have ascribable causes.

True hyperfunction, on the other hand, is usually due to a cancerous type of condition in which hormone production has become partially or totally autonomous. Hypersecretion may be due to hyperplasia of an endocrine organ or cell type, or it may be the result of an ectopic tumor. Typically, ectopic tumors produce polypeptide hormones that, in appropriate cases, may overstimulate thyroid- or steroid-producing organs.

Another form of hyperfunction is the result of hypofunction. For example, in congenital adrenal hyperplasia, the deficit in cortisol in the blood and consequent diminished negative feedback leads to hypersecretion of ACTH from the pituitary and to adrenal hyperplasia. Treatment is straightforward—replacement of the missing hormone in physiologic amounts.

The Role of Genes

What role does heredity play in the etiology of endocrine disease? In some types, none; in others, it is important. For example, if one (homozygous) identical twin has adult-onset diabetes, there is about a 95% chance that the other twin also will have it.

The most noteable recent advance in the discovery of hereditary involvement in endocrinopathies is that of the major histocompatibility complex (MHC) on the short arm of human chromosome 6. Even though the details of the complex are still being elucidated, it is undoubtedly one of the major developments in human biology in the last two decades.

Although the subject of the MHC more properly belongs in an immunology textbook, an overview, at this point, will orient the novice. The MHC codes for several groups, namely, cell-surface antigens (transplantation antigens), three components of complement, and two enzyme systems (red cell glyoxalase I and adrenal 21-hydroxylase) (Fig. 1.8).

Transplantation antigens are controlled by four loci: *HLA-A, HLA-B, HLA-C,* and *HLA-D(DR)*, each with a large number of alleles. The nomenclature is confusing because, like Topsy, it just grew. International workshops have attempted standardization, but not systematization. Moreover, the nomenclature is not static. As more defined antisera become available, certain antigens may be further subdivided.

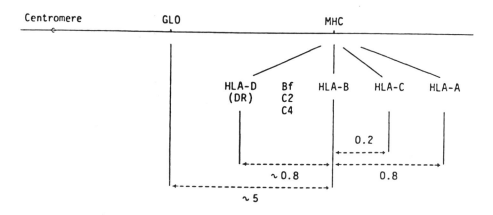

Figure 1.8 The major histocompatibility complex on the short arm of human chromosome 6: Bf, properdin factor B; C2, C4, second and fourth complement components; GLO, red cell glyoxalase I. The locus for 21-hydroxylase is very close to *HLA-B*. The distances are derived from recombination rates in family studies (*Sources*: From Farid and Bear, 1981, with permission).

Antigens HLA-A, B, and C are the classic transplantation antigens tested on lymphocytes by complement-dependent cytotoxicity. Over 70 antigens have already been identified. The HLA-D loci, on the other hand, are identified by functional assay of lymphocytic interaction (mixed lymphocytic culture). There are also antigenic specificities related to HLA-D antigens (D-related; DR) which are demonstrated serologically on bone marrow (B) peripheral lymphocytes.

The structure of the gene products is known. There are three general groups consisting of the HLA-A, B, and C antigens, the HLA-D antigens and the HLA-DR antigens. The HLA-A, B, C, and DR antigens are said to be transmembrane proteins of the cellular plasma membrane; the significance of this observation is obscure. Antigens HLA-A, B, and C are more widely distributed than are the HLA-D and DR antigens, being found in all nucleated cells. (There is some disagreement over their presence on sperm and placental trophoblastic cells.)

The genes of the HLA system produce an extraordinary amount of genetic variability in human populations. For example, the known alleles of the HLA-A, B, C, and D loci could generate more than 3×10^8 genetically different people. In practice, there appears to be some grouping of gene frequencies on the basis of race. While HLA-A2 occurs at high frequency in all populations, A1, A3, A28, A29, Aw30, and Aw32 are very low in Japanese subjects, and A11 is very low in Africans. On the other hand, Aw42 and Aw43 are perhaps specific to Africans and Dw12 to Japanese. Such selection may extend to certain ethnic groups.

An additional complication to associating gene frequency with a disease is linkage disequilibrium. This is the tendency for alleles at different HLA loci to occur more frequently than chance would predict. Not all alleles are involved, only eight or nine showing significant linkage disequilibrium in Caucasians.

Although certain endocrine diseases are associated statistically with increased gene frequency of certain alleles, the interpretation of the correlation is still uncertain. In general, it is assumed that certain alleles may predispose an individual to certain diseases, which will become manifest in the presence of certain environmental factors. Proving such an assumption in human populations, however, is extraordinarily difficult. Furthermore, simple genetic models are inadequate in such circumstances. If inheritance is not monogenic, or if penetrance is reduced, demonstration of genetic factors becomes most difficult.

Techniques

When an endocrinopathy is suggested by the patient's history or by clinical observations, one must document one's suspicions with laboratory findings. Such tests should initially test an *entire system* by the application of an appropriate stress. For example, the oral glucose tolerance test is one of the oldest and most commonly applied. The ingestion of a large amount of glucose places a severe stress on the body's ability to dispose of glucose (to glycogen and triglycerides). An appropriate response indicates that all components of the system are operative. An inappropriate response indicates an inadequacy in one (or more) of the components of the system. Although lack of insulin would be a prime suspect, the fault could also lie with one of four or five other hormones. "Organ" tests would then be used to find the culprit.

In hyperfunction, one should administer an inhibitory substance (rather than a stress) to ascertain the degree of autonomy of the deranged organ. For example, administration of dexamethasone should suppress the release of pituitary ACTH and adrenal cortisol. If cortisol is not suppressed (and ACTH is), then the secretory activity of the adrenal is autonomous.

Organ tests are selective and usually consist of supplying a stimulatory hormone and measuring the expected product of that stimulation in the blood. Thus, one would expect an increase in thyrotropin (and prolactin) after administration of thyrotropin-releasing hormone.

Serum or Plasma Versus Urine Sampling

Serum or plasma hornomal levels are now usually determinable by RIA, and this is the method of choice in most situations. For those hormones with short half-lives and episodic secretion, a single sample (or even two samples) may produce misleading information. Urine represents an automatic integrator and, *if it is collected reliably*, may provide an important alternative source of information.

Treatment

When there is no, or minimal, function left in a hormonal organ or tissue, there is no alternative but to administer replacement doses of the last hormone made by the system (the one that will affect the target tissues), thus maintaining normal body responses. One must then be alert to a change in demand by the body. If the secretory activity of the tissue is not too severely compromised, one can alleviate the demand for hormone by minimizing stress. For example, some mild diabetics can go without medication by applying rigid dietary control, i.e., restricting the ingestion of calories.

Hormone resistance is one form of hypofunction. It is a state in which the body fails to respond normally to a hormone, i.e., supraphysiologic or even pharmacologic amounts of the hormone must be administered to normalize a biological response. Insulin resistance is common, but examples of resistance to other hormones also exist.

Explanations of hormone resistance usually lie in aberrant receptors or postreceptor reactions. Little is known about the latter, but the former may now be divided into two categories: reduced affinity and reduced number of receptors. In either, an increased concentration of hormone, whether endogenous or exogenous, may correct the deficiency, provided the lesion is not too severe.

In hyperfunction, the most usual recourse is surgical removal or radiologic destruction of part or all of the gland, i.e., the patient is deliberately made hypofunctional. In some instances, as with the thyroid, the physician may intervene medically.

SUMMARY

Endocrinology is the study of hormones and of the endocrine or ductless glands of tissues that secrete them. As a science, it is about 100 years old, but because progress is exponential with time, most of the scientific advances have occurred in the last 50 years.

Even though ancient civilizations recognized and used the effects of castration, it was not until the late nineteenth century that reversal of the effects of castration by administration of a lipid,

testicular extract, was demonstrated. The first hormone, secretin, was isolated in 1901, insulin in the early 1920s, and many
steroid hormones in the 1930s. Since then, a steady procession of
new hormones has brought us to the verge of understanding the
regulation of bodily functions.

Endocrinology is fascinating for several reasons. One of the
most compelling is its interdisciplinary nature. One cannot truly
understand endocrinology without some grasp of anatomical and
histological relationships. As the effects of hormones at the
organ, tissue, and cellular levels are discovered, the physiological
principles underlying the regulation of many bodily functions are
elucidated. Discovery of how hormones act at a molecular level is
today allowing us to understand the fundamental basis of many
aspects of life.

Classically, hormones are *minute* quantities of substances
that are *secreted* directly into the blood, *transported* to a remote
target organ where they produce *specific effects*. A hormone may
have more than one target organ and may produce multiple effects. Hormones and neural impulses act in a coordinated, integrated fashion to control all bodily functions. Humoral and
neural control of *metabolism* is the emphasis of this text.

Recently, we have become aware of substances that do not
meet all of these requirements, in that they act *locally*. Depending
upon the type of action, these substances are classified as
paracrine or neurocrine. Their appearance in blood seems to be
adventitious because there is no correlation between concentration and stimulus for secretion.

Mature, circulating polypeptidic hormones all have undergone posttranslational modification. All, of course, were synthesized with a signal peptide at the NH_2-terminus. Most large
peptides have an additional sequence inserted which makes the
prohormone inactive; it is usually removed in the secretion
granule or vesicle before secretion. A few are synthesized as
multigene products, that is, a large polypeptide containing the sequences of two or more hormones. The mature forms are usually
flanked by basic dipeptides in the precursor sequences.

Because the daily production of a hormone is normally quite
small, measured in micrograms or milligrams, and because there
are only a few dozen hormones controlling the metabolism of the
entire body, biological amplification must exist. Presumably this

requires a cascade of enzymatic reactions, although I must admit that this is largely a guess. The mechanism of action of only two hormones, glucagon and epinephrine, is known at the molecular level, and these two do act through a cascade.

Hormone secretion is *not* constant. The control of secretion is complex, and it is still incompletely understood. Some adjectives describing secretion are pulsatile, diurnal, ultradian, episodic, and homeostatic. More than one descriptor may be applicable to a given hormone. For example, the rhythm of secretion for several hormones is sleep-entrained so that the secretion pattern is diurnal. Normally secretion of these hormones is turned off, and secretion occurs episodically. These episodes are more frequent and more intense in the morning than in the late afternoon and evening, thereby producing a diurnal rhythm.

The secretion of all hormones is regulated by *homeostasis*. This term refers to our bodies' need for a relatively constant internal milieu. Any perturbation in the system is sensed and relayed in a series of positive-feedforward reactions (hormonal secretions) and one negative-feedback reaction that cancels the perturbation; the system is thereby restored to its initial state, and hormone secretion ceases. Because our external environment changes, sometimes drastically, the body must compensate by changing the setpoint of the system. The interplay of stimulus, negative feedback, and setpoint may be quite complex.

In the blood, most hormones are loosely associated with or bound to plasma proteins, most notably albumin. Steroid and thyroid hormones are, however, exceptions. In addition to binding loosely to albumin, they bind *tightly* to certain specific β-globulins, making the bulk of the hormone incapable of diffusing through capillary and cellular membranes. (Binding is noncovalent and reversible.) Bound hormone is, therefore, physiologically inactive and metabolically inert.

All the classic hormones are present in blood circulating through all of the body tissues. What, then, makes a specific tissue a target for a given hormone? The answer, in one word, is receptors, highly specific tissue proteins with a very high affinity for one hormone and no, or very little, affinity for all the others. (As you will learn later, this statement is an oversimplification.) For polypeptidic hormones and epinephrine, these receptors are located on the exofacial side of the cellular plasma membrane while those for steroid and thyroid hormones are found intracellularly.

Binding to a cell's exterior dictates that there must be an intracellular "messenger" to relay the information carried on the hormone to the intracellular machinery. Although we still do not know the "second" messenger for some hormones, most notably insulin, we already know of four, namely, cAMP, Ca^{2+}, diacylglycerol, and inositol triphosphate. These, in turn, activate three different protein kinases: cAMP-dependent protein kinase, Ca^{2+}–calmodulin-dependent protein kinase, and Ca^{2+}–phospholipid/diacylglycerol-dependent protein kinase (protein kinase C). Even though we do not know the subsequent steps in most cases, it is already clear that the protein kinases interact in a sort of check-and-balance system. The net result, presumably, is the enhancement of homeostasis.

The interactions between hormones, their receptors, and adenylate cyclase, the generator of cAMP, are complex. Adenylate cyclase has two different regulatory subunits, one being stimulatory and the other inhibitory. Hormone–receptor complexes interact with one or the other. Each regulatory subunit is itself a tripeptide with differing α-subunits and identical β- and γ-subunits. Both require magnesium and GTP for activity, although the affinities of the two for magnesium differ. The details of this complex interaction are not yet physiologically clear.

It is premature to make categorical statements, but results so far strongly suggest that hormones acting through second messengers modify enzymatic activity by posttranslational modification, such as phosphorylation–dephosphorylation reactions. This mode of operation has the advantage of speed, responses being seen in about 1 min, and a gain that is considerably greater than that produced by allosteric modification. As a result, a certain aspect of metabolism can be rapidly turned on (or off).

Some of these same hormones have trophic actions; that is, they cause the target tissue to grow. Even though we have no ideas whatsoever concerning the mechanism(s) of this type of response, the difference in time scales (minutes vs. days) suggests very strongly that the mechanisms are different from those regulating metabolism directly.

Steroid and thyroid hormones, on the other hand, being lipids, diffuse readily into cells. In target tissues, they bind to intracellular receptors and turn on cellular machinery to synthesize enzymes that produce the observed physiological effects. The time scale here is also long, ranging from many hours to a day.

All steroid hormones are derived from a common precursor, cholesterol, in a series of repetitive reactions. Moreover, even though steroidogenic tissues are capable of de novo synthesis of cholesterol, in fact, most of it is imported on LDL. All of the steroid hormones contain, as an essential element, the same tetracyclic, cyclopentanoperhydrophenanthrene ring system found in cholesterol. (A hormone that is a derivative of vitamin D is an exception; see Chap. 7.) Corticosteroids and progesterone, which contain 21 carbons, have a two-carbon atom side chain; androgens contain 19 carbons and estrogens 18 carbon atoms.

SUPPLEMENTAL BIBLIOGRAPHY

The bibliography given at the end of each chapter is very incomplete because I make no pretense of covering everything. Indeed, an up-to-date library on endocrinology would contain many volumes and take more time to read than most of us have to devote to the subject. Rather, I have selected this bibliography to provide you with a ready entry into selected areas of current interest. Most of the papers are recent, and *their* lists of references will allow you to probe an area quickly and in depth.

APUD

Fujita, T and S Kobayashi. Paraneuronal cells in the GEP endocrine system. In *Gut Hormones* (SR Bloom, ed), Churchill Livingstone, Edinburgh, 1978, pp 414–422.

Pearse, AGE. Common cytochemical and ultrastructural characteristics of cells producing polypeptide hormones (the APUD series) and their relevance to thyroid and ultimobranchial C cells and calcitionin. *Proc R Soc London (Biol) 170*:71–80, 1968.

Pearse, AGE. The cytochemical and ultrastructure of polypeptide hormone producing cells of the APUD series and the embryonic, physiologic and pathologic implications of the concept. *J Histochem Cytochem 17*:303–313, 1969.

Calmodulin

Means, AR and JG Chafouleas. Calmodulin in endocrine cells. *Annu Rev Physiol 44*:667–682, 1982.

Rasmussen, H. The calcium messenger system. *New Engl J. Med 314*: 1094–1101; 1164–1170, 1986.

Watterson, DM and FF Vincenzi (eds). Calmodulin and cell functions. *Ann NY Acad Sci 356*:1–444, 1980.

Clinical Aspects

Catt, K and M Dufau. Introduction: The clinical significance of peptide hormone receptors. *Clin Endocrinol Metab 12*: xi, 1983.

Farid, NR and JC Bear. The human major histocompatibility complex and endocrine disease. *Endocr Rev 2*:50–86, 1981.

Hershman, JM. *Endocrine Pathophysiology: A Patient-Oriented Approach.* Lea & Febiger, Philadelphia, 1982, 316 pp.

Lever, EG. GA Medeiros-Neto, and LJ DeGroot. Inherited disorders of thyroid metabolism. *Endocr Rev 4*:213–239, 1983.

Rabin, D and TJ McKenna. *Clinical Endocrinology and Metabolism.* Grune & Stratton, New York, 1982, 652 pp.

Spiegel, AM, P. Gierschik, MA Levine, and RW Downs, Jr. Clinical implications of guanine nucleotide-binding proteins as receptor-effector couplers. *N Engl J Med 312*:26–33, 1986.

Verhoeven, GFM and JD Wilson. The syndrome of primary hormone resistance. *Metabolism 28*:253–289, 1979.

Wilson, JD and DW Foster. (eds). *Williams Textbook of Endocrinology.* 7th ed, WB Saunders, Philadelphia, 1985, 1413 pp.

Prohormones and Preprohormones

Cooke, NE, D Coit, J Shine, JD Baxter, and JA Martial. Human prolactin: cDNA structural analysis and evolutionary comparisons. *J Biol Chem 256*:4007–4016, 1981.

Docherty, K and DF Steiner. Post-translational proteolysis in polypeptide hormone biosynthesis. *Annu Rev Physiol 44*:625–638, 1982.

Esch, F, P Bohlen, N Ling, R Benoit, P Brazeau, and R Guillemin. Primary structure of ovine hypothalamic somatostatin-28 and somatostatin-25. *Proc Natl Acad Sci USA 77*:6827–6831, 1980.

Gainer, H, JT Russell, and YP Loh. The enzymology and intracellular organization of peptide precursor processing: The secretory vesicle hypothesis. *Neuroendocrinology 40*:171–184, 1985.

Goodman, RH, JW Jacobs, WW Chin, PK Lund, PC Dee, and JF Habener. Nucleotide sequence of a cloned structural gene coding for a precursor of pancreatic somatostatin. *Proc Natl Acad Sci USA 77*:5869–5873, 1980.

Hobart, P, R Crawford, LP Shen, R Pictet, and WJ Rutter. Cloning and sequence analysis of cDNAs encoding two distinct somatostatin precursors found in the endocrine pancreas of anglerfish. *Nature* 228:137–141, 1980.

Kronenberg, HM, BE McDevitt, JA Majzoub, J Nathans, PA Sharp, JT Potts, Jr, and A Rich. Cloning and nucleotide sequence of DNA coding for bovine preproparathyroid hormone. *Proc Natl Acad Sci USA* 76:4981–4985, 1979.

Lewis, RV, AS Stern, S Kimura, J Rossier, S Stein, and S Udenfriend. An about 50,000 dalton protein in adrenal medulla: A common precursor of [met]- and [leu]enkephalin. *Science* 208:1459–1461, 1980.

Lingappa, VR and G Blobel. Early events in the biosynthesis of secretory and membrane proteins. *Recent Prog Horm Res* 36:451–475, 1980.

Martial, JA, RA Hallewell, JD Baxter, and HM Goodman. Human growth hormone: Complementary DNA cloning and expression in bacteria. *Science* 205:602–607, 1979.

Maurer, RA, CR Erwin, and JE Donelson. Analysis of 5' flanking sequences and intron–exon boundaries of the rat prolactin gene. *J Biol Chem* 256:10524–10528, 1981.

Nilson, JH, AR Thomason, S Horowitz, NL Sasavage, J Blenis, R Albers, W Salser, and FM Rottman. Construction and characterization of a cDNA clone containing a portion of the bovine prolactin sequence. *Nucleic Acids Res* 8:1561–1573, 1980.

Pradayrol, L, H Jornvall, V Mutt, and A Ribet. *N*-Terminally extended somatostatin: The primary structure of somatostatin-28. *FEBS Lett* 109:55–58, 1980.

Russell, JT, MJ Brownstein, and H Gainer. Trypsin liberates an arginine vasopressin-like peptide and neurophysin from a M_r 20,000 putative common precursor. *Proc Natl Acad Sci USA* 76:6086–6090, 1979.

Shally, AV, W-Y Huang, RCC Chang, A Arimura, TW Redding, RP Millar, MW Hunkapillar, and LE Hood. Isolation and structure of prosomatostatin: A putative somatostatin precursor from pig hypothalamus. *Proc Natl Acad Sci USA* 77:4489–4493, 1980.

Seeburg, PE, HJ Shine, JS Martial, JD Baxter, and HM Goodman. Nucleotide sequence and amplification in bacteria of a structural gene for rat growth hormone. *Nature* 270:486–494, 1977.

Swift, GH, J-C Dagorn, PL Ashley, SW Cummings, and RS MacDonald. Rat pancreatic kallikrein mRNA: Nucleotide sequence and amino acid sequence of the encoded preproenzyme. *Proc Natl Acad Sci USA* 79:7263–7267, 1982.

Ullrich, A, J Shine, J Chirgwin, R Pictet, E Tischer, WJ Rutter, and HM Goodman. Rat insulin genes: Construction of plasmids containing the coding sequences. *Science* 196:1313–1319, 1977.

Receptors and Hormone Action

Aurbach, GD. Polypeptide and amine hormone regulation of adenylate cyclase. *Annu Rev Physiol 44*:653–656, 1982.

Birnbaumer, L, J Codina, R Mattera, RA Cerione, JD Hildebrandt, T Sunyer, FJ Rojas, MG Caron, RJ Lefkowitz, and R Iyengar. Regulation of hormone receptors and adenylyl cyclases by guanine nucleotide binding N proteins. *Recent Prog Horm Res 41*:41–94, 1985.

Cohen, P. The role of protein phosphorylation in the hormonal control of enzyme activity. *Eur J Biochem 151*:439–448. 1985.

Gershengorn, MC. Thyrotropin-releasing hormone action: Mechanism of calcium-mediated stimulation of prolactin secretion. *Recent Prog Horm Res 41*:607–646, 1985.

Ivarie, RH, JA Morris, and NL Eberhardt. Hormonal domains of response: Actions of glucocorticoid and thyroid hormones in regulating pleiotropic responses in cultured cells. *Recent Prog Horm Res 36*:195–235, 1980.

Kelly, RB. Pathways of protein secretion in eukaryotes. *Science 230*:25–32, 1985.

King, WJ and GL Greene. Monoclonal antibodies localize oestrogen receptors in the nuclei of target cells. *Nature 307*:745–747, 1984.

Lefkowitz, RE, MG Caron, and GL Stiles. Mechanisms of membrane-receptor regulation. *N Engl J Med 310*:1570–1579, 1984.

Parthasarathy, R and F Eisenberg, Jr. The inositol phospholipids: A stereochemical view of biological activity. *Biochem J 235*:313–322, 1986.

Sibley, DR and RJ Lefkowitz. Molecular mechanisms of receptor desensitization using the β-adrenergic receptor-coupled adenylate cyclase system as a model. *Nature 317*:124–129, 1985.

Tomlinson, S, S MacNeil, and BL Brown. Calcium, cyclic AMP and hormone action. *Clin Endocrinol 23*:595–610, 1985.

von der Ahe, D, S Janich, C Scheidereit, R. Renkawitz, GS Beato, and M Beato. Glucocorticoid and progesterone receptors bind to the same sites in two hormonally regulated promoters. *Nature 313*:706–709, 1985.

Walter, P, S Green, G Greene, A Krust, J-M Bornert, J-M Jeltsch, A Staub, E Jensen, G Scrace, M Waterfield, and P Chambon. Cloning of the human estrogen receptor cDNA. *Proc Natl Acad Sci USA 82*:7889–7893, 1985.

Walters, MR. Steroid hormone receptors and the nucleus. *Endocr Rev 6*:512–543, 1985.

Welshons, WV, ME Lieberman, and J Gorski. Nuclear localization of unoccupied oestrogen receptors. *Nature 307*:747–749, 1984.

Techniques

Andersson, S. Secretion of gastrointestinal hormones. *Annu Rev Physiol 35*:431–452, 1973.

Eisenbarth, GS and RA Jackson. Application of monoclonal antibody techniques to endocrinology. *Endocr Rev 3*:26–39, 1982.

Keane, PM, J Stuart, J Mendez, S Barbadoro, and WHC Walker. Rapid, specific assay for plasma cortisol by competitive protein binding. *Clin Chem 21*:1474–1478, 1975.

Schrader, WT and BW O'Malley. *Laboratory Methods for Hormone Action and Molecular Endocrinology,* 9th ed., Houston Biological Associates, Houston, 1985.

Sonksen, PH (ed). Radioimmunoassay and saturation analysis. *Br Med Bull 30*:1–103, 1974.

2

Hormones: An Overview

General Description   47
Neuroendocrinology   49
Clinical Aspects   62
    Hypopituitarism   62
    Hyperpituitarism   63
Summary   63
Supplemental Bibliography   64

GENERAL DESCRIPTION

Remember how difficult it was to associate names and faces when you were introduced to a large number of people, but how everything came into focus as you met them individually? You will have the same problem here as I introduce you to hormones. The names are suggestive of their function, but sometimes, as you will learn in later chapters, the function is much broader than the name implies, or the function may be species-specific.

There are two popular ways in which to categorize hormones; namely, by source or by function. I will do both.

An additional burden for the student is the recent introduction of a revised nomenclature for many polypeptide hormones. It is so new that it is still not widely used; hence, one must know both nomenclatures. In addition, the names are frequently so long and so cumbersome that initials are widely used, usually based on the older classification system.

The hypothalamus is now recognized as being the "master gland," a role once assigned to the pituitary. By the ablative–replacement approach, many biological activities are recognized in the hypothalamus. Until an entity is isolated, synthesized, and shown to duplicate the endogenous activity, it is called a "factor" (F). Afterward, it is promoted to full recognition as a hormone (H).

The gut is the largest endocrine organ in the body. Secretin, a gastrointestinal (GI) hormone, was the first hormone to be characterized (1901). Accordingly, it is curious that, until very recently, investigations into the gastrointestinal hormones appeared exclusively in gastroenterological journals rather than in endocrine journals. Today, there is a general recognition of the interdependence of the gastrointestinal and the so-called classic hormones.

The most active areas of identification are those of gastrointestinal hormones, neurohormones, and growth factors. A few of the names listed under GI tract (Table 2.1) have not yet been awarded full hormonal status (see Table 1.4). In addition, there are several growth factors, used more or less extensively in tissue culture technology, that could possibly be hormones. Moreover, certain oncogenes and growth factors are related, thus providing a linkage between normal and abnormal growth. As you can see, endocrinology is a dynamic and exciting area in which to work!

Classification according to function (Table 2.2) is perhaps more useful because one can actually conceptualize the interrelationship between apparently disparate hormones arising from several sources. On the other hand, I cannot fit all hormones directly into such a scheme—some actions are still too poorly defined, and others are too peripheral. These would obscure, rather than illustrate, points of view.

The most complicated systems are those that start with a CNS input and involve a series of three endocrine organs before producing targeted responses (Fig. 2.1). The negative feedbacks that are operative will be discussed in detail in the appropriate sections; in general, they follow the pattern shown in Figure 1.1. The reasons for the complexities are still not apparent, although it is obvious that there are several levels for interaction. For example, we already know that thyrotropin-releasing hormone (TRH) promotes the release of prolactin (PRL) as well as thyroid-stimulating hormone (TSH), and that somatostatin (SRIH) inhibits the release of TSH as well as the release of somatotropin (STH). The benefit that ensues to the whole organism, however, is still completely obscure.

The release of STH and PRL is controlled by dual, opposing hypothalamic hormones, one promoting release, the other inhibiting it (Fig. 2.2). Note, that these two pituitary hormones have no endocrine target organs, at least in the ordinary sense of the word. I say this because STH does promote hepatic synthesis of somatomedins, but negative feedback by their inhibition of STH secretion is not established.

There are three endocrine systems that are metabolite driven, and the neural imputs that exist are peripheral, serving to modify the metabolite input (Fig. 2.3). Two of these systems (calcium and glucose), having both a positive and a negative control, are tightly regulated. All, of course, have the property of correcting the imbalance that generated the initial signal, in ways more complicated than those shown.

NEUROENDOCRINOLOGY

Figures 2.1 and 2.2 point to the centrality of the central nervous system (CNS) in endocrinology. Hence, it is now appropriate that we discuss the interface between the two.

Neuroendocrinology is the branch of endocrinology that investigates the mechanisms by which neural inputs control endocrine secretion, i.e., the setpoint. To my knowledge, these signals, at the level of the secretory cells, are always positive (stimulatory) and not subject to negative feedback in the usual sense. When, however, the condition generating the neural signal is satisfied, the signal ceases.

The CNS includes, in addition to the cerebellum and cerebrum, areas of more immediate interest to neuroendocrinologists, such as the third ventricle, the median eminence, the infundibular stalk, and the neurohypophysis (posterior pituitary) (Fig. 2.4). Most of the CNS except for the median eminence, the infundibular stalk, and the neurohypophysis lies behind the "blood–brain barrier," a phrase that implies lack of free passage of some chemicals, chiefly drugs. The third ventricle is filled with cerebrospinal fluid which is apparently in dynamic equilibrium with the tissues that it bathes. Because of technical difficulties, reports on this fluid are fragmentary.

Messages are received by the CNS from all parts of the body over complex neural networks. No neuron apparently runs directly from a somatic receptor to the brain; they are interrupted by a series of junctions (synapses) that require release of monoaminergic neurotransmitters, such as dopamine, norepinephrine, serotonin,

Table 2.1 A List of Hormones by Source

Gland	Old name	New name	Abbreviation
Hypothalamus	Growth hormone release-inhibiting hormone	Somatostatin-14	GRIH/SRIH
		Somatostatin-28	GRIH/SRIH
	Growth hormone-releasing factor	Somatocrinin	GRF/SRF
	Prolactin release-inhibiting hormone	Dopamine	—
	Prolactin-releasing factor	Prolactoliberin	PRF
	Adrenocorticotrophic hormone-releasing hormone	Corticoliberin	CRH
	Thryoid-stimulating hormone-releasing hormone	Thyroliberin	TRH
	Lutenizing hormone-releasing hormone	Gonadoliberin	GnRH(LHRH)
	Follicle-stimulating hormone-releasing hormone	Gonadoliberin	GnRH(FSHRH)
	Melanocyte-stimulating hormone release-inhibiting factor[a]	Melanostatin[a]	MRIF
	Melanocyte-stimulating hormone-releasing factor[a]	Melanoliberin[a]	MRF
Adenohypophysis	Growth hormone	Somatotropin	GH/STH
	Prolactin	—	PRL
	Adrenocorticotrophic hormone	Corticotropin	ACTH
	Thyroid-stimulating hormone	Thyrotropin	TSH
	Luteinizing hormone	Luteotropin	LH
	Follicle-stimulating hormone	Folliculotropin	FSH

Gland	Hormone	Chemical name	Abbreviation
Intermediate lobe (pars intermedia) (not present in humans)	Melanocyte-stimulating hormone	—	MSH
Neurohypophysis	Antidiuretic hormone	Vasopressin	ADH
	Milk letdown hormone	Oxytocin	—
Thyroid	Thyroxine	3,3′,5,5′-Tetraiodothyronine	T_4
	—	3,3′,5-Triiodothyronine	T_3
	Thyrocalcitonin	Calcitonin	—
Parathyroid	Parathyroid hormone	—	PTH
Adrenal cortex	Cortisol/hydrocortisone	11β,17,21-Trihydroxy-4-pregnene-3,20-dione	[b]
	Aldosterone	11β,21-Dihydroxy-3,20-dioxo-4-pregnen-18-al	
	Dehydroepiandrosterone	3β-Hydroxy-5-androsten-17-one	
	Corticosterone	11β,21-Dihydroxy-4-pregnene-3,20-dione	
Adrenal medulla	Adrenaline	Epinephrine	—
	Noradrenaline	Norepinephrine	—
	Met-and Leu-enkephalin	—	—
Ovary	Estradiol-17β	1,3,5(10)-Estratriene-3,17β-diol	E_2
	Relaxin	—	—
	Inhibin	Folliculostatin	—
Corpus lutum	Progesterone	4-Pregnene-3,20-dione	Pg
Testes	Testosterone	17β-hydroxy-4-androsten-3-one	T
	Inhibin	Folliculostatin	—

(continues)

Table 2.1 (Continued)

Gland	Old name	New name	Abbreviation
Kidney	Dihydroxyvitamin D	1α,25-Dihydroxycholecalciferol	(OH)₂CC
	Erythropoietin	—	—
Liver	Sulfation factor	Somatomedin	SM
GI tract	Secretin	—	—
	Gastrin	—	—
	Pancreozymin/cholecystokinin	—	CCK
	Gastric inhibitory peptide	—	GIP
	Motilin	—	—
	Substance P	—	—
	Vasoactive intestinal peptide	—	VIP
	Chymodenin	—	—
	Somatostatin	—	—
	Bombesin	—	—
	Glucagon	—	—
Pancreas	Glucagon	—	—
	Insulin	—	—
	Somatostatin	—	—
Heart	Atrial natriuretic factor	—	ANF
Blood	Angiotensin II(III)	—	—

^aThere is no pituitary intermediate lobe in humans.
^bAdrenocortical hormones (and their metabolites) have two arbitrary alphabetical designations; the key to their use is usually included in the article employing them.

Table 2.2 A List of Hormones by Function

Function	Major hormones involved[a]
General growth	STH, somatocrinin, somatostatin, somatomedin
Osseous growth	Above + PTH, calcitonin, $(OH)_2CC$
Muscle growth	Testosterone
Basal metabolic rate	TRH, somatostatin, TSH, T_4, T_3
Salt–water metabolism	ADH, (renin), angiotensin II/III, aldosterone, ANF
Reproduction	GnRH, LH, FHS, PRL, E_2, T, Pg, DHT, DHEA, folliculostatin, hCG, antimullerian hormone, hCS, relaxin
Regulation of metabolism	Insulin, glucagon, epinephrine, ACTH, CRH, glucocorticoids,, GIP, many GI hormones

[a]This list is suggestive rather than exhaustive. Because of the interrelatedness of endocrine systems and the permissive nature of thyroid and glucocorticoid hormones, each category could be enlarged.

or γ-aminobutyric acid (GABA), to carry the electrical impulse across the synaptic gap. Moreover, each synapse is receiving both positive and negative signals and, therefore, is acting to integrate information that it is receiving. There may be two or three synapses cascaded, each with a different monoaminergic transmitter, before the neural message reaches the brain.

Pharmacologists have developed agonists and antagonists that are more or less specific for monoaminergic neurotransmitters (Table 2.3). By using these in various ways, neuroendocrinologists have been able to deduce which amines are probably involved in a given situation (Table 2.4) and, sometimes, with painstaking anatomical dissection and histological analyses, to identify the specific ganglia and nuclei involved. Given the chemical and anatomical complexities, you should understand the lack of definite information.

The hypothalamus is a small portion of the brain that is virtually inaccessible (see Fig. 2.4), lying as it does beneath the rest of the brain. Even when it is exposed, there are few topographic features to use in identifying areas. Nevertheless, the *rat* hypothalamus has been stereotaxically mapped using electrodes that can deliver a

```
                                              adenohypoph-   --
CNS-----> hypothalamus----------->  adenohy-  ------------  |--
                releasing           pophysis  seal hormone  |--
                hormone                                      --

ACTH
--------->  adrenal cortex  -------->  cortisol + corticosterone
TSH                                    + DHEA
--------->  thyroid         -------->  T4 + T3
FSH/LH
--------->  gonads          -------->  estradiol/testosterone
LH
--------->  corpus luteum   -------->  progesterone
```

Figure 2.1 The "three-tiered" endocrine systems involving the hypothalamus, the adenohypophysis, and a target endocrine organ.

```
                    releasing hormone          adenohypoph-              STH
                                                                     ,---|--->
CNS--->hypothalamus----------------> adenohy-  -----------------
                    release-inhibiting    pophysis   seal hormone
                    hormone                                          `---|--->
                                                                        PRL
```

Figure 2.2 The "two-tiered" endocrine systems involving only the hypothalamus and the adenohypophysis. Note that STH and PRL secretion are controlled by both releasing hormones and release-inhibiting hormones, perhaps as a substitute for the lack of negative-feedback control.

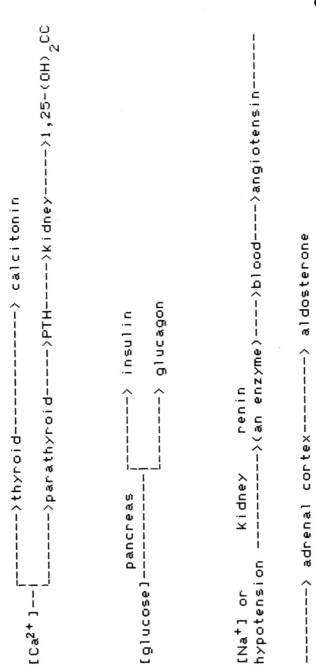

Figure 2.3 Metabolite-driven endocrine systems.

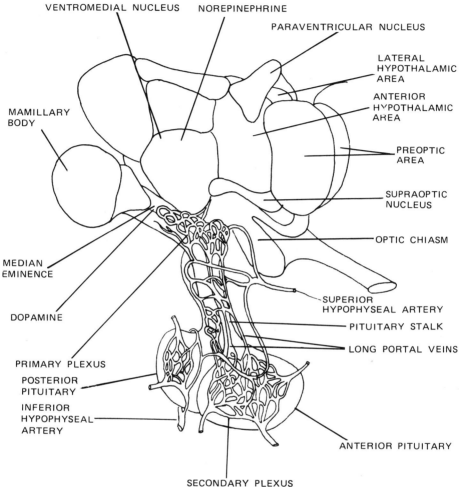

Figure 2.4 A representation of the hypothalamus and pituitary including the portal circulation from the former to the adenohypophysis.

very small stimulatory current or a much larger cauterizing current. A change in biological function is then correlated with a histological volume of damage by the latter current. In this way, more than 10 hypothalamic nuclei have been identified (Fig. 2.5).

Table 2.3 Specific[a] Agonists and Antagonists of Monoaminergic Transmitters

Function	Agonist	Antagonist/blocker
Adrenergic		
α	Clonidine Phenylephrine	WB4104 Ergotamine Phentolamine Phenoxybenzamine
β	Hydroxybenzylisoproterenol (−)Isoproterenol	Propranolol Dichlorisoproterenol
Dopaminergic	Apomorphine Bromocriptine	(+)Butaclamol Haloperidol α-Flupenthixol
Serotoninergic	—	Cyproheptadine Methysergide
GABAergic	Muscimol Bicuculline	Picrotoxin

[a]"Purity" of pharmacological action, like purity of chemicals, is a theoretical concept. A given drug has a predominant action, but there are usually side reactions, especially at high dosages. Another important factor in whole-animal experiments is the ability to pass through the blood–brain barrier. The drugs listed have not been categorized in this way.

Table 2.4 Neurotransmitter Effects on Pituitary Hormone Secretion in Man

Neurotransmitter	STH	PRL	TSH	ACTH	LH/FSH
Norepinephrine					
α	↑	—	—	↑	—
β	↓	—	—	↓	—
Dopamine	↑	↓	↓	(↓)	↓(↑)
Serotonin	↑	↑	(↓)	↑	U
GABA	↑	↑	U	U	U
Acetylcholine	↓	U	U	U	U
Enkephalin	↑	↑	(−)	(↓)	(↓)

↑ stimulates; ↓ suppresses; — no effect; ( ) suggestive effect; U unknown.
Source: From Frohman, 1980, with permission.

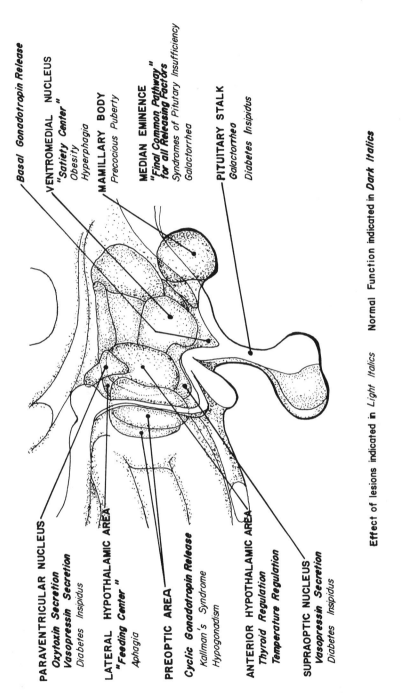

Basal Gonadotropin Release

VENTROMEDIAL NUCLEUS
"Satiety Center"
Obesity
Hyperphagia

MAMILLARY BODY
Precocious Puberty

MEDIAN EMINENCE
"Final Common Pathway"
for all Releasing Factors
Syndromes of Pituitary Insufficiency
Galactorrhea

PITUITARY STALK
Galactorrhea
Diabetes Insipidus

PARAVENTRICULAR NUCLEUS
Oxytoxin Secretion
Vasopressin Secretion
Diabetes Insipidus

LATERAL HYPOTHALAMIC AREA
"Feeding Center"
Aphagia

PREOPTIC AREA

Cyclic Gonadotropin Release
Kallman's Syndrome
Hypogonadism

ANTERIOR HYPOTHALAMIC AREA
Thyroid Regulation
Temperature Regulation

SUPRAOPTIC NUCLEUS
Vasopressin Secretion
Diabetes Insipidus

Effect of lesions indicated in *Light Italics*   Normal Function indicated in **Dark Italics**

Figure 2.5 Approximate location of hypothalamic nuclei with both their normal function and the effects of lesions.

The pituitary, a three-part organ, except in man, hangs from the infundibular stalk. Each part of the pituitary has two or three names; the anterior pituitary or adenohypophysis (pars distalis); the intermediate lobe (pars intermedia), which is missing in primates; and the posterior pituitary or neurohypophysis (pars nervosa) (see Fig. 2.4). Some of the names describe anatomy while others hint at function.

In the hypothalamus, there are peptidergic neurons in addition to monoaminergic neurons. Some of these neurons arise in a hypothalamic nucleus, travel through the median eminence and down the infundibular stalk, terminating in the neurohypophysis. Two hormones, vasopressin and oxytocin, are synthesized in the supraoptic nucleus (SON) and paraventricular nucleus (PVN) along with a stoichiometric amount of a carrier neurophysin. In an arrangement unique to the neurohypophysis, they are transported along the axon and deposited in secretary granules in the posterior pituitary.

The adenohypophysis receives its hypothalamic, hypophysiotropic hormones through a portal system. Within the upper infundibular stalk and median eminence, the superior hypophyseal artery divides into capillary tufts, making contact with nerve endings of the hypothalamic peptidergic neurons. The capillary tufts drain into portal veins that traverse the stalk (pars tuberalis) before breaking up into sinusoids in the adenohypophysis. This arrangement delivers the hypophysiotropic hormones to their target cells without dilution by the general circulation. Thus, a minute quantity of hypothalamic hormone can have a rather large effect.

Initially, hypophysiotropic hormones were believed to be limited to the hypothalamus. We now know that this is not true. Not only are the "hypothalamic" hormones of mammals present in other parts of the brain and gut (gastroenteropancreatic tissues), but they are phylogenetically ancient substances with the unaltered peptide present in species that do not possess a pituitary. Thus, we may surmise, for example, that TRH, as a releasing hormone for TSH secretion, is a recent evolutionary event and that the primitive role for this peptide represents some aspects of neuronal function. Frog skin is rich in TRH as well as neural peptides. [A gonadoliberin GnRH)-like material present in frog sympathetic ganglia functions as a neurotransmitter.] In evolutionary transition, TRH is unable to stimulate thyroid function in amphibia or fish despite being present in high concentration in the hypothalamus and brain of these species. Thus, it appears that hypothalamic peptides (TRH, GnRH, somatostatin, vasopressin, oxytocin, and probably others) initially arose with a paracrine or neurocrine function (see Chap. 1) and that only in later evolution did they acquire the role of regulating pituitary secretion.

Another corollary of this portal delivery system is the need for several adenohypophyseal cell types, each with receptors for the appropriate hypophysiotropic hormone(s). Based on histological stains, three categories of cells have long been recognized: acidophils, basophils, and chromophobes. Immunostaining, however, has shown that there are five cell types for six hormones. Somatotropin and PRL belong to the acidophil series and ACTH, TSH, and the gonadotropins (FSH and LH) are located in the basophil series (Table 2.5). When these cells become hypersecretory, they discharge their granules and become chromophobic.

Table 2.5 Cytology of the Human Adenohypophysis

Hormone	Cell name	Stain	%	Comments
Acidophils				
STH	Somatotrope	Eosin or orange G	50	Tumors in acromegaly
PRL	Lactotrope	Erythosin or carmoisine	15–20	Hyperplasia with estrogen excess
Basophils				
ACTH	Corticotrope	PAS[a]	—	Decrease in Addison's disease
TSH	Thyrotrope	PAS[a] Aldehyde thionin	10	Hypertrophy in myxedema
FSH	Gonadotrope ⎫ PAS[a]			Degranulation
	⎬ +		10	in hypogonadism
LH	Gonadotrope ⎭ aldehyde thionin			

[a]The periodic acid-Schiff (PAS) stain is characteristic of glycoproteins. Note that 1-39 ACTH is not a glycoprotein whereas proopiomelanocortin is.

CLINICAL ASPECTS

In this section, I shall discuss hypothalamopituitary disease from a general perspective, reserving specific details to individual chapters.

Hypopituitarism

Inappropriately low secretion of hypophyseal hormones may be caused by either pituitary or hypothalamic disease; the latter is classified as secondary. The failure may be isolated to one or more cell types or may involve all cell types; the latter is called panhypopituitarism. For reasons that are not understood, the frequency of the various hypophyseal endocrinopathies is different. A deficiency of vasopressin (diabetes insipidus) is most frequently seen followed by gonadal dysfunction, hypothyroidism, and, least frequently, by hypocortisolism.

The pituitary is susceptible to infarction, especially during the peripartum period when blood loss and shock may lead to panhypopituitarism (Sheehan's syndome). This condition is readily recognizable because many bodily functions are affected: failure of lactation and all of the consequences of gonadal failure, adrenocortical insufficiency, thyroid deficiency, and inadequate vasopressin secretion (see appropriate chapters for details). Fortunately, Sheehan's syndrome is becoming increasingly rare as better obstetrical care becomes available.

Secondary hypopituitarism, as a result of hypothalamic damage, was suspected long before the isolation of hypothalamic hormones. The causes of hypothalamic damage may be a fracture at the base of the brain, basal meningitis, or irradiation of tumors of the head and neck region. The secretion of STH, of TSH, and/or of ACTH from the pituitary may fail, but PRL secretion may rise (suppression of the PRL release-inhibiting hormone, dopamine).

Idiopathic hypopituitarism, whether unitropic or global, is often secondary to hypothalamic dysfunction. This can be readily demonstrated by striking increases in serum concentrations of pituitary hormones following administration of the appropriate hypothalamic-releasing hormone.

Hypopituitarism may also have a nutritional origin. Extreme weight loss (30% or more of ideal body weight), as seen in prolonged starvation or anorexia nervosa, may produce a functional disease reversible upon refeeding.

Hyperpituitarism

As you should now be able to predict, there are three generic types of hyperpituitarism. Tumors may cause selective hyperactivity of specific adenohypophyseal cell types, target organ failure may remove feedback control of pituitary–hypothalamic secretion, or a tumor of the hypothalamus may cause hypersecretion of a specific hypothalamic hormone, leading to overstimulation of the associated endocrine system. The last two are examples of secondary hyperpituitarism.

SUMMARY

A few years ago, a new system of nomenclature of polypeptidic hormones was introduced in an effort to systematize their naming. Although this change was desirable, the names are still long, and everyone reverts to letter abbreviations that are based on the old system.

The neural and humoral endocrine systems are integrated at the level of the hypothalamus. In addition, neurocrine peptides are distributed through the brain, although no one has yet discerned a reason for their existence.

The hypothalamus makes two types of peptides. The neurohypophyseal peptides, oxytocin and vasopressin (antidiuretic hormone), are transported intraaxonally and stored in the posterior pituitary.

The hypophysiotropic hormones are transported to nerve endings in the median eminence, where they are picked up by a portal system and delivered, undiluted by the systemic circulation, to the anterior pituitary. This organ, which has a different embryological derivation from the posterior pituitary, has five different cell types elaborating six hormones. The somatotropes, under the influence of somatocrinin and somatostatin, synthesize and release somatotropin or growth hormone. The prolactotropes synthesize and release prolactin in response to prolactoliberin and dopamine. Both of these cell types have no chemical, negative-feedback control, but instead have dual (one positive and one negative) hypothalamic control.

The other three cell types have a humoral negative-feedback control, as well as hypothalamic control. Thus, the thyrotropes synthesize and release thyrotropin in response to thyroliberin and somatostatin, as well as thyroxine and other hormones. The adrenocorticotropes synthesize and release adrenocorticotropin in response to corticoliberin and cortisol–corticosterone. And the gonadotropes synthesize and release folliculotropin and luteotropin in response to gonadoliberin and folliculostatin or a gonadal steroid, respectively.

As the names imply, the adenohypophyseal hormones regulate the synthesis and release of yet another hormone from their endocrine target organs as well as having a trophic action on that organ. Thus, thyrotropin acts on the thyroid to promote the synthesis and release of thyroxine and triiodothyronine; adrenocorticotropin acts on the adrenal cortex to promote the synthesis and release of cortisol and of corticosterone; folliculotropin promotes the maturation of ovarian follicular follicles; and luteotropin promotes gonadal steroidogenesis, ovulation, growth of the corpus luteum, and synthesis and release of progesterone.

Thus, a number of critical endocrine systems function under a complex control with central nervous system input and three levels of endocrine control. Other systems involving Na^+–K^+, Ca^{2+}–HPO_4^-, and carbohydrate–lipid metabolism are wholly or partially independent of hypothalamoadenohypophyseal control.

SUPPLEMENTAL BIBLIOGRAPHY

General

Tepperman, J. *Metabolic and Endocrine Physiology*, 4th ed. Year Book Medical Publishers, Chicago, 1980, 335 pp.

Neuroendocrinology

Frohman, LA. Neurotransmitters as regulators of endocrine function. In *Neuroendocrinology* (DT Krieger and JC Hughes, eds). Sinauer Associates, Inc., New York, 1980, pp 44–57.
Jackson, IMD and WW Vale. Extrapituitary functions of hypothalamic hormones: A symposium. *Fed Proc 40*:2543–2569, 1981.
Krieger, DT and JC Hughes (eds). *Neuroendocrinology*. Sinauer Associates, Inc., New York, 1980, 352 pp.

Krieger, DT. The hypothalamus and neuroendocrinology. In *Neuroendocrinology* (DT Krieger and JC Hughes, eds), Sinauer Associates, Inc., New York, 1980, pp 3–12.

Krieger, DT. The hypothalamus and neuroendocrine pathology. In *Neuroendocrinology* (see DT Krieger and JC Hughes, eds), Sinauer Associates, Inc., New York, 1980, pp 13–22.

3

Nutrition and Regulatory Polypeptides of the Gastrointestinal Tract

Introduction   67
The Gastrin Family   71
    Gastrins   71
    Cholecystokinin   74
The Secretin Family   76
    Secretin   76
    Gastric inhibitory peptide   79
    Vasoactive intestinal peptide   81
    Glucagon/Enteroglucagon   82
The Gastrin-Releasing Peptide Family   83
    Gastrin-releasing peptide   83
    Substance P   85
Pancreatic Polypeptide   85
Somatostatin   87
Motilin   89
Neurotensin   92
Clinical Aspects   92
Summary   93
Supplemental Bibliography   95

INTRODUCTION

The gut or alimentary canal (Fig. 3.1) constitutes the largest endocrine organ in the body. Unlike other endocrine organs, endocrine cells of the gut are distributed along the surface of the gastrointestinal mucosa with their mucosal surface exposed to the lumen of the tract. Thus, they are able to react promptly to secretagogues present in the gut.

So far, all of the cells producing gastrointestinal hormones possess amine-handling properties and, therefore, belong to the amine precursor uptake and decarboxylation (APUD) series. All are derived embryologically from the neural crest. Thus, it should not be surprising that the gut releases a mixture of polypeptides having endocrine, paracrine, or neurocrine functions. Some have more than one type of function (Table 3.1).

67

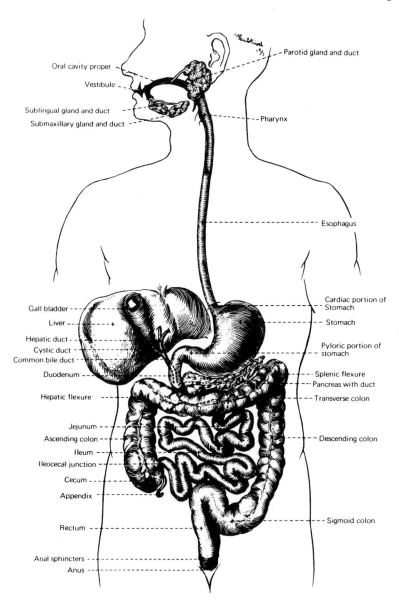

Figure 3.1 The digestive system showing the alimentary canal and accessory organs. The liver and gallbladder are turned up and to the right (*Source*: *Basic Physiology and Anatomy*, Chaffee and Creiskeimer, Lippincott, 1969, with permission).

Table 3.1 Location and Function of Established Gut Regulatory Peptides

Cell type	Peptide	Location	Mode	Established actions
G	Gastrin	Antrum, upper small intestine	E	↑ Gastric acid secretion
D2	PP	Pancreas	E	↓ Pancreatic enzyme release and gallbladder contraction
S	Secretin	Duodenum, jejunum	E	↑ Release of pancreatic HCO_3^-
I	CCK	Small intestine	E,N	↑ Contraction of gallbladder and release of pancreatic enzymes
EC2	Motilin	Small intestine	E	↑ Gut motility
K	GIP	Small intestine	E	↑ Secretion of insulin (man); ↓ Release of gastric acid (dog)
?	Neurotensin	Ileum	E, N	?
EG	Enteroglucagon	Ileum, colon	E, N	Trophic to gut
D	Somatostatin	All areas	E, P, N	↓ Release and action of many peptides
H(D1)	VIP	All areas	N	↑ Muscle relaxation, vasodilation, excretion
EC1	Substance P	All areas	N	Sensory, vasodilatory; stimulates muscle contraction
P	GRP	All areas	P, N	↑ Release of peptides
B	Insulin	Pancreas	E	Regulates anabolic reactions
A	Glucagon	Pancreas	E	↑ Gluconeogenesis and lipolysis

Abbreviations used: PP, pancreatic polypeptide; CCK, cholecystokinin (pancreozymin); GIP, gastric inhibitory peptide; GRP, gastrin-releasing peptide; VIP, vasoactive intestinal peptide; ↑stimulated; ↓inhibits; E, endocrine; N, neurocrine; P, paracrine.

"Regulatory" accurately describes their function, irrespective of mechanism of action.

All the peptides covered in this chapter have a common function; namely, promotion of cellular nutrition in the broadest sense. This represents the spectrum of digestion of ingested food, orderly propulsion of chyme through the gastrointestinal tract, and disposition of processed food to the major storage forms of the body (glycogen, triglycerides, and protein). Possibly, even satiety is controlled. All of this is accomplished in a coordinated manner by the regulatory peptides, each working in its own way, to ensure smooth and efficient utilization of ingested food. When this coordinated action is lost through a disease process, pathologic manifestations follow. Some of these are discussed in the section on clinical aspects, but mostly, science has not yet progressed far enough to assign a mechanism to each disease state.

The lack of scientific progress is due to the diffuse nature of endocrine tissue in the gut, making typical ablation–replacement experiments impossible. Moreover, in the absence of ablation, there is no deficit in some body function that can be corrected by administration of a tissue extract, i.e., there is no good bioassay. Instead, a function, not necessarily physiologic that gives adequate sensitivity serves as a bioassay in a large-scale purification. Thus, there is no assurance that the "pure" peptide once obtained is physiologically relevant. A great deal more work is required to test the significance of a large investment of time and money.

Because there are many hormones, there should be many different cell types, like there are in the pituitary. On the basis of structure, 12 cell types have been recognized in the gut and five in the pancreas. By immunocytochemistry, specific polypeptides can be assigned to a specific cell type. Some cell types have not yet been linked to a specific polypeptide, whereas others contain two or more, requiring subclassification (see Table 3.1).

The distribution of peptides in the gut is variable. The neural peptides tend to be distributed throughout the stomach, small intestine, and colon, and some, including vasoactive intestinal peptide (VIP), cholecystokinin (CCK), and substance P, are also found in pancreatic neurons. The endocrine peptides tend to be more restricted. Thus, endocrine cells containing CCK, gastric inhibitory peptide (GIP), motilin, and secretin are found only in the upper small intestine; gastrin cells only in gastric antrum and upper duodenum; and cells containing glucagon, insulin, and pancreatic polypeptide (PP) only in the pancreas. Moreover, the neurocrine substances are found in the CNS as well as in the peripheral nervous system, lung, thyroid, and adrenal. The role that these substances play in each tissue is not clear.

THE GASTRIN FAMILY

Gastrins

The gastrin family (Fig. 3.2) contains only two members—the gastrins and cholecystokinin-pancreozymin (CCK). The COOH-terminal pentapeptide in both hormones is identical, which probably accounts for overlapping biological activities and for the ability of CCK to serve as both a weak agonist and a competitive inhibitor of gastrin action.

All of the biological activity of gastrin resides in the COOH-terminal tetrapeptide, which is called tetragastrin or, sometimes, simply tetrin. It is the synthetic pentagastrin that is commercially available, however. The rest of the chain presumably affects the rate of destruction or removal of the hormone because G-17 and G-34 have different half-lives in blood: namely, 6 and 40 min, respectively, The rest of the chain must also affect biological activity in some way because G-17 is five to six times more potent than equimolar concentrations of G-34.

Gastrins I and II differ in the sulfation of tyrosine-12 of gastrin-17. Because all of the bioactivity resides in gastrin residues 13 to 17, sulfation plays no role in bioactivity. (Compare, however, CCK.)

The mRNA coding for gastrin is about 620 nucleotides long, suggesting a gastrin precursor peptide of about 200-amino acid residues. A large precursor of gastrin has been proposed but never isolated. Partial sequence analysis of the gastrin mRNA indicates an NH$_2$-terminal extension connecting to the G-34 form through a His-Arg-Arg link. Partial hydrolysis by a trypsinlike enzyme would thus produce gastrin-34, whereas more complete hydrolysis would yield gastrin-17.

The preponderant form of gastrin in gastric antral mucosa and in gastrinomas (Zollinger-Ellison tumor) is G-17, whereas in blood it is G-34 (one-third is G-17). Because G-17 is more potent than G-34, bioactivity is principally due to G-17.

```
            1                    5                   10                     15
G34  pyroglu.leu.gly.pro.gln.gly.pro.pro.his.leu.val.ala.asp.pro.ser.lys.lys.
CCK      lys.ala.pro.ser.gly.arg.val.ser.met.ile.lys.asn.leu.glu.ser.leu.
          1            5                   10                      15


                                                  (H)     (I)
                                               (SO3H)(II)
                                                  |         34
G34  glu.gly.pro.trp.leu.glu.glu.glu.glu.ala.tyr.gly.trp.met.asp.phe.NH2
            20              25              30                     34
G17   1            5               10              15          17


                                                       (H)     (I)
                                                    (SO3H)(II)
                                                       |         33
CCK  asp.pro.ser.his.arg.ile.ser.asp.arg.asp.tyr.met.gly.trp.met.asp.phe.NH2
            20              25              30                          33
                                                       SO3H
```

Figure 3.2 The gastrin family. G17 starts at residue 18 or G34 and is identical with residues 18 to 34 of G34. Note the Lys-Lys sequence at positions 16,17 of G34. Gastrin II is G17 sulfated at Tyr-12; gastrin I has no sulfate. G34 also occurs in sulfated and nonsulfated forms. Identities in CCK and gastrins are underlined.

72

The principal stimulus for gastrin release is feeding, especially that of a high-protein meal. It is also stimulated by antral distention and vagal (cholinergic) stimulation. Gastrin-releasing peptide (GRH; see p. 83), as the name implies, causes the release of gastrin, but its physiological importance is still unknown.

One action of gastrin at physiologic concentrations is the regulation of gastric acid secretion (Table 3.2), which is an extremely complex, incompletely understood process involving three major stimulants: acetylcholine (vagal), gastrin, and histamine. Parietal cells have separate receptors for gastrin and for histamine; the action of the latter can be blocked by cimetidine, a histamine (H_2)-receptor antagonist. Gastrin alone has little effect on acid secretion unless there is a basal level of histamine present. In other words, there is a marked synergism. At any rate, the net effect under appropriate conditions is the release of hydrochloric acid which, in turn, completes a negative-feedback loop and inhibits gastrin release.

Several hormones besides gastrin influence gastric acid secretion. Secretin is a potent noncompetitive inhibitor of gastrin-mediated acid secretion and a weak inhibitor of gastrin release. Patients with gastrinomas, however, exhibit paradoxic responses to intravenous secretin in that gastrin levels increase, usually by more than 50%. Gastric inhibitory peptide is also a powerful inhibitor of gastric acid secretion in dogs, an effect from which its name is derived. Studies in humans, however, have failed to show convincing suppression. Other members of the secretin family have similar actions.

Table 3.2   Actions of Gastrins

Physiological action
    stimulation (with histamine) of gastric acid secretion
    stimulation of antral smooth muscle activity
Nonphysiological actions*
    stimulates lower esophageal sphincter tone
    relaxes pyloric sphincter
    stimulates pancreatic enzyme secretion
    increases intestinal motor activity
    modestly stimulates pancreatic bicarbonate and water secretion
    trophic action on gut mucosal cell

---

*Actions seen when the concentration of hormone in the blood exceeds the physiological range.

Cholecystokinin

The other member of the gastrin family is cholecystokinin (CCK) (see Fig. 3.2). (This hormone was formerly also called pancreozymin.) Work with CCK has lagged because of problems in the development of a satisfactorily specific and sensitive radioimmunoassay (RIA). These problems are related to the poor immunogenicity of the hormone, its lack of ready iodination (there is only one tyrosine, and it is sulfated; iodination presumably occurs on histidine-20), its lack of stability after iodination, and the variability in specificity of immunoassays under development. Use of the Bolton-Hunter reagent [N-hydroxysuccinimidyl ester of 3-(p-hydroxyphenyl)propionic acid] has apparently solved two problems: namely, those of iodination and of stability of the iodinated hormone derivate (Fig. 3.3).

All of the bioactivity of CCK resides in the COOH-terminal decapeptide; in fact, it is ten times more potent than the intact hormone. The only tyrosine in CCK lies within this decapeptide, and it must be sulfated for biological activity. Synthetic CCK26-33 (CCK8) having two to ten times the bioactivity of the intact hormone is now available. The concentration of CCK8 in the intestine is similar to that of CCK33, with the former accounting for most of the immunoreactive CCK in gut neurons.

The physiologic stimuli for release of CCK are still unresolved because of difficulties with the assay of circulating CCK. Most recent efforts report the *difference* between an assay that uses a broad spectrum of immunoactivity, which will, *of course*, include the gastrins, and another that uses a highly specific gastrin assay. Subjects eating a standard breakfast responded with increases in serum CCK8 immunoactivity of 5–10 fmol/ml from undetectable fasting levels. There was no clear evidence of increases in other forms of CCK!

The products of protein and fat digestion are clearly physiologic stimuli for CCK release. In humans and the dog, intraduodenal tryptophan and tyrosine are good stimulants; methionine and valine are also effective in humans, but not in dogs. Clearly, much more needs to be done.

Cholecystokinin includes a wide variety of biological effects (Table 3.3), most of which are probably nonphysiologic. Again, without a good assay, it is difficult to tell. The assays used to monitor the isolation of CCK were the stimulation of gallbladder

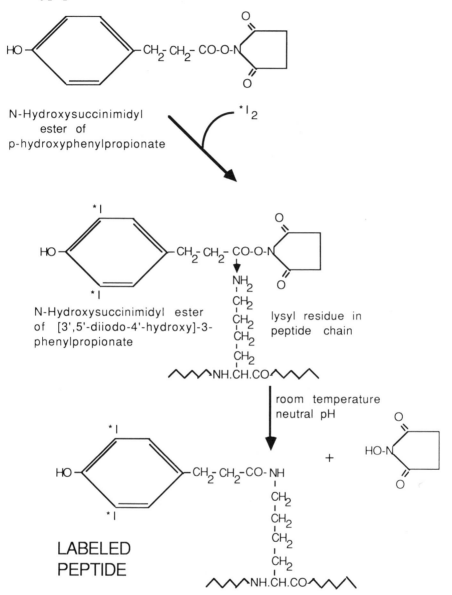

Figure 3.3 Labeling of proteins using the Hunter-Bolton reagent, which is the *N*-hydroxysuccinimidyl ester of 3-(*p*-hydroxyphenyl)propionic acid. This reagent reacts readily with free amino groups at neutral pH and room temperature. Its phenolic ring is usually iodinated with radioactive iodine before the reaction with a polypeptide, thereby avoiding exposure of the polypeptide to oxidizing conditions.

Table 3.3 Actions of Cholecystokinins

Physiological actions
stimulations of release of pancreatic enzymes
stimulation of gallbladder contraction
Nonphysiological actions
stimulates release of pepsin
stimulates activity of Brunner's gland
stimulates release of hepatic bicarbonate and water
enhances secretin-mediated release of pancreatic bicarbonate
competitively inhibits gastrin-mediated release of gastric acid
has a trophic action on the pancreas
may participate in induction of satiety

contraction, important for the digestion of fat; and the release of enzymes from the pancreas, which is crucial for the digestive process. The latter action led to the designation of pancreozymin. Only after the determination of structure and synthesis were complete did the investigators involved realize that they had isolated the same hormone, that is, CCK!

Secretin and CCK potentiate each other's action on the exocrine pancreas.

Effects on the CNS are a recent and controversial discovery. There are CCK receptors (binding affinity, ca. 10^{-9} M^{-1}) in many parts of the (mouse) brain, and fasting significantly increases the number of receptors in the olfactory bulb and the hypothalamus; the latter is known to regulate appetite.

THE SECRETIN FAMILY

Secretin

The secretin family consists of secretin, glucagon, GIP and VIP (Fig. 3.4). Seventeen of 27 amino acids in secretin are homologous with one or more of the others. Homology is greater for glucagon (13) than for the NH_2-terminal portion of GIP (9) or VIP (8).

The chemistry of secretin, the oldest hormone (1902), is still simple—no precursor forms have been found (do not assume there are none), and no fragment of the 27-amino acid polypeptide containing the biological activity has been detected. Secretinlike

	1				5					10					15
VIP	his.ser.asp.ala.val.phe.thr.asp.asn.tyr.thr.arg.leu.arg.lys.
Secretin	his.ser.asp.gly.thr.phe.thr.ser.glu.leu.ser.arg.leu.arg.asp.
Glucagon	his.ser.gln.gly.thr.phe.thr.ser.asp.tyr.ser.lys.tyr.leu.asp.
GIP	tyr.ala.glu.gly.thr.phe.ile.ser.asp.tyr.ser.ile.ala.met.asp.

					20					25					30
VIP	gln.met.ala.val.lys.lys.tyr.leu.asn.ser.ile.leu.asn.NH₂
Secretin	ser.ala.arg.leu.gln.arg.leu.leu.gln.gly.leu.val.NH₂
Glucagon	ser.arg.arg.ala.gln.asp.phe.val.gln.trp.leu.met.asn.thr
GIP	lys.ile.arg.gln.gln.asp.phe.val.asn.trp.leu.leu.ala.gln.gln.gln

					35					40
GIP	lys.gly.lys.lys.ser.asp.trp.lys.his.asn.ile.thr.gln

Figure 3.4 The secretin family: VIP, vasoactive intestinal peptide; GIP, glucose-dependent insulinotropic polypeptide. Identities are underlined. The amino acid code is given in Appendix C.

biological activity is present in extracts of rat brain; it has not been rigorously identified.

The physiologic stimuli for secretin release are still under investigation; an RIA sentive enough for this work was only recently devised. The major stimulus is a proximal duodenal pH of 4.5 to 5.0, or less, following ingestion of a meal. Neutralization of gastric acid by antacid or suppression of acid secretion by cimetidine abolishes the rise in plasma secretin level. Protein, fat, glucose, alcohol, and nicotine do not stimulate secretin release. It is likely that bile is also not a stimulant because persons with achlorhydria have no postprandial rise in plasma secretin even though bile function is normal.

Secretin has a plethora of biological actions attributed to it (Table 3.4). However, only two have now been established as being physiologic. They are the promotion of pancreatic water and electrolyte excretion and the inhibition of both gastrin secretion and gastrin-induced gastric acid excretion. Thus, secretin is an enterogastrone, at least in the dog. (An enterogastrone is an

Table 3.4   Actions of Secretin

Physiological actions
   stimulation of release of pancreatic water and bicarbonate
   inhibition of gastrin secretion
   inhibition of gastrin-induced release of gastric acid
Nonphysiological actions
   reduction of lower esophageal pressure
   stimulation of release of pepsin
   stimulation of mucous excretion
   reduction of gastric motility
   reduction of gastrin-mediated DNA synthesis
   increased blood flow and oxygen consumption in pancreas
   stimulation of pancreatic enzyme release
   stimulation of pancreatic RNA synthesis
   stimulation of insulin secretion
   stimulation of activity of Brunner's gland
   decreased motility of duodenum, jejunum, and colon
   stimulation of renal excretion of water, sodium, and potassium
   increased cardiac output
   increased splanchnic blood flow
   increased lipolysis

enteric substance that inhibits gastric acid production.) Patients with gastrinomas exhibit paradoxic responses in that serum gastrin levels increase.

The half-life of secretin in the circulation is quite short (ca. 3 min), perhaps because the head, lower extremities, and mesentery, in addition to the kidney, contribute to its clearance.

Gastric Inhibitory Peptide

Although GIP, a newer hormone first isolated in 1970, is usually an acronym for "gastric inhibitory polypeptide," it could also be called "glucose-dependent insulinotropic polypeptide"; these two names aptly describe its important functions. Two such dissimilar actions raise the possibility of impurity, especially because the structure and properties have not yet been confirmed by synthesis. Indeed, the preparation whose sequence is given (Fig. 3.4) contains about 5% impurity as shown by high pressure liquid chromatography (HPLC) and isotachophoresis.

With the caveat that further purification may alter the description of responses (Table 3.5), let us examine what is now known. Gastric inhibitory peptide was originally isolated and characterized as an inhibitor of gastric acid secretion in (denervated) Heidenhain pouch preparations in dogs. In humans, however, the evidence does not support an enterogastrone role for GIP.

The incretin effect of GIP in man is, on the other hand, well established. Oral glucose produces a larger insulin response than intravenous glucose, indicating a gastrointestinal mediator of insulin release. In 1932 the term *incretin* was coined to designate this agent. It was not until 1973, however, that the incretin action of GIP was discovered; more definitive experiments were reported in 1978 (see Fig. 3.5).

The principal stimulants for GIP release are carbohydrate and fat ingestion, with the latter being more potent in the basal state. After consumption of oral glucose, serum glucose, GIP, and insulin concentrations are all variable. To provide a reproducible system, the glucose-clamp technique was used in which glucose was infused over a period of 2 hr; plasm glucose, GIP, and insulin were measured. Midway through the infusion, an oral glucose load of 40 g/m² was administered which produced concomitant increases in

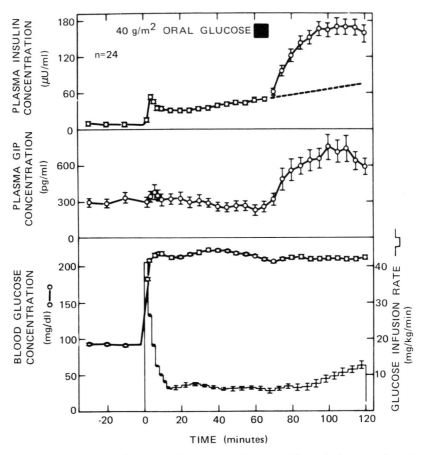

Figure 3.5 Hyperglycemic clamp experiment with oral glucose showing mean ± SEM for 24 subjects. The dashed line represents the expected plasma insulin concentration had oral glucose not been given (*Source: J Clin Invest 62*: 155, 1978, by copyright permission of The American Society of Clinical Investigation, from an article by DK Andersen, D Elahi, JC Brown, JD Tobin, and R Andres).

plasma GIP and insulin (see Fig. 3.5). In extensions of this technique, infusion of pharmacologic quantities of GIP (in place of oral glucose) still produced increased insulin release. At the other end of the scale, there appears to be a glucose threshhold of ca. 2000 mg/L required for expression of GIP's insulinotropic activity.

Table 3.5 Actions of GIP

Physiological actions
  stimulation of insulin secretion
  inhibition of gastric acid secretion (dogs, not man)
Nonphysiological or insufficiently studied actions
  stimulation of glucagon secretion (counterproductive)
  stimulation of small-intestinal excretion
  reduction of lower-esophageal sphincter pressure
  stimulation of mesenteric blood flow
  stimulation of lipoprotein lipase activity
  interactions with other GI hormones

Other aspects of GIP's incretin action are less well understood. Feedback control appears to be correlated more with hyperglycemia than with hyperinsulinemia, with glucose somehow facilitating metabolic clearance of GIP. The mechanism of action of GIP on the pancreatic β-cell is not understood, and the presence of GIP receptors on the β-cell has not been demonstrated. It is presently assumed that GIP interacts with the β-cell through a nonglucose pathway. For example, GIP exerts an additive effect with arginine infused at 7.5 g/m². When the arginine infusion was increased to 15 g/m², however, GIP was no longer insulinotropic (see Chap. 9 for a description of insulin secretion).

Vasoactive Intestinal Peptide

Vasoactive intestinal peptide (VIP), a decade after its isolation from porcine duodenum, is known to have a much wider distribution and broader range of actions than its name implies. It should be viewed as a neural peptide rather than as a true hormone. This peptide is present throughout the gastrointestinal tract, from the salivary glands, to the rectum, to the pancreas. It is also widely distributed in peripheral and central neural tissues, especially in the caudate nucleus. In a few cases, the synaptosomes have been shown to contain the highest concentrations. Human placenta and cord blood contain immunoreactive VIP in concentrations 100 and three times, respectively, that in normal plasma.

The physiologic stimuli inducing release of VIP include the following:

1. Oxytocin (in dogs)
2. Vagal and mechanical stimulation (in animals)
3. Intraduodenal administration of hydrochloric acid or ethanol (in humans)

The ubiquitousness of VIP, preponderantly in neurons, and its ability to influence many bodily functions indicate that VIP probably serves a neurocrine function. Functions that may be mediated or modulated by VIP include:

1. Vasodilation in salivary and sweat glands and in the skeletal, splanchnic, coronary, and cerebral circulations
2. Regulation of gastric, intestinal, and pancreatic secretion
3. Mediation of the nonadrenergic inhibitory system in the lower esophageal sphincter, the airways, and possibly elsewhere
4. Stimulation of prolactin release and, possibly, also of other hypothalamic–pituitary hormones
5. Participation in certain fetal or neonatal responses as suggested by the elevated content of VIP in placenta and cord blood

Glucagon/Enteroglucagon

The pancreatic α-cell contains a 29-amino acid hormone called glucagon (see Fig. 3.4). Antibodies produced against this antigen react with substances, called glucagonlike immunoreactivity (GLI), or enteroglucagon, present in certain cells of the intestine. Intestinal extracts contain GLIs that are heterogeneous in both size and isoelectric point. Of the two dominating molecular species, only the larger (10 kDa), called glicentin, has been purified and partially sequenced. It contains a large NH_2-terminal extension and a COOH-terminal octapeptide commencing with a Lys-Arg dipeptide. The properties of synthetic, COOH-terminal 37-amino acid sequence of glicentin mimic in every way those of glucagon extended at its COOH-terminus with the COOH-terminal octapeptide of glicentin and of the smaller (4-kDa) impure gut GLI. The octapeptide completely inhibits binding of the 37-amino acid peptide to antiglucagon–24-29 antisera, but not to antiglucagon–11-15 antisera nor to hepatic glucagon receptors. Thus, the COOH-terminal regions of pancreatic proglucagon and glicentin are virtually identical.

Plasma concentrations of GLIs increase after a meal, the magnitude of the rise being directly related to the size of the meal and the composition of the food. They also increase very markedly after birth when neonates switch from placental to oral feeding; this rise is not seen if neonates are placed on intravenous feeding.

THE GASTRIN-RELEASING PEPTIDE FAMILY

The gastrin-releasing peptide family contains two neuropeptides, gastrin-releasing peptide (GRP) and substance P.

Gastrin-Releasing Peptide

Recently, GRP was isolated from porcine nonantral gastric tissue and sequenced. It is homologous to bombesin, a neuropeptide first isolated from frog skin. In fact, synthetic oligodeoxyribonucleotides corresponding to amphibian bombesin were used as hybridization probes to screen a cDNA library from a human pulmonary carcinoid tumor rich in immunoreactivity to GRP. Sequencing of the recombinant plasmids showed that hGRP mRNA encodes a precursor of 148 amino acids containing the usual signal sequence (23 amino acid residues) followed by GRP (27 amino acid residues) and a carboxyl extension. Later a second nucleotide was isolated, with 19 fewer bases, that showed a reading-frame shift (Fig. 3.6).

In an amazingly short time, the sequences of GRP from four species were reported (see Fig. 3.6). The COOH-terminal heptapeptides from these four, as well as bombesin, are identical. In addition, there is extensive homology among the four that diminishes at the NH_2-terminus.

Gastrin-releasing peptide and bombesin have similar biological effects. Infusion of nanogram amounts of either peptide into dogs or humans increases plasma immunoreactive levels of gastrin, pancreatic polypeptide (PP), glucagon, GIP, and insulin. The GRP is widely distributed throughout the neural system, gastrointestinal tract, and pulmonary tract. Within the CNS, GRP causes hypothermia and hyperglycemia and stimulates

```
                 20               40
I/II  MRGSELPLVL  LALVLCLAPR  GRAIVPLPAGG  GTVLTKMYPR  GNHWAVGHLMIG  KKSTGESSS
                                                                              60
p                 IA VSV      A                                       INH₂
c                 IA V G Q    D                                       INH₂
a                 IA QP       SPA    I     S                          INH₂
ab                I                  *EQRL  NQ                         INH₂
SP                                          R  PKPQQFFGLM.NH₂


                 80              100               120
I/II  VSERGSLKQQ  LREYIRWEEA  ARNLLGLIEA  KENRNHQPPQ  PKALGNQQPS  WDSEDSSNFK

                       140
1     D......LVD  SLLQVLNVKE  GTPS

II    DVGSKGKVGR  LSAPGSQREG  RNFQLNQQ
```

Figure 3.6 Amino acid sequences of two human progastrin-releasing peptides showing the result of a reading-frame shift in mRNA and a comparison of four GRPs of (h)uman, (p)orcine, (c)anine, and (a)vian origin and of amphibian bombesin(ab) (shown in box). Only differences from hGRP are shown. Note the high degree of homology, especially at the COOH-termini. The COOH-terminal glycine (in the box) serves to amidate the adjacent methionine before release of GRP: SP, substance P; *Q, pyroglutamic acid. The single-letter amino acid code is given in Appendix C.

84

the sympathetic nervous system. Aside from tumors, the highest levels in humans are found in neonatal lung.

Virtually nothing is known about the physiologic role of GRP. It will be interesting to find out what regulates the release of GRP and what role GRP plays in the release of gastrin and other gastrointestinal hormones.

Substance P

Substance P (SP) has some homology with GRP (see Fig. 3.6). It inhibits stimulated, but not basal, gastric, and pancreatic secretions induced by either exogenous or endogenous stimulants. This is probably a direct action of SP on gastric and pancreatic glands because no changes in serum insulin, gastrin, or pancreatic polypeptide levels were seen. Thus, the structural homology with GRP is not reflected functionally. Substance P also stimulates intestinal contractile activity under basal conditions, but it does not affect that induced by a meal. All the actions of SP are mimicked by SP 6–11, indicating that the bioactivity of SP is contained in a COOH-terminal fragment.

PANCREATIC POLYPEPTIDE

Pancreatic polypeptide (PP), a putative hormone containing 36 amino acids (Fig. 3.7), is anomalous in several respects. First, it was not isolated and characterized by virtue of its biological action. Second, its isolation was not a problem because it is present in pancreatic islet cells at about the same concentration as insulin. And third, because of its abundance and its crystallization (like insulin) as a zinc salt, its crystallographic structure is known at 1.4 Å resolution. Hence, it was named from its source rather than from an action.

Pancreatic polypeptide-producing cells are located on the periphery of the islets in the head of the pancreas, to the exclusion of glucagon-producing cells which occur at the periphery of the islets in the tail of the pancreas. It is stored in membrane-enclosed granules in D2 cells. Because of its high concentration, PP has been isolated in pure form from several species and sequenced.

Biologically, PP concentrations in serum rise in response to eating, protein being the most potent stimulus. The rapidity of

Pancreatic Polypeptide

APLEPVYPGD NATPEEMAEY AADLRRYINM LTRPRY.NH₂

Motilin

FVPIFTYGEL QRMQEKERNK GQ

Neurotensin

pyro-ELYENKPRRP YIL

Figure 3.7 Amino acid sequences of human pancreatic polypeptide, porcine motilin, and bovine neurotensin. The sequences of pancreatic polypeptide from other mammalian species do not differ much from that of bPP (number of changes denoted in parentheses: oPP(1), pPP(1), and hPP(4) differ only at amino acid residue numbers 2, 6, 10, 11, and 23. The amino-acid single-letter code is given in Appendix C.

the response (3 min) suggests that the initial secretory phase may be neurally mediated. On the other hand, the prolonged response (6–8 hr) of the second part of the biphasic response may involve a different mechanism. *Infusions* of amino acids or triglycerides have no significant effect on hPP levels, whereas infusion of glucose has a suppressive effect. Infusion of bPP into human subjects and into dogs at concentrations in the physiologic range reveal that PP has anti-CCK actions, i.e., it inhibits pancreatic enzyme excretion and bile flow. It also suppresses plasma motilin concentrations. Such a postprandial response appears counterproductive, but it may be that this "hormone" plays a conservatory role, ensuring a continued supply of pancreatic digestive enzymes and bile.

As usual, pharmacologic studies in the dog show activities in addition to those already discussed.

1. Stimulation of basal gastric acid excretion
2. Inhibition of pentagastrin-stimulated acid excretion

There are no reports of metabolic effects of PP in mammals. In chickens, aPP may influence hepatic glycogenolysis and either tissue glucose utilization or hepatic lipogenesis.

SOMATOSTATIN

Somatostatin, initially isolated from hypothalami and named for its effect on the release of somatotropin from the pituitary, was subsequently found to be ubiquitous and to have a number of biological actions. Regardless of source, the peptide has two forms, one containing 14 amino acid residues (S14) and the other having 28 (S28). The ratio of the two varies with the source.

Even though S28 has the form of a prohormone, i.e., an NH_2-terminal tetradecapeptide terminating in Arg-Lys, tests of both natural and synthetic A28 in dogs showed that the putative prohormone is as active, or nearly as active, as S14 in inhibiting gastrointestinal secretory actions, such as gastric and pancreatic excretion and release of gastrin, insulin, and pancreatic polypeptide. Because a prohormone is customarily characterized as weakly active or devoid of activity, Pradayrol's group no longer refers to S28 as a prosomatostatin.

Schally's group did, however, discover some differences. Whereas S14 strongly reduced intestinal blood flow and oxygen consumption and stimulated intestinal mobility (at 0.25 nmol/kg/hr), S28 was devoid of such activity.

From general principles, one would expect a larger precursor to exist, and indeed, three groups have identified two separate precursors of somatostatin. Even though they agree that the connecting peptide is large and attached to the NH_2-terminus of somatostatin, they differ concerning size and nucleotide sequence, except for the last 24 codons.

The sequence of somatostatin from only a few species is available, nevertheless, comparison of anglerfish and porcine somatostatin indicates extensive conservation (Fig. 3.8). It is odd that catfish somatostatin is so different.

The assay of somatostatinlike immunoreactivity in plasma or serum is presently unreliable owing to a combination of circumstances. Because S14 contains no tyrosyl residues for labeling with iodine, alternative approaches must be used. In addition, plasma at neutral pH contains peptidases directed toward the

```
                    1                          5                           10                                    15
Anglerfish     ...gly.arg.gln.arg.gly.pro.leu.leu.ala.pro.arg.glu.arg.lys.ala.
Porcine        H₂N.ser.ala.asn.ser.asn.          .ala.met.
Catfish                                           .ala.met.
Hypothalamic                      H₂N.asp.asn.thr.val.      .ser.lys.pro.leu.
                                                                           H₂N.


                    20                   25        28
anglerfish     gly.cys.lys.asn.phe.phe.trp.lys.thr.phe.thr.ser.cys
porcine        ala.        .met.      .tyr.            .ser.ser.      .ala.
catfish        ala.                                                  .ala.
hypothalamic
```

Figure 3.8 Comparison of amino acid sequences of somatostatin isolated from anglerfish islets, porcine intestine, catfish islets, and mammalian hypothalami. Only differences from anglerfish islet somatostatin are noted. Note the complete identity of somatostatin-14 from mammalian hypothalami, anglerfish islets, and porcine intestine (*Source*: From Goodman, RH, JW Jacobs, WW Chin, PK Lund, PC Dee, and JF Habener, *Proc Natl Acad Sci USA* 77:5872, 1980).

NH_2-terminus. Thus, synthetic ^{125}I-labeled-Tyr-1-Tyr-1-S14 is rapidly cleaved. No one appears to have used the Hunter-Bolton reagent, which the presence of two lysines suggests. Furthermore, the circulating forms of somatostatinlike immunoactivity are unknown.

Two different approaches to the resolution of this problem, namely, solvent extraction to remove peptidases and assay at low pH (<6.0) to inactivate peptidases, have still not led to a consistent set of values. There is also a distinct possibility that somatostatin has predominantly a paracrine–neurocrine role and that plasma concentrations represent adventitious leakage.

The multiple and seemingly unrelated inhibitory activities of somatostatin have led to the proposal that, at least under some circumstances, it represents a paracrine regulator. In support of this hypothesis, Larsson (1981) has reviewed the histological evidence. In the gut and the pancreas (excepting the guinea pig), somatostatin D cells have long cytoplasmic processes that terminate on putative effector cells. This hypothesis is still tenuous. Short-range communication through gap junctions is another possibility. (There is no doubt that somatostatin also has an endocrine function; see Chap. 4).

A summary of stimulators and inhibitors of release of somatostatinlike immunoactivity (SLI) is given in Table 3.6. Note that insulin and SLI have similar responses to glucose, arginine, leucine, α-ketoisocaproic acid, gastrointestinal peptides, β-adrenergic agonists, and antidiabetic drugs. In general, the SLI response is less than that of insulin, thus making somatostatin a low-level brake. In the stomach, VIP, secretin, glucagon, and especially GIP strongly stimulate SLI secretion in a dose-dependent manner. Both basal and stimulated SLI secretions are inhibited by cholinergic and adrenergic agonists.

Somatostatin exerts a wide spectrum of effects (Table 3.7). Currently, it would require prescience to subdivide these effects into physiological and nonphysiological. Receptors for somatostatin have so far been demonstrated only in the pituitary and brain.

MOTILIN

Motilin is a 22–amino acid peptide (see Fig. 3.7) present in high concentrations in the upper intestine. Radioimmunoassay is

Table 3.6 Substances Affecting Secretion of Somatostatinlike Immunoactivity from Isolated Pancreatic Islets or Perfused Pancreases of Stomachs

Pancreas		Stomach	
Stimulators	Inhibitors	Stimulators	Inhibitors
Metabolites and analogues			
glucose	Glyceraldehyde		
leucine	Mannoheptulose		
arginine			
α-ketoisocaproic acid			
Peptides and neurotransmitters			
CCK	β-Endorphin	GIP	Acetylcholine
GIP	Epinephrine	Secretin	Substance P
secretin	Somatostatin analogues	VIP	Met-enkaphalin
gastrin		Glucagon	
VIP		Isoproterenol	
glucagon		Epinephrine	
isoproterenol			
actylcholine			
Ions and nucleotides			
Calcium	Magnesium		
Sodium			
Popassium			
cAMP			
Drugs			
tolbutamide	Morphine		
glibenclamide	Metabolic blockers		
theophylline			

Source: Modified from CHS McIntosh and RA Pederson. In *Gut Hormones* (SR Bloom and JM Polak, eds.). Churchill Livingstone, Edinburgh, 1981, pp 362–365.

relatively easy, and this has been used to detect the results of processing extracts and plasmas. Motilin exists in two molecular forms in human gut extracts as well as in plasma, but the molecular weights of the two forms have not been reported.

Table 3.7 Biological Actions of Somatostatin

Inhibition of basal and stimulated STH and TSH secretion under normal conditions; inhibition of STH in acromegaly

Inhibition of prolactin and ACTH in pathological conditions

Inhibition of TRH release from hypothalamic fragments

Inhibition of basal and stimulated release of insulin, glucagon, and PP by direct action on the respective cells

Inhibition of secretion of all GI hormones examined (gastrin, secretin, CCK, GIP, VIP, motilin, enteroglucagon)

Inhibition of calcitonin release

Inhibition of renin release

Inhibition of TSH-stimulated secretion of T_3 and T_4

Inhibition of gastric acid and pepsin, pancreatic bicarbonate and enzymes, and salivary amylase

Inhibition of gastric and biliary motility; inhibition of electrically evoked release of acetylcholine from the myenteric plexus; inhibition of splanchnic blood flow

Behavioral changes in the rat; inhibition of spontaneous electrical activity of neurons in many parts of the brain; inhibition of firing of myenteric neurons

Impaired absorption of glucose, xylose, amino acids, triglycerides, and ions, e.g., calcium

Stimulation of sodium chloride absorption by rabbit intestine

Impaired platelet aggregation

Source: From YC Patel, HH Zingg, D Fitz-Patrick, and CB Srikant, In *Gut Hormones* (SR Bloom and JM Polak, eds.) Churchill Livingstone, Edinburgh, 1981, p 340.

Release of motilin after a meal is dependent upon its composition; fat is a potent stimulant, whereas oral glucose inhibits release. Distention of the stomach, either by mechanical means or by ingestion of a large volume of water, is also a good stimulant. Release does not appear to be under cholinergic control because atropine is ineffective in inhibiting the rise provoked by gastric distention. Basal motilin release is, however, atropine sensitive. Somatostatin and PP infusions cause a substantial suppression of motilin release, whereas bombesin stimulates it. Whether or not these substances are involved in physiologic regulation is not known.

Exogenous infusions of motilin closely mimicking physiologic levels accelerated gastric emptying and produced higher plasma glucose and insulin levels if the stomach had contained glucose. With glucose, this gives the appearance of a negative feedback because glucose inhibits motilin release. With fat, however, other factors must override motilin; it is well known that fatty meals are processed more slowly than carbohydrate or protein meals.

NEUROTENSIN

Neurotensin is a 13–amino acid peptide (see Fig. 3.7) originally isolated from bovine hypothalami. An identical substance was later found in bovine and human small intestine, and structurally related peptides can be extracted from many tissues. Results from the use of NH_2-terminal-directed and COOH-terminal-directed antisera suggest that there may be a neurotensin family sharing COOH-terminal homologies.

Infusion of neurotensin into the femoral vein of dogs at a rate of 4–60 pmol/kg/min produced dilation of the mesenteric vascular bed, inhibition of gastric smooth muscle contraction, and inhibition of gastric acid secretion. In vitro, neurotensin at 5 nM produces a half-maximal contraction of isolated guinea pig ileal smooth muscle. Which, if any, of these actions is physiologically important remains to be determined.

CLINICAL ASPECTS

The Zollinger-Ellison syndrome is due to a pancreatic tumor secreting gastrin in large amounts. As a result, there is a heavy and continuous excretion of gastric juice, as one would expect. Because gastric acid does not reach the tumor, negative feedback is absent. Also, secretin, normally a weak inhibitor of gastrin secretion, paradoxically increases serum gastrin levels (see p.73 and p.79).

The usual clinical symptom of Zollinger-Ellison syndrome is severe and intractable peptic ulceration. Sometimes the contents of the small intestine become acidic, thereby inactivating the pancreatic enzymes and producing steatorrhea (fatty stools). Fortunately, this syndrome is rare. Medical treatment aims at the suppression of excretion of gastric acid (HCl) by the use of the H_2-receptor antagonist, cimetidine (Tagomet).

There are several types of malabsorption. Any compromise in function of the intestinal mucosa will, of course, produce the syndrome. Celiac disease and tropical malabsorption are two forms. Even though the mucosal atrophy in the latter is generally milder than in celiac disease, it usually affects the entire small intestine uniformly, and malabsorption is, therefore, more severe. Plasma enteroglucagon response to a test meal appears to be exaggerated in both these diseases. Plasma motilin concentrations were also increased in tropical malabsorption, but both GIP and insulin release were reduced. Long-term treatment of celiac patients with a gluten-free diet appeared to reduce their response to nearly that of normal subjects.

SUMMARY

If one defines nutrition, not in terms of what one eats, but rather in terms of the basic building blocks that must be absorbed from the intestine, then the gastrointestinal hormones play an essential role in nutrition.

As a group, they are somewhat different from many of the hormones described in Chapter 2. First, they are secreted from many, many tiny bits of tissue scattered along selected segments of the gastrointestinal tract. And then, in retrospect, it is apparent that most, if not all, of them are also found in the CNS. And finally, there are several impure fractions with ascribable biological functions, which implies that more gastrointestinal hormones await isolation and characterization.

In this chapter, I describe 12 gastrointestinal hormones involved, directly or indirectly, in digestion. Gastrin and cholecystokinin are related. The former is a gastric hormone released in response to eating, especially a protein meal. The antral distention and vagal stimulation accompanying eating also stimulate the release of gastrin. (Gastrin-releasing peptide, a new hormone, is a powerful stimulant of gastrin release, but its physiologic role in digestion is not yet clear.) The hormone promotes the release of hydrochloric acid which has two actions: it turns secretion of gastrin off, and it provides the optimal pH for pepsin activity, which initiates protein hydrolysis in the stomach. Cholecystokinin, on the other hand, acts on the gallbladder and pancreas to promote release of bile and of pancreatic enzymes, respectively. The bile promotes emulsification of ingested fats, which greatly accelerates lipase action on them to produce fatty acids, monoglycerides, and glycerol. Pancreatic enzymes promote an increased rate of hydrolysis of all foodstuffs. The secretagogues for CCK are not well studied, but certainly the products of protein and fat digestion are physiologic stimuli.

The secretin family includes secretin, glucagon, glucose-dependent insulinotropic polypeptide or gastric inhibitory polypeptide, and vasoactive intestinal peptide. Secretin, the first hormone isolated, is released in response to a proximal duodenal pH of 4.5 to 5.0 or less. It promotes the release of pancreatic water containing sodium bicarbonate which neutralizes the acidic chyme and establishes an intestinal pH optimal for all the intestinal enzymes. It also inhibits both gastrin secretion and gastrin-induced gastric acid excretion.

Although glucagon is a pancreatic peptide containing 29-amino acid residues, enteroglucagon may be a family of related peptides that cross-react with antiglucagon antisera. One, called glicentin, is large (10 kDa) and contains a COOH-terminal octapeptide similar to that of glucagon.

Gastric inhibitory peptide (GIP) has different actions in dogs and in humans. In the dog, it inhibits gastric acid secretion, whereas in humans, it is a potent secretogogue for insulin. This difference may reflect the fact that the dog is a carnivore, whereas man is an omnivore. The principal stimulants for GIP release are ingested carbohydrate and fat.

Vasoactive intestinal peptide (VIP) is a neurohormone present in many tissues outside the gastrointestinal tract. The physiological stimuli inducing VIP release are oxytocin (in dogs), vagal stimulation (in animals), and intraduodenal hydrochloric acid (in man). It influences many bodily functions.

Although substance P has some homology with gastrin-releasing peptide, it has no overlapping functional activity. It inhibits stimulated, but not basal, gastric and pancreatic secretions induced by either exogenous or endogenous stimulants. It also stimulates intestinal contractile activity under basal conditions, but not that induced by a meal.

Pancreatic polypeptide is an abundant, putative hormone. Its serum concentration rises in response to eating, especially a protein meal. It has anti-CCK actions, inhibiting pancreatic enzyme release and bile flow. It also suppresses plasma motilin concentrations.

Somatostatin is an ubiquitous substance. In the hypothalamoadenohypophyseal system, it has an acknowledged endocrine function. Elsewhere, however, it probably acts as a paracrine hormone. Two forms (at least) exist, a 14- and a 28-amino acid peptide, and both are active. At the present time, the physiological and nonphysiological effects cannot be separated.

Motilin is a 22-amino acid peptide present in high concentrations in the upper intestine. It exists in two molecular forms, but these have not been characterized. Its release is powerfully stimulated by a fatty meal or gastric distention and inhibited by ingestion of glucose. Motilin accelerates gastric emptying.

Neurotensin, a 13-amino acid peptide, is probably a member of a widely distributed family. Infusion of neurotensin at very low concentrations produces dilation of the mesenteric vascular bed and inhibition of gastric smooth muscle contraction and gastric acid excretion. Its physiological role is not known.

SUPPLEMENTAL BIBLIOGRAPHY

General

Bloom, SR and JM Polak. Gut hormones. *Adv Clin Chem 21*:177–244, 1980.

Bloom, SR and JM Polak (eds). *Gut Hormones*. Churchill Livingstone, Edinburgh, 1981, 605 pp.

Dockray, GJ. Comparative biochemistry and physiology of gut hormones. *Annu Rev Physiol 41*:83–95, 1979.

Ferri, G-L, TE Adrian, MA Ghatei, DJ O'Shaughnessy, L Probert, YC Lee, AM Buchan, JM Polak, and SR Bloom. Tissue localization and relative distribution of regulatory peptides in separated layers from the human bowel. *Gastroenterology 84*:777–786, 1983.

Grossman, MI. Neural and hormonal regulation of gastrointestinal function: An overview. *Annu Rev Physiol 41*:27–33, 1979.

Loonen, AJM and W Soudijn. Peptides with a dual function: Central neuroregulators and gut hormones. *J Physiol(Paris) 75*:831–850, 1979.

Modlin, IM, A Sank, and D Albert. Current aspects of gut hormones. *J Surg Res 30*:602–618, 1981.

Polak, JM and SR Bloom. Regulatory peptides: Key factors in the control of bodily functions. *Br Med J 286*:1461–1466, 1983.

Clinical

Besterman, HS, GC Cook, DL Sarson, ND Christofides, MG Bryant, M
    Gregor, and SR Bloom. Gut hormones in tropical malabsorption. *Br
    Med J 2*:1252–1255, 1979.
Creutzfeldt, W. Clinical significance of gastrointestinal hormones. *Intl
    Cong Series, Excerpta Med 500*:471–474, 1980.
Kilander, AF, G Doteval, G Lindstedt, and P-A Lundberg. Plasma entero-
    glucagon related to malabsorption in coeliac disease. *Gut
    25*:629–635, 1984.

The Gastrin Family

Dockray, GJ. Cholecystokinin. In *Gut Hormones* (SR Bloom and JM Polak,
    eds). Churchill Livingstone, Edinburgh. 1981, pp 228–239.
Noyes, BE, M Mevarech, R Stein, and KL Agarwal. Detection and partial
    nucleotide sequence analysis of gastrin mRNA by using an oligode-
    oxynucleotide probe. *Proc Natl Acad Sci USA 76*:1770–1774, 1979.
Saito, A, JA Williams, and ID Goldfine. Alterations in brain cholecystokinin
    receptors after fasting. *Nature 289*:599–600, 1981.
Sankaran, H, CW Deveney, ID Goldfine, and JA Williams. Preparation of
    biologically active radioiodinated cholecytokinin for radio-receptor
    assay and radioimmunoassay. *J Biol Chem 254*:9349–9351, 1979.
Soll, AH and JH Walsh. Regulation of gastric acid secretion. *Annu Rev
    Physiol 41*:35–53, 1979.

The Gastrin-Releasing Peptide Family

Lezoche, E, N Basso, and V Speranza. Actions of bombesin in man. In
    Gut Hormones (SR Bloom and JM Polak, eds). Churchill Livingstone,
    Edinburgh, 1981, pp 419–424.
Powell, D and P Skrabanek. Substance P. In *Gut Hormones* (SR Bloom
    and JM Polak, eds). Churchill Livingstone, Edinburgh, 1981, pp
    396–401.
Spindel, ER, MD Zilberberg, JF Habener, and WW Chin. Two prohor-
    mones for gastrin-releasing peptide are encoded by two RNAs differ-
    ing by 19 nucleotides. *Proc Natl Acad Sci USA 83*:19–23, 1986.
Walsh, JH, JR Reeve, and SR Vigna. Distribution and molecular forms of
    mammalian bombesin. In *Gut Hormones* (SR Bloom and JM Polak,
    eds). Churchill Livingstone, Edinburgh, 1981, pp 413–418.

Motilin

Christofides, ND and SR Bloom. Motilin. In *Gut Hormones* (SR Bloom and
    JM Polak, eds). Churchill Livingstone, Edinburgh, 1981, pp 273–279.

Neurotensin

Carraway, RE. Variants of neurotensin. In *Gut Hormones* (SR Bloom and JM Polak, eds). Churchill Livingstone, Edinburgh, 1981, pp 300–305.

Hammer, RA and SE Leeman. Neurotensin: Properties and actions. In *Gut Hormones* (SR Bloom and JM Polak, eds). Churchill Livingstone, Edinburgh, 1981, pp 290–299.

Pancreatic Polypeptide

Blundell, TL, JE Pitts, IJ Tickle, SP Wood, and C-W Wu. X-ray analysis (1.4 A resolution) of avian pancreatic polypeptide: A small globular protein hormone. *Proc Natl Acad Sci USA 78*: 4175–4179, 1981.

Chance, RE, NE Moon, and MG Johnson. Human pancreatic polypeptide (HPP) and bovine pancreatic polypeptide (BPP). In *Methods of Hormone Radioimmunoassay* (BM Jaffee and HR Behrman, eds). 2nd ed, Academic Press, New York, 1979, pp 657–672.

Floyd, JC,Jr, AI Vinik, B Glaser, SS Fajans, and S Pek. Pancreatic polypeptide. *Intl Cong Series Excerpta Med 500*:490–495, 1980.

Schwartz, TW, RL Gingerich, and HS Tager. Biosynthesis of pancreatic polypeptide. *J Biol Chem 255*:11494–11498, 1980.

The Secretin Family

Andersen, DK. Physiological effects of GIP in man. In *Gut Hormones* (SR Bloom and JM Polak, eds). Churchill Livingstone, Edinburgh, 1981, pp 256–263.

Andersen, DK, D Elahi, JC Brown, JD Tobin, and R Andres. Oral glucose augmentation of insulin secretion. *J Clin Invest 62*:152–161, 1978.

Brown, JC, M Dahl, S Kwauk, CHJ McIntosh, M Muller, SC Otte, and RA Pederson. Properties and actions of GIP. In *Gut Hormones* (SR Bloom and JM Polak, eds). Churchill Livingstone, Edinburgh, 1981, pp 248–255.

Brown, JC, CHS McIntosh, H Koop, M Muller, SC Otte, and RA Pederson. GIP. *Intl Cong Series, Excerpta Med 500*:475–481, 1981.

McCulloch, J. PAT Kelly, R Uddman, and L Edvinsson. Functional role for vasoactive intestinal polypeptide in caudate nucleus: A 2-deoxy [^{14}C]glucose investigation. *Proc Natl Acad Sci USA 80*:1472–1476, 1983.

Maxwell, V, A Schulkes, JC Brown, TE Solomon, JH Walsh, and MI Grossman. Effect of gastric inhibitory polypeptide on pentagastrin-stimulated acid secretion in man. *Dig Dis Sci 25*:113–116, 1980.

Misra, P. The newer hormones of the gastrointestinal system. In *Perspectives in Clinical Endocrinology* (WB Easman, ed). SP Medical and Scientific Books, New York, 1980, pp 387–417.

Said, SI. VIP overview. In *Gut Hormones* (SR Bloom and JM Polak, eds).
Churchill Livingstone, Edinburgh, 1981, pp 379–384.

Somatostatin

Konturek, SJ, J Tasler, J Jaworek, W Pawlik, KM Walus, V Schusdziaara,
CA Meyers, DH Coy, and AV Schally. Gastrointestinal secretory,
motor, circulatory and metabolic effects of prosomatostatin. *Proc
Natl Acad Sci USA* 78:1967–1971, 1981.

Larsson, L-I. Somatostatin cells. In *Gut Hormones* (SR Bloom and JM
Polak, eds). Churchill Livingstone, Edinburgh, 1981, pp 350–353.

Noe, BD. Synthesis of one form of pancreatic islet somatostatin predominates. *J Biol Chem* 256:9397–9400, 1981.

Shields, D. In vitro biosynthesis of somatostatin: Evidence for two distinct preprosomatostatin molecules, *J Biol Chem 255*: 11625–11628,
1980.

Vaysse, N, L Pradayrol, C Susini, JA Chayvialle, and A Ribet. Somato-
statin-28: Biological actions. In *Gut Hormones* (SR Bloom and JM
Polak, eds). Churchill Livingstone, Edinburgh, 1981, pp 358–361.

4

Growth

Introduction   99
The Somatomammotropin Family   100
Regulation of Somatotropin Secretion   103
    Somatocrinin   103
    Somatostatin   106
    Secretion of Somatotropin   106
Growth Factors   107
    Somatomedins   107
    Epidermal growth factor and urogastrone   113
    Platelet-derived growth factor   114
    Mechanism of action   117
    Nerve growth factor   117
    Fibroblast growth factor   118
Clinical Aspects   121
Summary   124
Supplemental Bibliography   125

INTRODUCTION

This chapter will consider the control of soft-tissue growth, whereas Chapter 7 will deal with skeletal growth as well as with aspects of calcium and phosphorus metabolism. Obviously, the two are interrelated.

We define growth as true hyperplasia, i.e., an increase in the number of cells. Therefore, the hormones, or growth factors, involved must be mitogenic, producing increased synthesis of DNA, RNA, and protein as a prerequisite for mitosis. Concurrently, there must be increased activity in a number of other areas. Increased phospholipid synthesis is required for the formation of new membranes. Increased synthesis of complex carbohydrates is needed for the manufacture of additional glycoprotein and proteoglycan; some of the latter will require sulfation.

99

Progress here has been as uneven as it has been in gastroenterological endocrinology (see Chap. 3). Even though clinical-grade hSTH somatotropin (growth hormone), was available two decades ago, it is now apparent that this material is a complex mixture containing at least two somatotropins (22 kDa, 20 kDa) with differing physiological properties. In addition, a number of lower-molecular-weight peptides contaminate some preparations of STH. Hence, the literature on the effects of STH is confusing because most investigators used preparations of unstated or unknown purity.

Other substances, called growth factors, have been isolated from unlikely sources, such as salivary glands, platelets, urine, serum, etc. As they were purified and sequenced, it became obvious that some of them are related, if not identical. Hence, once again, we must ask whether these growth factors belong to the endocrine or paracrine families. And, again, we can expect that this decade will produce results that both clarify and obfuscate.

THE SOMATOMAMMOTROPIN FAMILY

The somatomammotropin family comprises the somatotropins (STH) or growth hormones (GH), the prolactins (PRL), and the placental lactogens (PL) or chorionic somatomammotropins (CS). They share structural similarities and overlapping functional characteristics. The existing members of the STH–PRL family are thought to be derived from a common ancestral gene that diverged about 4×10^8 years ago to give rise to separate STH and PRL families. The CSs appear to have diverged differently in primates than in rodents and ungulates, the former arising from STH genes, whereas the latter came from PRL genes.

Because of the interest in growth, this family has been extensively studied, especially in homeothermic species. The genes of several mammalian species, as well as those of the chicken, consist of five exons, the amino acids encoded by exon I and part of exon II being contained in the signal sequence. (This family has no prohormone form.) The PRL genes are much larger than those for STH (10–12 kb vs. 2 kb) because of larger introns.

The STHs have two disulfide loops, and the PRLs have three. The integrity of neither the small NH_2-terminal loop distinctive to PRLs nor the COOH-terminal loop, common to all, is required for bioactivity. Reduction of the disulfide bond in the large loop followed by alkylation produces variable results. The large loop can, however, be cleaved proteolytically in the region between residues 134 and 150 of hSTH without loss of bioactivity.

The bioactivity of many polypeptide hormones resides in a small fragment. Considerable energy has been invested in a search for such a fragment for this family. Degradative, hybridization, and synthetic techniques, in general, show that activity resides in the NH_2-terminal two-thirds of the molecules, that portion encoded by exons II–IV. Although the remainder of the molecule may not be essential, it is important because without it the NH_2-terminal portion has low potency.

Nicoll, Mayer, and Russell (1986) performed a sophisticated analysis of the amino acid sequences of STH of eight mammalian species and the chicken, and of PRL of seven mammalian species (see Appendix F). Homologies, both between and within the two groups, were distributed throughout the molecules, although there were a few clusters. In spite of an elaborate analysis, they were unable to discern any pattern of homologous amino acids to guide future research, nor were they able to explain paradoxes, such as the reason why hCS, with 85% identical sequence homology with hSTH, is essentially inactive in assays for STH, whereas chicken STH with only a 56% homology has appreciable activity.

The large number of differences among species in amino acid sequences has some very practical consequences. First, because of species specificity, one must carefully select replacement STH. For example, only primate STH is biologically effective in humans. Therefore, treatment of children having short stature resulting from a pituitary deficiency of STH requires the use of *human* STH, which obviously is difficult to obtain. The use of STH produced by recombinant DNA techniques is now alleviating this limitation. And second, STH is antigenic. This restricts attempts at long-term treatment or studies because of loss of effectiveness, as well as occasionally producing complications associated with activation of immune mechanisms.

In spite of the implications of the foregoing discussion, human pituitary somatotropin, as classically prepared, is a mixture of polypeptides (for an excellent review, see Lewis et al., 1980). Human somatotropin makes up as much as 10% of the dry weight of a human pituitary—nearly 8 mg per gland. About 80–90% of this is the hSTH1–191 described earlier. Several other related polypeptides exist—one is probably a genetic variant and others are probably posttranslational modifications. Data for each are still fragmentary.

The hSTH1–191 contains four cysteines that form two disulfide bridges: Cys-53 to Cys-165 and Cys-182 to Cys-189. The pituitary contains an enzyme(s), still incompletely characterized, that may nick hSTH in the region between Arg-134 and Asn-149, converting the molecule into a two-chain structure—a large NH_2-terminal peptide (F1) and a smaller COOH-terminal peptide (F2). The cleaved form retains growth-promoting activity, but reduction of the disulfide bonds markedly lowers activity, with F2 having no activity, and F1 only one-tenth the activity of the intact hormone. The physiological importance of the cleaved form is still uncertain.

For nearly half a century, the pituitary has been known to contain diabetogenic activity (production of hyperglycemia and hyperinsulinemia in a fasted dog 10 hr after injection of a test substance), and STH has been thought to be the substance responsible. Highly purified hSTH, however, is only weakly active in this manner. When clinical-grade hSTH is chromatographed, a mixture of at least five low-molecular mass (5 to 10 kDa) peptides contains most of the diabetogenic activity.

Additionally, there is an α-amino-acetylated form of hSTH, accounting for 5% of hSTH in pituitaries, and an interchain disulfide dimer that is inactive as a growth promoter unless it is reduced and carbamido-methylated (formation of the adduct hSTH-S-CH_2-CO-NH_2). Still other forms are seen during electrophoresis of clinical-grade hSTH in urea-containing gels.

There is also a structural variant of hSTH having 15 fewer amino acid residues (deletion of residues 32 to 46)(20 kDa) than does intact hSTH (22 kDa). This 20-kDa variant, constituting 5 to 10% of hSTH, is found in every gland (>50) examined so far. It has been overlooked because it exists as a dimer in pituitary extracts and is routinely discarded. In fact, sodium dodecyl sulfate (SDS) electrophoresis, a technique seldom used in investigations of hSTH, is the only good means of detecting this variant. While 20-kDa STH retains full growth-promoting ability, it has only 20% of the diabetogenic activity of the 22-kDa form.

REGULATION OF SOMATOTROPIN SECRETION

Somatocrinin

Hypothalamic extracts contain two opposing activities related to the secretion of adenohyphohyseal STH: a somatotropin-releasing factor (SRF or somatocrinin) and a somatotropin release-inhibiting hormone (SRIH or somatostatin) (see Fig. 3.8). The former was isolated in 1982 from ectopic tumors (because its low concentration in the hypothalamus made its isolation from that source logistically nearly impossible; it was sequenced and synthesized simultaneously by two groups (those of Guillemin and of Vale). Three peptides were isolated: hpSRF-44-NH$_2$, the amide of the mature hormone, hpSRF-40, and hpSRF-37 (Fig. 4.1). [In this section *only*, the second lower-case letter represents the organ from which the polypeptide was isolated: h, hypothalamus; p, pancreas.] The shorter forms are believed to be alternative processing products of the precursor polypeptide, although proteolytic degradation products cannot be excluded. The ratio of the three products varies markedly from tumor to tumor.

Armed with experience and two radioimmunoassays of different epitope specificities, human hypothalamus was shown to contain two substances separable by high-pressure liquid chromatography (HPLC) that coeluted with hpSRF-40 and hpSRF-44-NH$_2$. One reacted with antibody directed against the amidated COOH-terminal sequence as well as with antibody directed against the central portion of hpSRF-44. The other reacted with only the latter. More recently, rat hypothalamic rhSRF was isolated from 80,000 hypothalami and characterized as a 43-amino acid peptide with a free carboxyl group. It has a 67% homology with the corresponding NH$_2$-terminal 43 residues in hpSRF1-44 (see Fig. 4.1).

Isolation was naturally accompanied by synthesis of the three peptides characterized as well as fragments thereof. Assay for the release of STH from normal rat adenohypophyseal cell monolayer culture showed that the COOH-terminal 20 amino acid residues, including amidation of the COOH-terminal carboxyl, are crucial to the bioactivity of hpSRF (Table 4.1).

Molecular cloning and analysis of cDNA coding for preproSRF-107 and preproSRF-108 established the primary

```
                1                   5                      10
hpSRF-44-NH2    tyr.ala.asp.ala.ile.phe.thr.asn.ser.tyr.arg.lys.val.
phSRF-44-NH2
bhSRF-44-NH2
rhSRF-43-OH     his.                                        .arg.ile.

                15                  20                     25
hpSRF-44-NH2    leu.gly.gln.leu.ser.ala.arg.lys.leu.leu.gln.asp.ile.
phSRF-44-NH2
bhSRF-44-NH2
rhSRF-43-OH                         .tyr.                   .his.glu.

                             30                  35
hpSRF-44-NH2    met.ser.arg.gln.gln.gly.glu.ser.asn.gln.glu.arg.gly.
phSRF-44-NH2                                         .arg.
bhSRF-44-NH2                     .asn.               .arg.
rhSRF-43-OH                      .asn.               .arg.       .gln.arg.

                40
hpSRF-44-NH2    ala.arg.ala.arg.leu.NH2
phSRF-44-NH2        .val.
bhSRF-44-NH2        .lys.val.
rhSRF-43-OH     ser.        .phe.asn.OH
```

Figure 4.1 The sequences of four somatocrinins. Note that the rat hypothalamic factor has one less amino acid residue than the others and that it is not amidated. Only differences from the hpSRF are shown. The sequence homology of rhSRF with hpSRF, VIP, glucagon, secretin, and GIP is 67, 43, 31, 30, and 14%, respectively.

Table 4.1 Relative Potencies of COOH-Terminal Deletion
Analogues of hpGRF-44-NH$_2$

Analogues	Potency	95% Confidence limits
hpGRF-44-NH$_2$	100	
hpGRF-44-OH	61	50–75
hpGRF-40-NH$_2$	49	38–62
hpGRF-40-OH	30	25–37
hpGRF-37-NH$_2$	28	23–33
hpGRF-37-OH	12	9–16
hpGRF-34-OH	17	12–25
hpGRF-31-OH	9	6–12
hpGRF-28-OH	6	4– 9
hpGRF-24-OH	0.01	—

GRF is equivalent to SRF.
Source: Modified from Guillemin et al., 1984, with permission.

structures of two precursors for hpSRF (Fig. 4.2). They contain
the sequence of hpSRF-44 flanked by basic processing units, a
signal sequence of 20 amino acid residues and a COOH-terminal
amidation signal (Leu-44–Gly). The two polypeptides differ by
serine-103.

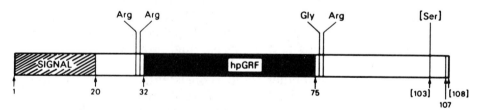

Figure 4.2 Schematic representation of preproSRF-107 and
preproSRF-108. The sequence of hpSRF-44 (in black, see Fig. 4.1) is flanked by processing sites consisting of basic amino acids. A glycine residue
immediately adjacent to the COOH-terminus of SRF mediates the amidation of SRF-44. A hydrophobic sequence of 20 amino acids at the NH$_2$-
terminus represents the signal sequence. Two cryptic sequences of 9
NH$_2$-terminal and 31 COOH-terminal amino acids make up the pro segment. Prepro-SRF-107 lacks the serine-103 (*Source*: From Guillemin et al.,
1984, with permission).

Somatostatin

As in the gastrointestinal tract (see Chap. 3), hypothalamic somatostatin comes in two sizes, S14 and S28, both of which are biologically active. Unlike the gastrointestinal tract, however, it is clear that here the peptides have an endocrine function, being released in the median eminence and transported in the portal circulation to the adenohypophysis where they bind to receptors on the somatotropes.

Secretion of Somatotropin

Somatocrinin, somatostatin, somatomedins, and prostaglandin E_2, all influence STH secretion. Cyclic AMP and calcium are both involved, but the detailed mechanisms are only now being investigated.

In vitro experiments show that $hpSRF-44-NH_2$ is a potent (sensitivity, 3 pM), fast-acting (30 sec), short-lived (5 min) stimulant of STH release and of cAMP production in the presence of calcium; a response is not dependent upon protein synthesis. There are parallelism and identical maximal responses seen in dose-response curves for SRF, 8-bromo-cAMP, and the phosphodiesterase inhibitor, isobutylmethylxanthine, further indicating the intermediacy of cAMP.

Somatocrinin is also rapid and short-lived in vivo. In anesthetized rats, there is a maximal STH response in 3 to 5 min; plasma STH concentrations return to baseline within 15 min. If the rats are conscious and freely moving, however, there is no consistent increase. Only when these animals were treated with antisomatostatin antibodies could a consistent, dramatic, and immediate release of STH be demonstrated. There is no apparent explanation for this observation. Humans respond a little differently. Normal, adult (unanesthetized) subjects maximally increase plasma STH concentrations in response to hpSRF-44 (0.1–10 μg/kg), in about 30 min and return to baseline in about 3 hr.

Studies of the interrelationships between prostaglandin E_2 (PGE_2) and SRF give entirely different results. The dose-response curves are divergent, and the maximal response to PGE_2 never reaches that for SRF. When the two are combined, there is excellent additivity at all concentrations.

As the names imply, there is antagonism between somatocrinin and somatostatin. Either somatostatin-14 or somatostatin-28 inhibits the response to SRF in a typical noncompetitive fashion, indicating that these two hormones act through different mechanisms. At a concentration of 1 nM, somatostatin-28 may be a slightly stronger inhibitor than somatostatin-14.

Other hormones also affect the response of pituitary cells to somatocrinin. Somatomedins (insulinlike growth factors; IGF-I and IGF-II) (see p. 107) can inhibit (0.1–1 nM) directly at the pituitary level, with the former being more effective. Pretreatment of pituitary cells with glucocorticoids or thyroid hormones enhances the response to hpSRF.

Insulin hypoglycemia, exercise, vasopressin, arginine, and L-dopa as well as sleep and stress cause an increased secretion of STH. The first four are mediated through α- and β-adrenergic receptor mechanisms in which the α-receptor is stimulatory and the β-receptor is inhibitory. Thus, neither epinephrine nor norepinephrine alone has an effect on growth hormone release in normal subjects. Inclusion of propranolol, a β-blocker, with a catecholamine produces an increased secretion of STH that can be inhibited by adding phentolamine, an α-blocker. These adrenergic effects are mediated by the brain.

Deep sleep (stage III or IV), which occurs within 1 or 2 hr after falling asleep, promotes STH secretion, perhaps by a serotoninergic mechanism. Administration of 5-hydroxytryptophan increases STH secretion, whereas cyproheptadine, a potent serotonin antagonist, blocks this response. Arginine-stimulated STH responses are also inhibited by cyproheptadine.

GROWTH FACTORS

Somatomedins

Costal cartilage from hypophysectomized rats shows no change in either sulfate-32 uptake upon exposure to STH in vitro or upon the addition of serum from hypophysectomized rats. Serum from rats treated with STH, however, stimulates sulfate uptake, indicating that STH stimulates skeletal growth indirectly through the generation of a circulating "sulfation factor," later renamed somatomedin.

Somatomedins (SM) are defined as having nonsuppressible insulinlike activity (NSILA) because their insulinlike actions are not blocked by antisera to insulin. Bioassays of insulinlike activity in plasma are six to ten times higher than radioimmunoassay (RIA) values and are only slightly suppressed by the addition of anti-insulin antisera. In fact, 93% of total insulinlike activity in the sera of fasting subjects is nonsuppressible. Extraction of plasma with acid ethanol removes 5 to 10% of NSILA. Two polypeptides were isolated from this extract and subsequently sequenced. They are now called insulinlike growth factors (IGF-I and II; formerly NSILAs I and II). Other workers following fibroblast multiplication-stimulating activity (MSA) isolated a polypeptide that is probably identical with IGF-II; SM-C and IGF-I are also identical (Table 4.2).

All of these factors appear to be regulated by STH, to be bound to carrier proteins of 70 and 120 kDa in plasma, and to cross-react with human serum carrier proteins, chick embryo fibroblasts, and rat adipocytes. This indicates a high degree of relatedness; yet there are important differences.

The sequences of only two somatomedins (IGF-I and II; Fig. 4.3) have been determined. They resemble proinsulin (86 amino acid residues) in having the constituents of the A and B chains with three intrachain disulfide bridges and a connecting peptide. The connecting peptide in IGF-I contains 12, IGF-II 8, and proinsulin 35 amino acid residues. The COOH-terminus of the A region of proinsulin is extended by eight residues in IGF-I and by six in IGF-II. Sequence homology is shared between IGF-I and IGF-II (62%), as well as insulin, nerve growth factor, and relaxin (Table 4.3), but not with STH. Somatomedins IGF-I and II contain 17 of the 19 invariant residues present in all of the insulins sequenced. Surface residues, however, differ from those of insulin, which may explain the lack of binding by anti-insulin antibodies.

Insulin has such important metabolic actions (see Chap. 9) that frequently its growth-promoting activity is overlooked. It is a component of every serum-free cell culture medium, albeit at rather high concentrations(1 μg/ml). The growth-promoting activity of insulin is not due to a contaminant because synthetic insulin shows the same response as the natural product. Rather, it occurs because the receptor for IGF-I/SM-C is closely related to that for insulin (Table 4.4). Both are tetrameric receptors having the composition

Table 4.2 Growth Factors (GF) of the PDGF, EGF, and Insulin Families

Growth factor	Source	Molecular mass (kDa)	Molecular structure
PDGF family			
platelet-derived GF (PDGF)	Human platelets	28–31	Two PC[a]
osteosarcoma-derived GF (ODGF)	Conditioned medium of U-2 OS cells	31	Two PC
glioma-derived GF	Conditioned medium of U-343 MGa C12 cells	31	Two PC
fibroblast-derived GF (FDGF)	Conditioned medium of SV40-transformed cells		
transforming protein of simian sarcoma virus	SSV-transformed cells	24	Two PC[b]
EGF family			
epidermal GF (EGF, urogastrone)	Urine (hEGF), salivary gland (mouse EGF)	6	One PC
transforming GF (TGF-α)	Transformed cells	7	Homologous with EGF
Insulin family			
Insulin	β-cells of islets of Langerhans	5.7	Two PC derived from proinsulin
insulinlike GF I (IGFI, somatomedin C)	Human plasma	6	Homologous with proinsulin
insulinlike GF II (IGF II)	Human plasma	6	Homologous with proinsulin
multiplication-stimulating activity (MSA)	Conditioned medium of rat liver cells	6	Rat equivalent to IGF II

[a]PC, polypeptide chain(s).
[b]Derived from p28[sis] precursor, amino acid sequence virtually identical with PDGF B chain.

```
Insulin     FVNQHLCGSH  LVEALYL  VC  GERGFFYTPK  T

IGF I        GPETLCGAE  LVDALQF  VC  GDRGFYFNKP  T

NGF          SSTHP VFH  MGE   FS  VC  DSVSVWVGDK  T

Relaxin  pESTNDFIKACGRE  LVR  LWVEIC  GSVS  WGR
                                          |_____
                                                                  |
Insulin     RREAEDLQVG  QVELGGGPGA  GSLQPLALEG  SLQKR            |
                                                                  |
IGF I        GYGSSSRRAP  QT                                      |
                                                                  |
NGF          TATNIKGKEV  TVLAEVNINN  SVFRQYFFET  KCRAS           |
                                                                  |
Relaxin      ----------  ----------  ----------  -----           |
                                           |_____|
                                           |
Insulin           GIVEQCCTSI  CSLYQLENYC  N

IGF I             GIVDECCFRS  CDLRRLEMYC  A

NGF               DPVESGCRGI  DSKH  WNSYC  T

Relaxin        RMTLSEKCCQVG  CIRKDIARLC


Insulin

IGF I        PIKPAKSA

NGF          TTHTFVKALT  TDEKQAAWRF  IRINTACVCV  LSRKATR

Relaxin
```

Figure 4.3 Comparison of the amino acid sequences of human proinsulin, IGF-I, NGF, and relaxin. Underlines indicate residues identical in at least two polypeptides. Deletions were inserted arbitrarily to increase identities. The connecting line between the half cystinyl (C) residues of the A and B segments represents the one disulfide bond conserved in all four hormones (*Source*: From Bradshaw, RA and HD Niall. *Trends Biochem Sci* 3:277, 1978, with permission).

α_2–β_2 with the α-subunit being ca. 135 kDa and the β-subunit being ca. 90 kDa; the α-subunit of the IGF-I receptor is slightly larger than that of insulin. Although the two share some antigenic determinants, monoclonal antibodies capable of distinguishing between

Table 4.3 Comparison of the A- and B-Chain Segments of the Insulin-Related Growth Factors

	Insulin	IGF-I/SM-C	NGF	Relaxin
Insulin		50	28	25
IGF-I/SM-C	25/50		14	26
NGF	14/50	7/50		17
Relaxin	12/48	12/47	8/46	

The ratios show identities to total positions compared for each pair. The whole numbers give these values as percentages. The comparisons were made starting and ending at a point where both proteins had the position occupied. Deletions were treated as nonidentities.

Table 4.4 Growth Factor Receptors

Receptor	Subunit composition	Molecular mass (kDa)	Activity
PDGF	One polypeptide chain	185	Tyrosine kinase
EGF	One polypeptide chain	170	Tyrosine kinase
Insulin	Two α-chains	135	Receptor binding
	Two β-chains	90	Tyrosine kinase
IGF I	Two α-chains	135	Receptor binding
	Two β-chains	90	Tyrosine kinase
IGF II	One polypeptide chain	250	Not known

the two receptors have been produced. Both receptors are associated with a specific tyrosine kinase activity, and both are synthesized as a single polypeptide (180 kDa), which is processed to produce an α–β-dimer. Thus, it is not surprising that IGF-I receptors have a low affinity for insulin.

The IGF-II receptors, on the other hand, are quite different. They consist of a single polypeptide chain (ca. 220 kDa), binding to IGF-II with a higher affinity than IGF-I and having no significant affinity whatsoever for insulin.

Thus, we can conclude that a tissue with IGF-I receptors will have a low affinity for insulin and will respond to micromolar concentrations of insulin, whereas tissues with high affinity for insulin possess insulin receptors and will respond to nanomolar quantities. Tissues having neither insulin nor IGF-1 receptors will be unresponsive to insulin.

There are, of course, tissues that fit each of these categories. The growth-promoting effects of insulin on human fibroblasts, chick embryo fibroblasts, rat myoblasts, mouse BALB/c 3T3 cells, and Chinese hamster lung fibroblasts are believed to be mediated by IGF-I receptors. On the other hand, the growth-stimulating effects of insulin on the cells of rat liver, human mammary tumor, and bovine adrenal cortex are produced through insulin receptors.

Somatomedins have numerous effects, both in vitro and in vivo (Table 4.5). The cartilage-stimulating activity is congruent

Table 4.5 Demonstrated Effects of Somatomedins

Effect	In vitro	In vivo
Cartilage-stimulating activity		
amino acid transport	+	
DNA and RNA synthesis	+	
protein synthesis	+	
Proteoglycan (chondroitin sulfate) synthesis	+	
collagen synthesis	+	
Insulinlike activity		
muscle		
amino acid transport	+	
sugar transport	+	+
glycogen synthesis	+	+
protein synthesis	+	+
energy		
sugar transport	+	
increased glucose turnover		+
glucose oxidation to CO_2	+	
hypoglycemia		+
lipogenesis	+	+
decreased lipolysis	+	+
Mitogenic activity		
cell replication in culture	+	
growth		+

with one of the two basic somatotropin assays; namely, the epiphyseal cartilage plate-widening assay (tibial line-widening assay). All of the steps in the synthesis of the organic matrix of bone are stimulated, including sulfation. Mitogenesis and muscle formation, the bases of the other basic somatotropin assay, namely, growth, are also stimulated. In vivo the metabolic effects mimic those of insulin, *the* anabolic hormone; consequently growth ensues.

Although most hormones exert a negative-feedback on their stimulatory source, negative-feedback of somatomedins on pituitary secretion of STH is not established.

Even though STH is necessary for somatomedin production, good nutrition is a prerequisite. We have all observed that youngsters grow well only if they receive an adequate, well-balanced diet. It makes ecological sense for the body to husband meager supplies for the maintenance of existing structures rather than investing in new ones during times of inadequate supply.

Other hormones may also be involved. Because PRL and hCS have extensive homology with STH, they have some growth-promoting activity. This may be important during pregnancy when STH concentrations in the plasma are normal or low, but that of hCS is elevated. For example, when pregnant rats are hypophysectomized, SM activity remains normal until parturition occurs.

Nonphysiologic amounts of glucocorticoids have a protein antianabolic effect. They have a direct inhibitory action on cartilage, cause some decrease in secretion of STH, and somehow interfere in the production or action (or both) of somatomedins. What happens during physiologic modulation of cortisol concentration is not known.

Androgens accelerate growth in both sexes, but somatomedins are probably not involved. The strongest evidence for this is the Laron-type dwarfism. These subjects have a congenital lack of somatomedins, yet they possess the pubertal growth spurt in response to the pubertal rise in androgens.

Thyroid hormones alter STH secretion in a direct relationship, but direct regulation of SM activity has not been established.

Epidermal Growth Factor and Urogastrone

During work on the isolation of nerve growth factor (NGF) from male mouse submaxillary glands, certain fractions produced unexpected results, such as premature opening of the eyelids and premature eruption of the incisors. The pure polypeptide, when administered to mice in microgram amounts, stimulates the pro-liferation and keratinization of epidermal tissues; hence, its name of epidermal growth factor (EGF). The sequence of the 53-amino acid residue, single-chain polypeptide is known (Fig. 4.4).

Nearly 50 years ago, it was observed that human urine con-tains a potent inhibitor of gastric acid secretion, which was named urogastrone (URO). Recently, two closely related polypeptides (β-and γ-urogastrone) were isolated and sequenced. β-urogastrone contains 53 amino acid residues, possesses the same three disulfide bridges as EGF, and has 70% homology with EGF, whereas γ-URO lacks a COOH-terminal arginine (see Fig. 4.4). Not unexpectedly, both possess the same intrinsic biological activities. More recently, the gene for hEGF (170 bp) was chemically syn-thesized and inserted into yeast to produce biologically active hEGF.

The sources of EGF–URO remain elusive. There must be sources other than the salivary glands because there is little sex difference in the serum concentration in spite of a 15-fold dif-ference in tissue concentration. Significant amounts of EGF–URO have been detected in mouse kidney, stomach, parotid, pancreas, small intestine, and liver (decreasing order). In humans, EGF–URO has been found in the submandibular salivary gland and in the glands of Brunner in the duodenum; it was undetectable in 18 other tissues.

The lack of fluctuation of the serum concentration suggests a paracrine function, yet the loci of action of EGF–URO (Table 4.6) are remote from identified sources. It should be appreciated that keratinization requires much more (0.5–6 μg/g body weight) pep-tide than does inhibition of gastric acid secretion (0.25 ng/g body weight), i.e., about 1000:1.

The receptor for EGF is being extensively studied as a model for the insulin receptor. It differs, however, in having only one polypeptide chain (see Table 4.4).

Platelet-Derived Growth Factor

Each human platelet contains about 1000 molecules of platelet-derived growth factor (PDGF) localized within α-granules. During clot formation or whenever platelets come into contact

```
        1             5                10
human   asn.ser.asp.ser.glu.cys.pro.leu.ser.his.asp.gly.trp.cys.
mouse   -------.tyr.pro.gly.-------.ser.---.tyr.---------------


        15            20               25
human   leu.his.asp.gly.val.cys.met.tyr.ile.glu.ala.leu.asp.lys.
mouse   ---.asn.gly.---------------.his.-------.ser.-------.ser.


        30            35               40
human   tyr.ala.cys.asn.cys.val.val.gly.tyr.ile.gly.glu.arg.cys.
mouse   ---.thr.---------------.ile.-------.ser.---.asp.--------


human   gln.tyr.arg.asp.leu.lys.trp.trp.glu.leu.arg.
mouse   ---.thr.-----------.arg.---------------------
```

Figure 4.4 Comparison of the amino acid sequences of human and mouse EGF; the former is also called urogastrone.

with a wettable surface, PDGF is released. Thus, human clotted blood serum contains 15–20 ng/ml of PDGF, whereas platelet-poor plasma contains only 1–2 ng/ml.

Connective tissue cells, such as fibroblasts, smooth muscle cells, and glial cells, require 1–2 ng/ml of PDGF for optimum growth in vitro. Supplementation of the cell culture medium with serum to a level of 10 to 20% satisfies this growth requirement. On the other hand, epithelial cells, lymphocytes, and endothelial cells have no requirement for PDGF and can grow in a medium supplemented with either plasma or serum.

From phylogenetic analysis, we can conclude that PDGF appeared suddenly or changed suddenly with the first chordates and has been functionally conserved ever since. This coincides with the appearance of the pressurized vascular system, and it is in accord with the known function of platelets in repairing damage to the vascular lining.

Pure, human PDGF is a basic (pI, 9.8), heat-stable (100°C) protein that can be resolved into several bands of activity upon SDS gel electrophoresis. The major species (PDGF-I, 31–35 kDa and PDGF-II, 28–32 kDa) are equally active in bioassays, radioreceptor assays, and radioimmunoassays. The reason(s) for the multiple products is not known. It may reflect microheterogeneity at

Table 4.6   Actions of Epidermal Growth Factor–Urogastrone

In vivo	In vitro
Cell proliferation	Cell proliferation
Keratinization	Enhanced keratinocyte growth
Enhanced ornithine and histidine decarboxylase	Increased activity of ornithine decarboxylase
Incisor eruption	Enhanced metabolite transport (uridine, aminoisobutyrate, glucose)
Inhibition of gastric acid secretion	Increased synthesis of DNA, RNA, and protein
Healing of ulcers	Increased membrane phosphorylation
Heptic triglyceride accumulation	Increased cyclic nucleotide levels (both cAMP and cGMP)
	Increased glycogen synthase activity Enhanced hyaluronic acid synthesis Enhanced fibronectin synthesis
	Increased cell binding to insolubilized concanavalin A
	Altered viral growth (cytomegalovirus reduced; herpes simplex type I increased)
	Inhibition of palate fusion
	Inhibition of acid secretion

Source: Modified from Hollenberg, 1979.

the structural gene level, partial degradation products generated during extraction and purification, or differing degrees of glycosylation.

Platelet-derived growth factor consists of a heterodimer linked by disulfide bonds (see Table 4.2). Amazingly, the amino acid sequence of the B-chain is virtually identical with the predicted sequence of the transforming protein p28[sis] of simian sarcoma virus, there being only three substitutions. This observation is an indication that normal and abnormal growth may, sometimes, be closely related.

The receptor for PDGF, like that for EGF, is a single polypeptide with intrinsic tyrosine kinase activity (see Table 4.4).

Mechanism of Action

The mechanism through which the growth-promoting factors or hormones act is still largely speculative, but now we have fragments of information that tantalize us. First, the data shown in Table 4.2 suggest that functional similarities may follow from structural similarities. Especially in the homology seen between p24^{sis} dimer and PDGF, one assumes that the viral gene product functions as a PDGF agonist, i.e., stimulates cell replication by interacting with the PDGF receptor. Indeed, SSV-transformed cells contain a growth factor in their cytoplasm that can be neutralized by PDGF antibodies.

Second, the regularity in structure of the receptors for growth-promoting substances may be important. So far, they appear to be transmembrane glycoproteins having three functional domains: a hormone-binding domain located exofacially, a lipophilic domain that inserts into the lipid bilayer, and a cytoplasmic domain containing in all cases but one a specific tyrosine kinase. At least seven retroviral oncogenes have also been isolated that possess tyrosine kinase activity. Even though no one yet knows the function of phosphorylation of tyrosine, its ubiquity is an indication of its importance. The retroviruses may have acquired the genes for tyrosine kinase so that they could perturb the regulatory network and cause uncontrolled activation of the cell cycle.

And last and most tentatively, oncogenes might somehow participate in the postreceptor pathways. The lack of evidence is a reflection of the state of knowledge, not of the invalidity of the hypothesis.

Nerve Growth Factor

The other growth factor isolated from male mouse submaxillary glands is nerve growth factor (NGF). It turned out to be related to proinsulin, IGF, and relaxin, a reproductive hormone (see Fig. 4.3 and Table 4.3). Nerve growth factor has 28% homology with insulin, 14% with IGF-I, and 17% with relaxin not including the connecting peptides. One of three disulfide bridges in proinsulin is preserved in all peptides, and all three are present in NGF.

In the salivary gland, NGF is stored as a 7S $\alpha\beta\gamma_2$-complex. The α-subunit is a 26 kDa peptide, the β-subunit is dimeric NGF (2.5S; noncovalently bonded), and the γ-subunits are arginine esteropeptidases of the serine family. Homozygous dystrophic mice have one-half the tissue concentrations of NGF as heterozygous mice.

In the blood, NGF is tightly bound to high–molecular-weight serum components that interfere in the RIA of NGF. The use of anti-mNGF antibodies to measure hNGF may also introduce another measurement error.

Nerve growth factor is thought to be a paracrine peptide that is synthesized and released from end organs of the sympathetic nervous system. It diffuses to nearby receptors on the termini of responsive neurons, is internalized, and is transported intra-axonally in a retrograde fashion to the cell bodies. Complexation of NGF with specific nuclear receptors induces specific enzymes, such as tyrosine hydroxylase and dopamine-β-hydroxylase, which leads to the principal biological activity of NGF, namely, proliferations of neurites and maintenance of the viability of responsive neurons. Nerve growth factor also produces some rapid metabolic responses, whereas the growth response requires 12 to 18 hr for expression.

A plasma membrane receptor for NGF has been isolated. It is a highly asymmetric 135 kDa protein that is visualized as spanning the bilayer with only a small segment in actual contact with the phospholipid components; portions extend into the water on either side of the membrane. It is not clear whether the isolated receptor is a high- or low-affinity type receptor. The nuclear receptor, which is saturable, remains insoluble in the nonionic detergent used to extract the plasma membrane receptor.

Fibroblast Growth Factor

For about two decades, investigators have been pursuing a mitogenic activity present in pituitary or brain extracts. Although, initially, fibroblasts were used in the assay (hence, the name fibroblast growth factor; FGF), it soon became apparent that such extracts were also potent stimulators of the proliferation of a number of different cell types including chondrocytes, adrenocortical cells, vascular smooth muscle cells, and vascular endothelial cells. Therefore, it became obvious that FGF activity includes several cell types that are closely, but not exclusively, connected by their derivation from the primary and secondary mesenchyme.

The in vivo physiologic function(s) of FGF remains unestablished. In addition to the effects noted, FGF can stabilize the phenotypic expression of cultured cells and even delay their senescence. Activities similar to those of FGF have been found in endothelium, corpus luteum, ovary, kidney, adrenal, retina, macrophages, and tumors. In vivo FGF can induce neovascularization, suggesting a functional similarity with tumor angiogenic factor and with corpus luteum angiogenic factor. It also promotes wound healing and limb regeneration. All these functional similarities suggest that there may be one or two common factors.

There are two pituitary FGFs, an acidic and a basic form, containing 140 and 146 amino acid residues, respectively, with a 55% homology between them. Their isolation was greatly facilitated by an exceptional affinity for heparin, enabling them to be purified several hundred thousand-fold on a Sepharose-heparin column. The sequence of the 146–amino acid residue peptide (Fig. 4.5) contains two highly basic clusters (bFGF18–22 and bFGF107–110), accounting for its affinity to heparin. There are no known proteins homologous to basic FGF, but there are three sequences that are similar to the cell recognition site of fibronectin. Sequences, bFGF37–40 (Asp-Gly-Arg-Val) and bFGF79–82 (Asp-Gly-Arg-Leu) are the inverse of the x-Arg-Gly-Asp-x sequence of fibronectin required for cell recognition. Sequence bFGF46–49 contains a conservative replacement of this series. The four cysteines are not involved in disulfide bridging. There is also an inverted repeat (with some conservative changes) of bFGF32–39 at bFGF46–53.

A number of fragments have been synthesized and tested for their ability to inhibit basal and FGF-stimulated cell growth; bFGF24–68-NH$_2$ was the most active. This fragment contains the inverted repeat as well as two of the inverted cell recognition sequences.

These same isolation techniques have also been applied to extracts of brain, corpus luteum, kidney, adrenal, retina, macrophages, and serum. Bovine brain extracts contain two FGFs. One is identical with that described previously, including an NH$_2$-terminal sequence of nine amino acids, whereas the second appears

```
        5                    10                    15
PRO.ALA.LEU.PRO.GLU.ASP.GLY.GLY.SER.GLY.ALA.PHE.PRO.PRO.GLY.

    ┌─────────────────┐
    |         20      |         25                    30
HIS.PHE|LYS.ASP.PRO.LYS.ARG|LEU.TYR.CYS.LYS.ASN.GLY.GLY.PHE.
    |_____|

                35                    40                    45
PHE.LEU.ARG.ILE.HIS.PRO.ASP.GLY.ARG.VAL.ASP.GLY.VAL.ARG.GLU.
        ------------------------------

                50                    55                    60
LYS.SER.ASP.PRO.HIS.ILE.LYS.LEU.GLN.LEU.GLN.ALA.GLU.GLU.ARG.
----------------------------

                65                    70                    75
GLY.VAL.VAL.SER.ILE.LYS.GLY.VAL.CYS.ALA.ASN.ARG.TYR.LEU.ALA.

                80                    85                    90
MET.LYS.GLU.ASP.GLY.ARG.LEU.LEU.ALA.SER.LYS.CYS.VAL.THR.ASP.

                95                    100                   105
GLU.CYS.PHE.PHE.PHE.GLU.ARG.LEU.GLU.SER.ASN.ASN.TYR.ASN.THR.

    ┌─────────────────┐
    |       110|      |         115                   120
TYR|ARG.SER.ARG.LYS|TYR.SER.SER.TRP.TYR.VAL.ALA.LEU.LYS.ARG.
    |_____|

                125                   130                   135
THR.GLY.GLN.TYR.LYS.LEU.GLY.PRO.LYS.THR.GLY.PRO.GLY.GLN.LYS.

                140                   145
ALA.ILE.LEU.PHE.LEU.PRO.MET.SER.ALA.LYS.SER
```

Figure 4.5 Primary structure of basic bovine fibroblast growth factor. The inverted repeat is dash underlined, the inverted fibronectin cell recognition sites are solid underlined, and the highly basic clusters are boxed.

to be acidic FGF. Human brain extracts contain an FGF that has the same NH_2-terminal sequence as basic bFGF. Other tissues contain one or both of these FGFs, sometimes in an NH_2-terminal truncated form that is believed to be an artifact. In the serum, FGF circulates as a 150-kDa molecule of unknown composition.

The widespread distribution of FGF suggests that it has a paracrine function. The expression of FGF activity depends very much upon its milieu. Thus, FGF in the pituitary plays a non-mitogenic role in the maintenance of prolactin and thyrotropin responsiveness, whereas in macrophages it may promote wound healing and, in the corpus luteum, angiogenesis.

CLINICAL ASPECTS

Hyposomatotropinemia leading to short stature (dwarfism) is not uncommon in children. The incidence (1:4000) is dependent upon the definition, for the height of a "normal" population follows a gaussian distribution. Height is markedly dependent upon parental genetices and nutrition as well as on the status of the thyroid and adrenal cortex (permissive hormones). Assuming that these other factors are not causative, two different stimulatory tests should be administered. If one of the two tests is positive, the pituitary is able to respond appropriately. (Use of somatocrinin may eventually provide a more direct measure of pituitary reserve of STH.) Administration of hSTH is the treatment of choice, although the human pituitary preparation has always been severely limited; recently, even that was withdrawn.

Recently, preliminary clinical testing of methionyl-hSTH (met-hSTH), an analog of hSTH made in *E. coli* by recombinant DNA techniques, was completed. Both American and European groups found it to be safe and effective. Interestingly, its major market is seen, not in the treatment of children for failure to grow, but in the treatment of obesity, because it increases lipolysis while preserving muscle mass.

A small fraction of "little people" are eusomatotropinemic. Laron-type dwarfs have a rarer defect, namely, an inability to produce somatomedins in response to growth hormone, either endogenous or exogenous. Until somatomedin becomes commercially available, there is little that can be done for such children. Androgens must be used judiciously because they are truly a double-edged sword; not only do they promote growth, but they also cause epiphyseal closure, thereby precluding further growth.

Hypersomatotropinemia is a rare disease leading to gigantism in children and acromegaly in adults, usually as a result of a pituitary adenoma. After closure of the epiphyses, linear growth is no longer possible. Instead, marked periosteal overgrowth leads to the widening of many bones. This is especially prominent in the feet, hands, and mandible. Enlargement of the abdominal viscera also occurs, and 25% of the patients have diabetes mellitus.

Other groups that have growth problems are girls with Turner's syndrome and both sexes with precocious puberty. Girls with Turner's syndrome (see Chap. 8) lack functional ovaries. Untreated, these girls are short during childhood, lack a pubertal growth spurt, and end up severely short (mean adult height, 147 cm). Administration of the synthetic estrogen, ethinyl estradiol, has a biphasic effect such that, whereas low doses stimulate bone growth, larger doses suppress it (Fig. 4.6). This same observation was made in a study of a small group of normal boys. Somatotropin and thyroid hormones are required for growth.

Children with central precocious puberty (see Chap. 8) have a different problem. The plasma concentration of their sex steroids is prematurely elevated, hence, they are growing more rapidly than their peers, and their bone age is advancing 2 years for each chronological year. As a consequence, greatly premature epiphyseal fusion will leave them very short as adults. The suppression of secretion of gonadotropins and sex steroids by administration of an agonist of luteinizing hormone-releasing hormone (LRH; see Chap. 8) decreased the rate of growth to a normal prepubertal rate and decreased the rate of bone maturation to one-half that of normal. Plasma STH and somatomedin C levels were elevated in these children, and they did not fall as a result of treatment in proportion to the decrease in rate of growth.

Insulin may act as an important regulator of growth during human fetal development. Infants born to poorly controlled diabetic mothers have a syndrome characterized by hyperinsulinemia; excessive size and weight for gestational age; excessive body fat; organomegaly involving heart, liver, and spleen; and hypertrophy of the umbilical cord. Some features, such as increased deposition of fat, glycogen, and protein, may be due to interaction of insulin with insulin receptors, whereas binding to IGF-I receptors may produce the excessive length and organ size. On the other hand, neonatal diabetes mellitus is characterized by retarded fetal growth, insufficient adipose tissue, and small muscle mass. The rare syndromes of pancreatic agenesis and congenital absence of the islets of Langerhans in which extreme

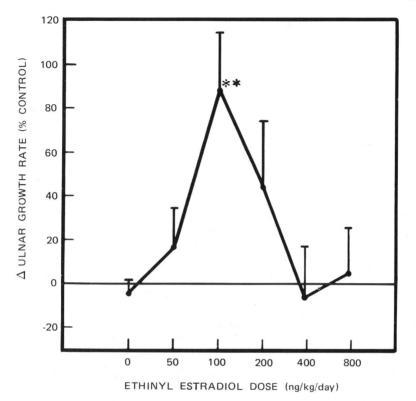

Figure 4.6 Relationship between dose of ethinylestradiol and ulnar growth rate (mean ± SE) in a group of girls with Turner's syndrome. The double asterisk indicates p < 0.025 as compared with the group receiving no treatment *Source*: Reprinted by permission of The New England Journal of Medicine *309*: 1104, 1983 from an article by JL Ross, MC Skerda, IM Valk, DL Loriaux and GB Cutler, Jr.

growth retardation, an absence of fat, and an absence of muscle mass are exhibited, provide an extreme example of this.

Leprechaunism, another rare syndrome, also demonstrates insulin's role as a growth factor. This disease is a heterogeneous group characterized by extreme insulin resistance in which the defect is abnormal binding (decreased affinity or decreased number of insulin receptors) or a postreceptor anomaly. The characteristic features are low birth weight, absence of subcutaneous fat, decreased muscle mass, characteristic facial features, hyperinsulinemia, insulin resistance, and early death.

SUMMARY

This chapter considers the control of soft tissue growth, deferring discussion of skeletal growth to Chapter 7. Growth is defined as hyperplasia, i.e., an increase in the number of cells. Thus, the hormones or growth factors involved must be mitogenic.

The somatomammotropin family comprises three members: somatotropin or growth hormone, prolactin, and placental lactogen or chorionic somatomammotropin. Because of extensive structural homology, the two pituitary hormones were difficult to separate and, indeed, even the existence of prolactin was hotly contested until 1973 when it was isolated in a pure form.

These three hormones naturally have certain common features. They are all large, have no prohormone form, have their active sites of bioactivity distributed over a large portion of the molecule, contain disulfide loops that are not essential for activity, and are somewhat immunogenic and quite species-specific. Growth hormone is a clinically important substance, and these properties have conspired to frustrate adequate treatment of short-statured children.

A great amount of physiological research was conducted in the past with somatotropin of unstated or unknown purity. In retrospect, the clinical-grade material used contained 20% or more of impurities, including two forms of the hormone (20 and 22 kDa), an acetylated form, and at least five smaller (5 to 10 kDa) peptides.

Secretion of STH is regulated by two hypothalamic hormones: somatocrinin promotes release, whereas somatostatin inhibits it. The former, which was recently isolated, is a 44–amino acid residue, amidated peptide with the COOH-terminal 20 residues containing the bioactivity. Somatostatin chemistry was discussed in Chapter 3.

The opposing actions of these two hormones on the pituitary somatotropes are modified by other hormones. The responses seen depend, somewhat, upon which species is being investigated and whether the observations are being made in vitro or in vivo.

In general, it seems that somatomedins inhibit, and glucocorticoids and thyroid hormones enhance, pituitary response to somatocrinin. Somatocrinin acts through an adenylate cyclase mechanism.

In intact humans, insulin hypoglycemia, exercise, vasopressin, arginine, L-dopa, sleep, and stress cause an increased secretion of STH. The first four act through α- and β-adrenergic receptors in which the α-receptor is stimulatory and the β-receptor is inhibitory. Sleep and arginine probably act through a serotoninergic mechanism.

The growth-promoting properties of somatotropin are mediated through the somatomedins, smaller peptides with a direct mitogenic action on several types of tissue. There are two somatomedins (A and C), which are also called insulinlike growth factors (IGF-I and IGF-II). The latter name calls attention to the fact that insulin, which one associates with the regulation of lipid and carbohydrate metabolism, is required for normal growth. Structurally, the somatomedins resemble proinsulin, and the receptors for IGF-I and insulin are both tetrameric, share some antigenic determinants, and possess a specific tyrosine kinase activity. The IGF-II is quite different.

Recently, a large number of "growth factors" have been described, named either for their source or for the target of their action. This chapter describes a few of the more actively investigated factors: epidermal GF or urogastrone, platelet-derived GF, nerve GF, and fibroblast GF. The physiological roles that these factors play in our bodies and their relationships to each other and to oncogenes now are areas of intense investigation. The result will surely be an improved understanding of the regulation of normal and abnormal growth.

SUPPLEMENTAL BIBLIOGRAPHY

Clinical

Bierich, JR, MB Ranke, P Beyer, et al. Therapie des hypophysaeren Zwergwuchses mit rekombinanten menschlichen Wachstumhormon, *Dtsh Med Wochenschr* 3:483-489, 1986.

Cutler, Jr, GB, FG Cassorla, JL Ross, OH Pescovitz KM Barnes, F Comite, PP Feuillan, L Laue, CM Fosterm D Kenigsberg, M Caruso-Nicoletti,

HB Garcia, M Uriarte, KD Hench, MC Skerda, LM Long, and DL Loriaux. Pubertal growth: Physiology and pathophysiology, *Recent Prog Horm Res 42*:443-465, 1986.

Essman, WB. Growth hormone dynamics in diabetes mellitus, In *Prospectives in Clinical Endocrinology* (WB Essman, ed) SP Medical and Scientific Books, New York, 1980, pp 305-341.

Kaplan, SL, GP August, SL Blethen, et al. Clinical studies with recombinant DNA-derived methionyl human growth hormone in growth hormone deficient children, *Lancet 03/29*:697-700, 1986.

Insulin

Strauss, DS. Growth-stimulatory actions of insulin in vitro and in vivo. *Endocr. Rev 5*:356–369, 1984.

Nonsomatotropin-Related Factors

Abraham, JA, A Mergia, JL Whang, A Tumolo, J Friedman, KA Hjerrild, D Gospodarowicz, and JC Fiddes. Nucleotide sequence of a bovine clone encoding the angiogenic protein, basic fibroblast growth factor. *Science 233*:545–548, 1986.

Bohlen, P, F Esch, P Brazeau, N Ling, and R Guillemin. Isolation and characterization of the porcine hypothalamic growth hormone releasing factor. *Biochem Biophys Res Commun 116*:726–734, 1983.

Bradshaw, RA and NV Costrini. Nerve growth factor: Structure, function and mechanism of action, In *Growth and Growth Factors* (K Shizume and K Takano, eds). University Park Press, Baltimore, 1980, pp 233–251.

Carpenter, G and S Cohen. Epidermal growth factor. *Annu Rev Biochem 48*:193–216, 1979.

Chan, CP and EG Krebs. Epidermal growth factor stimulates glycogen synthase activity in cultured cells. *Proc Natl Acad Sci USA 82*:4563–4567, 1985.

Esch, F, P Bohlen, N Ling, P Brazeau, and R Guillemin. Isolation and characterization of the bovine hypothalamic growth hormone releasing factor. *Biochem Biophs Res Commun 117*:772–779, 1983.

Heldin, C-H and B Westermark. Growth factors: Mechanism of action and relation to oncogenes. *Cell 37*:9–20, 1984.

Hollenberg, MD. Epidermal growth factor-urogastrone, a polypeptide acquiring hormonal status. *Vitam Horm 37*:69–110, 1979.

Ishii, S, Y-H Xu, RH Stratton, BA Roe, GT Merlino, and IT Pastan. Characterization and sequence of the promoter region of the human epidermal growth factor receptor gene. *Proc Natl Acad Sci USA 82*:4920–4924, 1985.

Phillips, LS and R Vassilopoulou-Sellin. Somatomedins, *N Engl J Med* *302*:371–380; 438–446, 1980.

Shooter, EM, BA Yankner, GE Landreth, and A Sutter. Biosynthesis and mechanism of action of nerve growth factor. *Recent Prog Horm Res* *37*:417–446, 1981.

Stiles, CD. The molecular biology of platelet-derived growth factor. *Cell* *33*:653–655, 1983.

Urdea, MS, et al. Chemical synthesis of a gene for human epidermal growth factor-urogastrone and its expression in yeast. *Proc Natl Acad Sci USA 80*:7461–7465, 1983.

Yankner, BA and EM Shooter. The biology and the mechanism of action of nerve growth factor. *Annu Rev Biochem 51*:845–868, 1982.

Zapf, J, ER Froesch, and RE Humbel. The insulin-like growth factors (IGF) of human serum: Chemical and biological characterization and aspects of their possible physiological role. *Curr Top Cell Reg 19*:257–309, 1981.

The Somatotropin Family and Related Hormones

Brazeau, P, N Ling, P Bohlen, F Esch, S-Y Ying, and R Guillemin. Growth hormone releasing factor, somatocrinin, releases pituitary growth hormone in vitro. *Proc Natl Acad Sci USA 79*:7909–7913, 1983.

Cooke, NE, D Coit, J Shine, JD Baxter, and JA Martial. Human prolactin: cDNA structural analysis and evolutionary comparisons. *J Biol Chem 256*:4007–4016, 1981.

Esch, FS, P Bohlen, NC Ling, PE Brazeau, WB Wehrenberg, and R Guillemin. Primary structures of three human pancreas peptides with growth hormone-releasing activity. *J Biol Chem 258*:1806–1812, 1983.

Guillemin, R, P Brazeau, P Bohlen, F Esch, N Ling, WB Ehrenberg, B Bloch, C Mougin, F Zeytin, and A Baird. Somatocrinin: The growth hormone releasing factor. *Recent Prog Horm Res 40*:233–286, 1984.

Lewis, UJ, RNP Singh, GFT Tutwiler, MB Sigel, EF VanderLaan, and WP VanderLaan. Human growth hormone: A complex of proteins. *Recent Prog Horm Res 36*:477–504, 1980.

Nicoll, CS, GL Mayer, and SM Russell. Structural features of prolactins and growth hormones that can be related to their biological properties. *Endocr Rev 7*:169–203, 1986.

Nilsson, A, J Isgaard, A Lindahl, A Dahlstrom, A Skottner, and OGP Isaksson. Regulation by growth hormone of number of chrondrocytes containing IGF-1 in rat growth plate. *Science 233*:571–574, 1986.

Thorner, MD, ML Vance, WS Evans, RM Blizzard, AD Rogol, K Ho, DA Leong, JLC Borges, MJ Cronin, RM MacLeod, K Kovacs, S Asa, E Horvath, L Frohman, R Furlanetto, GJ Klingensmith, C Brook, P

Smith, S Reichlin, J Rivier, and W Vale. Physiological and clinical studies of GRF and GH. *Recent Prog Horm Res 42*:589–632, 1986.

Spiess, J, J Rivier, M Thorner, and W Vale. Sequence analysis of a growth hormone releasing factor from a human pancreatic islet cell tumor. *Biochemistry 21*:6037–6040, 1982.

Spiess, J, J Rivier, and W Vale. Characterization of rat hypothalamic growth hormone-releasing factor. *Nature 303*:532–535, 1983.

Zezaluk, KM and H Green. The generation of insulin-like growth factor-1-sensitive cells by growth hormone action. *Science 233*:551–553, 1986.

5

Thyroid Hormones

The Hypothalamo-Adenohypophyseal-Thyroidal System   129
    Thyrotropin-releasing hormone   129
    Thyrotropin   130
    Triiodothyronine and thyroxine   132
Thyroid Hormone Biosynthesis   134
    Iodide   134
    Thyroglobulin   135
    Triiodothyronine and thyroxine   140
Clinical Aspects   144
    Methods   144
    Metabolism   145
    Hypofunction   147
    Hyperfunction   149
Summary   150
Supplemental Bibliography   152

THE HYPOTHALAMO-ADENOHYPOPHYSEAL-THYROIDAL SYSTEM

The thyroid system consists of the CNS, hypothalamus, anterior pituitary, thyroid gland (except C cells), and target tissues. In homiothermic species, the system plays an important role in the regulation of metabolism of the body, often referred to as the "basal metabolic rate" (BMR). In all vertebrate species, this system is required for general growth and development and for differentiation of the nervous system. Activation of the thyroid system by a change in core body temperature is a relatively primitive type of reaction seen in homiothermic animals and in the human newborn, but not in adult humans.

Thyrotropin-Releasing Hormone

Thyrotropin-releasing hormone (TRH), a tripeptide, is made in the hypothalalamus in the form of a multiple-copy precursor.

129

Temperature-sensitive neurons terminating in the thyrotropic area, located between the paraventricular nucleus and the median eminence, are responsible for its synthesis. The neurotransmitters controlling thyrotropin (TSH) release are still controversial, but the most consistent findings favor stimulatory β-noradenergic and inhibitory dopaminergic pathways with some species variability. In normal humans, L-dihydroxyphenylalanine (L-Dopa) has no effect on basal TSH levels, but it does inhibit TRH-induced TSH release. The mechanisms controlling TRH release in adult humans remain obscure.

Thyroid-releasing hormone, pyroGlu-His-Pro-NH$_2$, is the simplest polypeptide hormone known and the first to be isolated from the hypothalamus. Every feature is essential for activity, even opening the pyro-glutamyl ring or removing the terminal amide nitrogen markedly suppresses activity. Only one change increases bioactivity, namely, the replacement of the imidazole N-H with N-CH$_3$. The half-lives of TRH in plasma are 3 and 7 min; 12 to 14% of a bolus injection may, however, be recovered unchanged in the urine. Most (80%) of the TRH in the body lies in extrahypothalamic areas of the brain. The function of this brain TRH is not known, but its wide distribution suggests that it may act as a neurotransmitter.

Thyrotropin

Thyrotropin (thyroid-stimulating hormone, TSH), is a dimeric glycoprotein (ca. 28 kDa containing 7–8% carbohydrate) consisting of dissimilar α and β subunits. The genes for these two subunits are located on different chromosomes, and they are independently regulated. The α subunits for TSH, folliculotropin (FSH), luteotropin (LH), and human chorionic gonadotropin (hCG) are made by the same gene in a pre-form. The signal sequence is cleaved cotranslationally, and two mannose chains having a high mannose content [(glucose)$_3$(mannose)$_9$(N-acetylglucosamine)$_2$] are transferred from dolichol pyrophosphate to appropriate asparagines [(Asp)-(x)-(Ser/Thr)] in the Golgi. After trimming off all glucoses and six mannoses, various other sugars (fucose, sialic acid, N-acetylgalactosamine, galactose, N-acetylglucosamine) are added sequentially to form "complex" polysaccharide chains.

The somewhat larger β-subunit is processed similarly, but it contains only one carbohydrate chain.

Although this process is somewhat complicated, it has its purposes. The high mannose content of the precursor forms induces conformational changes required for α–β-subunit combination, and it protects the subunits from intracellular proteolysis and aggregation. The final complex carbohydrate moities confer intrinsic biological activity and protect the secreted hormone from proteolysis, i.e., it decreases its metabolic clearance rate.

Synthesis of the two subunits is not coordinated; that of the β subunit is rate-limiting on the formation of hormone. In other words, much more α-subunit is made, and it and the mature hormone, but never the free β-subunit, are secreted into the vascular system. Thyroid hormone deficiency selectively stimulates TSH–β-subunit apoprotein synthesis as well as carbohydrate synthesis of both α and β-subunits in cultured rat pituitaries. Thus, hypothyroidism alters the rate-limiting step in TSH assembly, as well as the carbohydrate structure of TSH, which may play important roles in its biological function. The effect of TRH on TSH biosynthesis, on the other hand, is limited to the incorporation of carbohydrate, thereby enhancing its intrinsic bioactivity.

Release of TSH from the pituitary thyrotropes is controlled mainly by TRH and thyroxine (T_4). The thyrotropes have plasma cell membrane receptors for TRH, but the mode of action of the TRH–receptor complex is not established. Calcium ions, as usual, are required to demonstrate an effect of TRH on TSH release in vitro. The thyrotropes also have cytosolic and nuclear receptors for T_3 and T_4. According to a recent experiment on rats, a 5'-deiodinase in the thryotrope converts T_4 to T_3, which binds to a nuclear acceptor and somehow inhibits release of TSH. Other investigators have shown, by the use of pituitary tumor cells in culture, that T_3, as well as TRH at relatively high concentrations, decreases the number of TRH receptors; the effects are additive. Thus, the pituitary thyrotropes differ from other target tissues of thyroid hormones in being more responsive to T_4 than to T_3.

Other hormones secondarily control TSH secretion. Dopamine exerts tonic inhibitory control in humans and other species. Thyrotropes have dopamine receptors, and dopamine concentrations in the median eminence and portal blood are high. There are also some dopaminergic influences on the hypothalamus.

Somatostatin may be a physiologic inhibitor of TSH secretion, in that injection of an antiserum to somatostatin increases both basal plasma TSH concentrations and the response to cold in rats. Pharmacological doses of cortisol will further suppress a pituitary response (rat or human) that has been maximally suppressed with T_3. On the other hand, estrogens appear to sensitize the pituitary response to TRH. In a primary culture, fibroblast growth factor in picomolor concentrations increases both the sensitivity of rat anterior pituitary cells to TRH and the amounts of TSH (and prolactin) released.

Thyrotropin action on the thyroid is twofold: it is a trophic hormone promoting cellular proliferation, and it is a thyrogenic hormone acting to stimulate the secretion of T_3 and T_4. Although TSH mildly stimulates iodide uptake and organification, its principal actions are centered on lysosomal degradation of thyroglobulin with release of T_4, T_3, 3,5-diiodotyrosine (DIT), 3-iodotyrosine (MIT), and other iodinated thyronines and on deiodination of MIT and DIT. (In the interests of conservation of iodide, it is natural that these two reactions are tightly coupled.)

Thyrotropin stimulates thyroidal adenylate cyclase; cAMP, through its action on cAMP-dependent protein kinases, promotes certain steps in thyrogenesis. Energy supply through glucose oxidation and the generation of peroxide are not, however, cAMP-dependent. Cyclic AMP somehow also mediates an increased synthesis of α_1-adrenergic receptors, which may increase by as much as tenfold. These receptors in response to catecholamines produce an increase in intracellular calcium which, in turn, promotes iodide transport. The physiological significance of this observation is still not clear. Prostaglandins are also somehow involved. The mechanism of the trophic action of TSH is completely obscure.

Triiodothyronine and Thyroxine

The thyroid makes several iodinated amino acids, all by posttranslational modification of tyrosine (Fig. 5.1). Hence, there is no trinucleotide code for any of them. The iodothyronines are formed by condensation of two iodinated tyrosines (see p. 140). Thyroxine, tetraiodothyronine (T_4), is the preponderant form in the thyroid and in the blood. In fact, however, it is a prohormone in most

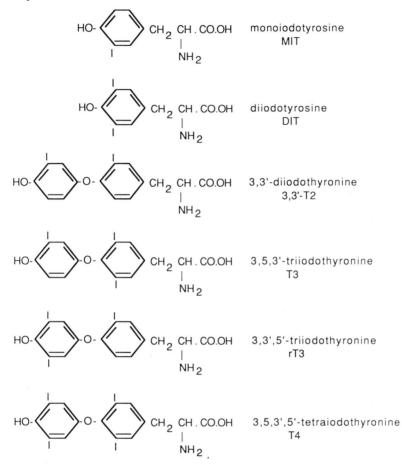

Figure 5.1 Structures of iodinated amino acid residues occurring in thyroglobulin by posttranslational modification of tyrosyl residues. Therefore, all the amino and carboxyl groups shown as free actually are involved in peptide bonds.

tissues except the anterior pituitary. In tissue, 3,5,3'-triiodothyronine (T_3), the true hormone, is the preponderant form because tissue receptors have a higher affinity for it. There are, of course, two isomeric triiodothyronines—the "other" one, 3,3',5'-triiodothyronine, is called reverse T_3 (rT_3). Reverse T_3 is probably an inactive degradation product of T_4. Food deprivation, carbohydrate restriction, and febrile illnesses lower plasma T_3 and increae plasma rT_3 concentrations. The fetal circulation has elevated levels of rT_3.

THYROID HORMONE BIOSYNTHESIS

Iodide

Nutrition

The endocrinology of the thyroid also has a nutritional aspect; iodide is a trace element. The dietary requirement for iodide is about 100 μg daily. More is not needed and is not necessarily better because excess iodide can block the iodide pump (see below). There is some danger today with the popularity of food additives that too much iodide may be ingested.

Uptake

To acquire iodide, the thyroid must accumulate it against a concentration gradient, an energy-requiring process. (This process is not unique to the thyroid because salivary glands, gastric parietal cells, and lactating mammary glands also concentrate iodide. The reason for this ability is not apparent in the first two cases, but the iodide transferred to the milk is vital to the neonate. None of these tissues can mimic the thyroid's ability to oxidize iodide and iodinate protein.) Hence, anything that interferes with ATP production, such as hypoxia, hypothermia, or ingestion of cyanide, will inhibit uptake. The iodide pump exhibits saturation kinetics and can be competitively inhibited by similar-sized monovalent anions, such as SCN^- or ClO_4^- as well as I^-. When working efficiently, the iodide pump can concentrate iodide from plasma at 10^{-7} M concentration by a factor of 25- to 100-fold. Thyrotropin acting through cAMP does not change the K_m of the iodide pump, but increases its V_{max}.

Efflux

Intracellular iodide (less than 0.25% of the total iodine in the gland) is not bound to anything and is free to diffuse out of the cell, and in fact, it does so at a rate of 40–50 μg daily in normal subjects. The rest of it is trapped in apical exocytotic vesicles by oxidation and immediate iodination of selected tyrosines of thyroglobulin (Tg; see p. 136).

Autoregulation

There are two types of controls on iodide transport. We have considered hormonal controls that act rapidly (in minutes). In addition, intrathyroidal iodine content produces autoregulation. Experimentally, autoregulation responses are demonstrated in hypophysectomized animals, either left untreated or given constant amounts of TSH. Such animals will concentrate iodide *if* the thyroidal iodide concentration is low, regardless of whether or not TSH is present. Relatively small doses of iodide depress the thyroid/serum ratio of iodide. In intact, iodine-deficient rats given an iodide supplement, TSH levels fall in proportion to the dose adminstered as iodide uptake and thyroid hormone synthesis increase. After 6 weeks of supplementation, however, radioiodine uptake is inversely correlated with dietary iodide intake, despite normal plasma concentrations of TSH, T_4, and T_3. Thus, autoregulation is a sluggish response modulated by a rapid TSH response.

Thyroglobulin

Structure

The thyroid is an unique endocrine organ in that it can store large quantities of hormone in the follicular colloid, enough to last for many weeks with no further synthesis. The substance stored is actually thyroglobulin (Tg), an enormous dimeric glycoprotein (19S, 660 kDa). The primary structure of bovine Tg was deduced, in 1985, from the sequence of its 8431-base cDNA. The 2750-amino acid monomer contains three types of repetitive sequences, each rich in cysteine. Over 75% of the Tg sequence is involved in these repetitive structures, indicating that this exceptionally large protein evolved from the serial duplication of a limited number of building blocks. The last 600 residues at the carboxyl end show no internal homology, are poor in cysteine, and contain a cluster of tyrosines, three of which are hormonogenic, i.e., produce T_3, or T_4, or both.

The bTg monomer contains 15 potential acceptor sites for *N*-glycosylation, less than the number actually seen. Thyroglobulin contains two types of chains linked through asparagine, the smaller (unit A, 1.8 kDa) containing *N*-acetylglucosamine, whereas the larger (unit B, 2.1–3.3 kDa) with a branched structure also contains sialic acid, fucose and galactose. The number of chains varies with the species (5 to 8 A's and 13 to 22 B's). A third type of unit, rich in galactosamine and attached to serine or threonine through *O*-glycosidic bonds, has been identified in human and guinea pig Tg. A fourth unit containing repeated glucuronic acid-galactosamine disaccharides attached through a galactosylxylosyl-serine linkage has been found only in hTg.

The synthesis of Tg occurs presumably in a well-defined sequence, although there is still uncertainty regarding the relationship between terminal glycosylation, iodination, and secretion into the follicular lumen. At any rate, noniodinated Tg, possessing 5500 amino acid residues including 144 tyrosyl residues, ends up in small exocytotic vesicles bordering the apical membrane of the cell where iodination takes place. When the thyroglobulin contains 1% by weight of iodine (a physiological amount), only about 10 of the tyrosyl residues occur in the form of MIT (monoiodotyrosine), 6 as DIT (diiodotyrosine), 5 as T_4, and fewer than 1 (statistically) as a T_3 residue. Thus, fewer than 20% of the tyrosyl residues in Tg are involved in iodothyronine metabolism. Thyroxine and T_3 are stored as *amino acid residues in thyroglobulin* until TSH signals for their release. Also, the normal thyroid gland releases many times more T_4 than T_3: the ratio of T_4/T_3 becomes smaller whenever the supply of iodine is limited.

Organification

The imposing name organification simply refers to the conversion of inorganic iodide to an organic form. The enzyme responsible for this conversion is thyroid peroxidase, a membrane-bound enzyme, that is somewhat unstable when it is removed from the membrane and purified. It has three substrates: iodide, Tg, and H_2O_2. The major products are Tg-bound MIT, DIT, T_3, and T_4, with smaller amounts of rT_3, $3,3'-T_2$, and monoiodohistidine (see Fig. 5.1). The intermediates are postulated to be free radicals. Both iodide and tyrosine can lose one electron, forming free radicals. The product formed from these short-lived intermediates depends upon their environment. In the presence of an excess of iodide, iodine forms:

$$2I^- \longleftrightarrow 2I \cdot \longleftrightarrow I_2$$

When tyrosine is the only substrate, bityrosine forms (Fig. 5.2A). When iodide and tyrosine (or MIT) are present, MIT (or DIT) forms (Fig. 2B).

This reaction is specific in the sense that only selected tyrosines are iodinated. Bovine Tg has 144 tyrosines and a theoretical uptake of 288 iodine atoms. In rat and man, maximal incorporation is seldom higher than 50 atoms, although in vitro, this number may be almost doubled. Thus, either many of the tyrosines of Tg are not accessible or the enzyme has some structural requirement. The major sites for hormonogenesis are Tyr-5, Tyr-2555, Tyr-2569, and Tyr-2748.

Thyroglobulin iodinated in vivo is quite heterogeneous. For example, Tg containing 40 to 50 iodine atoms can be fractionated, by sucrose density-gradient or isopycnic ultracentrifugation, into samples containing 26 to 70 iodine atoms. In severe iodine deficiency or upon treatment with antithyroid drugs (see later discussion), the iodine content may be less than one atom of iodine per molecule of Tg (on the average).

Coupling

Thyroid peroxidase also catalyzes intramolecular coupling of MIT and of DIT to produce thyronines. This postulate implies that certain iodotyrosine residues are so aligned that two of them can interact with the enzyme to produce coupling. Again, a free radical intermediate is postulated (Fig. 5.3). The coupling of two DITs produces T_4, whereas MIT and DIT residues interact to form T_3 and rT_3. Coupling is apparently dependent upon the level of iodination as uniodinated thyronine or monoiodothyronine have never been found in Tg, nor have diiodothyronines with both iodines located in one ring.

Most of the MIT and DIT residues are apparently so situated that they never couple. Only a few (about five) molecules of T_4 and one-tenth as much T_3 form in each molecule of Tg at normal iodination levels. If there is a low degree of iodination, relatively more T_3 and less T_4 form.

Thiourea compounds, such as propylthiouracil or methimazole, are used clinically to decrease iodination and coupling. They apparently act by competing with iodide for sites on the peroxidase, being oxidized in place of iodide. Propylthiouracil also inhibits peripheral deiodination of T_4 to T_3 (see p. 141).

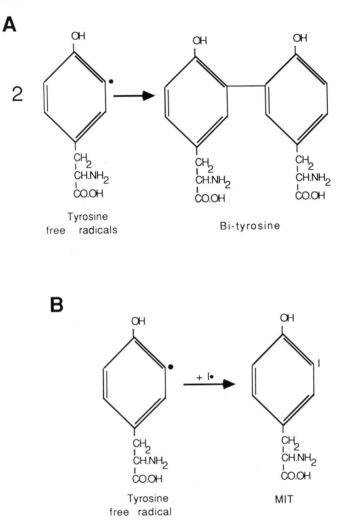

Figure 5.2   Reactions of tyrosyl free radicals. (A) If a tyrosyl free radical first encounters another tyrosyl free radical, a bityrosyl residue will form. (B) If a tyrosyl free radical first encounters an iodine free radical atom (or a free monoiodotyrosyl radical), then a monoiodotyrosyl residue (or a diiodotyrosyl residue) will form.

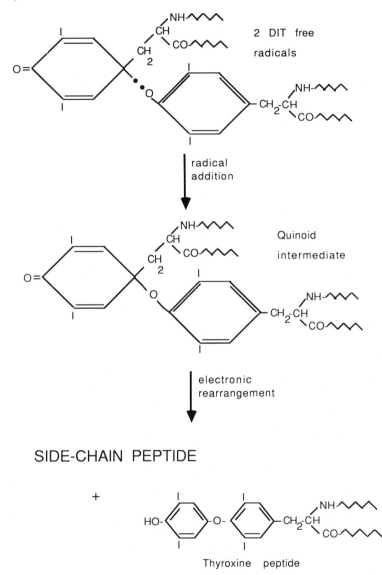

Figure 5.3 Reactions of iodotyrosyl free radicals in thyroglobulin to form iodothyronyl residues. Reactions are limited by steric considerations involving two iodotyrosyl residues and the thyroid peroxidase. Therefore, most iodotyrosyl residues never react. The reaction may involve two molecules of DIT, or two of MIT, or one each of MIT and DIT.

Storage

Thyroglobulin, whether iodinated or not, is extruded into the lumen of the follicle where it forms the colloid. In the adult, there are apparently two pools of thyroglobulin—an old and a new. The old pool is more or less static, whereas the new pool turns over rapidly. The last made is the first used.

Triiodothyronine and Thyroxine

Release

Thyrotropin controls usage of colloid which is ingested by pinocytosis. After fusion with lysosomes, the Tg is completely digested. The hormones are secreted while a NADP-requiring dehalogenase removes the iodine from MIT and DIT for reutilization. The pathways of iodine metabolism are summarized in Figure 5.4

Transport

Thyroid hormones are transported in blood bound to specific proteins (Table 5.1). Thyroxine-binding globulin (TBG) is a trace (0.25 μM) glycoprotein constituent of blood that has an extremely high affinity for T_4. This protein (60 kDa) has been isolated by several investigators, but there is no agreement on its composition. Only the first 19 residues have been sequenced.

Thyroxine-binding prealbumin (PA) is an unusually stable molecule (55 kDa; 5μM), made of four identical subunits containing no carbohydrate; it has 127 amino acid residues in each subunit. The four subunits are arranged tetrahedrally with major interactions between their pleated sheets such that a double trumpet-shaped molecule with an open channel through the center is formed. The two T_4-binding sites are located at the widened open ends. (The PA also binds retinol-binding protein, the carrier protein for vitamin A.) PA29–48 has significant homology with TBG.

Albumin (69 kDa; 0.7 mM) has much less affinity for T_4 but a much higher concentration than the other two binding proteins. As a consequence of the binding of these three plasma proteins, nearly all thyroid hormone in plasma is bound, only about 0.03% of T_4 and 0.4% of T_3 being unbound or free (Table 5.2 and 5.3). It is

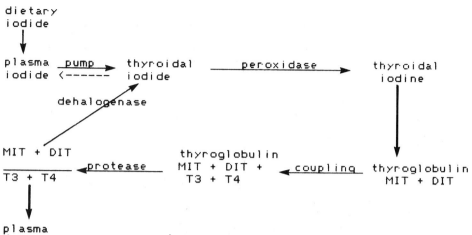

Figure 5.4 Summary of the metabolism of iodide and synthesis of thyroid hormones.

this tiny unbound fraction that is responsible for the peripheral metabolic status, the inhibition of TSH secretion, and hepatic and renal clearance of T_3 and T_4.

Estrogens, especially at the concentrations found in pregnancy, increase TBG and decrease PA plasma levels, whereas androgens have an opposing effect. Pharmacological quantities of glucocorticoids decrease TBG and increase PA plasma levels.

Production of Triiodothyronine

Thyroxine is now believed to be a prohormone. It is converted peripherally, mostly in the liver, to T_3 by a dehalogenase. Prophylthiouracil inhibits this enzyme except in the pituitary. Triiodothyronine is about five times more potent biologically than T_4. Hence, despite the preponderance of T_4 in the plasma, in biological value free T_3 outweighs free T_4, i.e., although the concentration of free T_3 is one-third that of free T_4, the fivefold greater potency of T_3 makes it, in one sense, dominant.

The production rate (PR) of a hormone is the total amount produced per unit time. It differs from the secretory rate (SR) whenever there is peripheral synthesis (outside the secretory gland). *Average* values of the production rate of T_4, T_3, and rT_3 in normal subjects are

Table 5.1   Affinites of the Thyroid Hormone-Binding Proteins for T$_4$ and T$_3$

	TBG (nM^{-1})	PA (nM^{-1})	HSA (μM^{-1})
T$_4$	6.0 (1)	32[a]	1.3[b]
T$_3$	0.33 (1)	2.5	0.2

[a]PA (prealbumin) has one high-affinity site and one low-affinity site (5.0 μM^{-1}) for T$_4$.
[b]HSA has one high-affinity site and several of lesser affinity.

88 (83–93), 30 (23–45), and 28 (17–52) μg/day (ranges given in parentheses). These values will change under altered physiologic or pathologic states. About 60% of T$_4$ is deiodinated to T$_3$ and rT$_3$, nearly equally. Eighty percent of T$_3$ and 97.5% of rT$_3$ come from deiodination of T$_4$, the balance being secreted from the thyroid.

Effects

Thyroid hormones are essential for normal growth and development and for normal metabolic activity in the adult mammal, including man. Our knowledge of the molecular events involved is primitive, and even at the level of the whole organism, there are still ambiguities. The latter probably arises because thyroid hormones have few direct effects, many actions being attributable to the modulation of activity of other hormones, such as insulin, glucagon, corticoids, and catecholamines.

Thyroid hormone is required for proper neural development (myelinization) during the neonatal period. In terms of neonatal screening, congenital hypothyroidism occurs more frequently than phenylketonurism and, if untreated, produces more severe mental retardation. Thyroid hormone is essential for postnatal growth. In addition to a direct component, there is also an indirect action because thyroid hormone is required for the adenohypophyseal synthesis of STH and possibly, also for the production of somatomedin.

Amphibian metamorphosis dramatizes the effects of thyroid hormone on differentiation. New organs, such as the legs, appear in the tadpole, whereas others, such as gills and tail, are absorbed. Urea cycle enzymes appear in the liver. During development of legs, thyroid hormone concentrations are low, but the target organ sensitivity is highest, associated with an

Table 5.2 Serum Values for Euthyroid People

	Total concentration (ng/ml)	Bound (%)	Unbound concentration (pg/ml)	Half-life (days)
T_4	45–115	99.97	14–35	7
T_3	1–2	99.6	5–10	1

Table 5.3 Distribution of Bound Hormone (%)

	TBG	TBPA	HSA
T_4	70	10	20
T_3	38	27	35

increased concentration of T_3 nuclear receptors. During the period of metamorphic climax when the gills and tail are absorbed, high concentrations of T_4 and T_3 exist in the plasma.

In warm-blooded animals, thyroid hormone causes an increase in oxygen consumption and heat production, which is expressed as an increase in the basal metabolic rate (BMR). All types of muscle, kidney, liver, and pancreas respond. On the other hand, a number of tissues are unaffected, namely, brain, dermis, lung, spleen, gonads and secondary sex organs, thymus, and lymph nodes. A few effects of thyroid hormone on fuel metabolism, which could conceivably explain some aspects of thyroid control of the BMR, will be described, but no satisfactory, holistic explanation is presently available.

The best documented example of direct control is mitochondrial FAD-linked α-glycerophosphate dehydrogenase which is stimulated quite specifically by thyroid hormone; RNA synthesis inhibitors block the response. This enzyme is part of the NADH shuttle, transferring NADH produced in the cytosol during glycolysis into the mitochondria where its energy can be converted into ATP by oxidative phosphorylation. (Older experiments purporting to show a direct action of thyroid hormone on mitochondria used nonphysiologic concentrations (1–10 μM) of hormone which produced mitochondrial swelling and uncoupling of oxidative phosphorylation.) In mammals, however, this enzyme is not as important as the malate–aspartate shuttle in transporting the energy being produced through glycolysis of glycogen and ingested carbohydrate.

Most effects produced by modulation of the activity of another hormone are complex and may vary with the organ and species being considered. For example, thyroid hormone potentiates insulin effects, increasing uptake and metabolism of glucose. It also increases hepatic metabolism of insulin, placing an increased demand on the pancreas. The net result is the postprandial hyperglycemia and abnormal response to glucose seen in hyperthyroidism. Again, the synthesis of glycogen is promoted at low concentrations of thyroid hormone (an insulin effect?), whereas glycogenolysis predominates at higher concentrations (a glucagon effect?).

Thyroid hormone is said to play a permissive role in the action of glucagon and catcholamines. This might occur through an increase in the number of adrenergic receptors or through a regulation of phosphodiesterase activity or both.

Response to thyroid hormones has an induction period of several hours, being longer for T_4 than for T_3, perhaps because of the requirement for deiodination of the former. The induction period presumably reflects the time required for nuclear binding and activation of transcription and translation of certain enzymes. Little is known about the first event, and virtually nothing about subsequent events.

Intracellular binding of thyroid hormones follows the steroid pattern. Although there are high-affinity binding proteins in the cytosol of responsive cells, transport into the nucleus does not require activation of the cytosolic protein–hormone complex. Therefore, the cytosolic binder appears to act as a concentrator, extracting hormone from the blood and presenting it to the nucleus. In keeping with the greater biological potency of T_3, the nuclear receptor–acceptor has a marked preference for T_3.

CLINICAL ASPECTS

Methods

Ideally, knowledge of the concentration of free (unbound) T_4 and T_3 in the plasma should readily discriminate euthyroidism from hyperthyroidism and hypothyroidism. This assay, however, is not widely available. Instead, total T_4 and sometimes total T_3 in plasma are measured by a direct (no extraction step) radioimmunoassay whereas a T_3 resin uptake affords an *index* of binding activity. The latter is somewhat complicated, and it is explained in the following.

Labeled T_3 ($^*T_3$) and a sponge containing particles of a resin having an affinity (and a large capacity) for T_3 and T_4 are incubated with a sample of plasma until equilibrium is attained. The sponge is removed and washed, and the radioactivity bound to it is counted (uptake) and expressed as a percentage of the radioactivity added.

Interpretation is complicated by the presence of two binding substances, TBG and resin, and two ligands, T_4 and $^*T_3$. The amounts of resin and $^*T_3$ are standardized, and the concentration of T_4 is known by RIA. Uptake is a function of the concentration of both TBG and T_4 (total T_3 is negligible compared to total T_4). The lowest uptakes of $^*T_3$ will occur with a combination of high [TBG] and low [T_4] because most of the $^*T_3$ will be bound to TBG. Conversely, the highest resin uptakes require a combination of low [TBG] and high [T_4], a condition that will leave few binding sites on the TBG available for $^*T_3$; the $^*T_3$ binds to the resin. Therefore, a high resin uptake is an *index* of a high unbound [T_3] and vice versa (Fig. 5.5).

The concentration of TSH in the serum or plasma is routinely measured by RIA. On the other hand, although an antibody to TRH exists, RIA of TRH is not routinely performed because of its lability in blood.

An in vivo test of thyroid function is the injection of a small quantity of iodide-131 (or iodide-123). The thyroid accumulates a radioactive isotope as readily as it does the natural one (iodide-127). The radioactive isotope emits an energetic γ-ray that can be detected by a solid crystal scintillation counter, allowing determination of uptake by placing a counter over the thyroid (Table 5.4). Furthermore, if a counter is provided with collimation and a scanning device, the thyroid can be viewed with considerable resolution (Fig. 5.6).

Metabolism

Thyroxine is converted in approximately equal amounts (about 40% each) to T_3 and rT_3. These, in turn, are deiodinated to form diiodothyronines (3,5-T_2, 3,3'-T_2, and 3',5'-T_2) (Table 5.5). All except T_4 and T_3 are biologically inactive and represent degradative catabolism of the active hormones. Other catabolic pathways

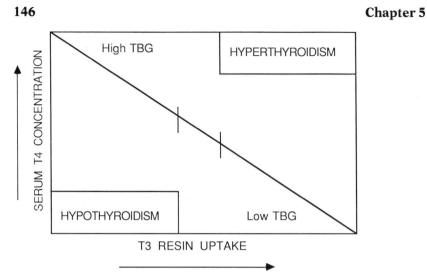

Figure 5.5 Interpretation of T_4 and T_3 resin uptake data.

Table 5.4 Radioisotopes Used to Image the Thyroid

	Radionuclide		
	^{123}I	^{131}I	^{99m}Tc
Mode of decay	Electron capture	β Minus	Isometric transition
Physical halflife	13.3 hr	8.06 days	6.03 hr
Decay constant	0.0533 hr^{-1}	0.0860 days^{-1}	0.1149 hr^{-1}
Photon energy (meV)	0.028 (0.867)	0.030 (0.046)	0.0186 (0.077)
Mean number per disintegration	0.159 (0.836) 0.529 (0.011)	0.080 (0.026) 0.284 (0.058) 0.364 (0.820) 0.637 (0.065) 0.723 (0.017)	0.1405 (0.879)
Relative cost	High	Low	Low
Absorbed dose[a] (rad/mCi)	7.5 (pure) 21 (impure)	800	0.18

[a]In an adult, assuming a thyroid uptake of 15% and a 19.6 g thyroid gland.
Source: From Gross, Shapiro, Thrall, Freitas, and Beierwaltes, *Endocr Rev 5*:222, 1984, with permission.

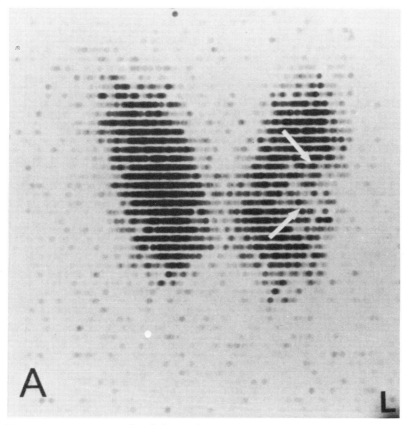

Figure 5.6 An example of thyroid scanning using iodide-131. The arrows denote an area of decreased isotope uptake in the midleft lobe, correlating with a palpable nodule in the left lobe (*Source*: From Gross, Shapiro, Thrall, Freitas, and Beierwaltes. *Endocr Rev 5*:224, 1984, with permission).

involve conjugation with glucuronic or sulfuric acid, the latter appearing to promote deiodination in the phenolic ring, as well as oxidative deamination and decarboxylation to the thyroacetic acid analogues.

Hypofunction

Thyroid disease is the second most common endocrinopathy (after diabetes mellitus) in the United States, the thyroid itself

Table 5.5 Iodothyronine Kinetics in Four Euthyroid Subjects

Measurement	T_4	T_3	rT_3	$3,3'\text{-}T_2$	$3',5'\text{-}T_2$
Concentration (ng/ml)	77 ± 9	1.1 ± 0.1	0.22 ± 0.002		
Concentration (pg/ml)					
from rT_3				4 ± 2	13 ± 4
from T_3				23 ± 4	—
MCR^a (L/day)		36.5 ± 1.6	130 ± 17	709 ± 116	266 ± 29
PR (μg/day)					
from rT_3		40.6 ± 2.1		3.2 ± 1.6	3.4 ± 1.1
from T_3				17.0 ± 4.5	—

[a]Corrected to 70-kg body weight.
Source: from Engler et al. *J. Clin Endocrinol Metab* 58:4, 1984, with permission.

being most often the cause. The clinical stigmata of hypothyroidism depend upon age. In the neonate, the disease is called cretinism, whereas in adults it is called myxedema.

Cretinism may be due to a nutritionally inadequate intake of iodide or to a congenital absence or deficiency in one of the enzymes involved in T_4 biosynthesis. The former was once common, for there are several areas in the world, the Great Lakes region being one, with inadequate iodide concentrations in the soil and, hence, in food derived from that soil. The prevalence of iodized salt and other food additives have largely eliminated this cause of hypothyroidism.

Although thyroid hormones only marginally affect the rate of metabolism of neural tissue and they are not considered to be "growth" hormones, failure of neural development producing severe mental retardation and failure to grow are two hallmarks of cretinism. The shame of cretinism is its needlessness because it is readily treatable by replacement therapy if it is detected in time. A contradiction in health care delivery is the failure of some states and countries to screen for it even though it is more common (1:6000 births) than phenylketonuria (1:12,000 births) which is widely screened. Treatment is most effective if it is started early, preferably before the age of 3 months. Failure to start therapy produces irreparable damage that is cumulative up to the age of about 2 years.

Myxedema, on the other hand, characterized as approaching a somnolent, vegetative state, is reversible. All the stigmata of a depressed basal metabolic rate are present: weak heart beat, mental and physical sluggishness, somnolescence, hypophagia, constipation, sensitivity to cold. Common causes are Hashimoto's lymphocytic thyroiditis, an autoimmune disease; idiopathic atrophy or aging; iatrogenic factors, such as surgery, x-irradiation, or iodine-131 treatment; or drugs, such as ingestion of excessive amounts of iodide, propylthiouracil, or lithium. Rarely, is TSH deficiency the cause.

Hyperfunction

Hyperthyroidism is characterized by all the sequelae of a high basal metabolic rate: increased cardiac output, tachycardia, a high rate of glucose absorption, restlessness, irritability, sleeplessness, anxiety, diarrhea, sensitivity to heat. The most common cause, called Graves disease, is associated with a diffusely enlarged thyroid. It is an immune disorder caused by the production of thyroid-stimulating IgG antibodies that bind to and activate TSH receptors. Serum T_4 and T_3 resin uptake assays, as well as radioactive iodide uptake, are used in making the diagnosis.

SUMMARY

The synthesis of thyroid hormones and the regulation of the basal metabolism of the body is summarized in Figure 5.7. In animals and the human newborn, core body temperature is sensed in the hypothalamic thyrotropic area that controls secretion of TRH. The factors controlling release in adult humans are not known. The TRH acts through plasma membrane receptors on the thyrotropes of the anterior pituitary. Thyrotropin release is positively controlled by TRH and negatively by T_4 and somatostatin. Estrogens sensitize the pituitary response to TRH, and pharmacologic doses of cortisol are suppressive. Fibroblast growth factor may increase the sensitivity of the pituitary to TRH.

Thyrotropin has both a trophic (mitogenic) action and a more rapid, thyrogenic action on the follicular cells of the thyroid; the latter is mediated through cAMP and prostaglandins. Thyrotropin stimulates all steps of thyrogenesis. It increases the activity of the iodide pump by increasing the number of transport molecules (V_{max}), the rate of organification or incorporation of iodide into the tyrosines of thyroglobulin, and especially, the rate of pinocytosis and degradation of thyroglobulin with the attendant release of T_3 and T_4.

Most T_3 and T_4 is transported in plasma bound to plasma proteins: thyroid-binding globulin, prealbumin, and albumin. It is only the tiny amount unbound that is able to cross cellular membranes and to be active physiologically. The bound fraction acts as a buffer or reservoir, constantly refilling the pool of unbound hormone by dissociation of bound hormone.

Except in the thyrotropes, T_4 acts as a prohormone, being converted to the more active T_3 by peripheral deiodination. The T_3 passes through the cellular membranes of target cells and interacts with nuclear components to initiate its actions.

Triiodothyronine basically acts to increase the basal metabolic rate (BMR), i.e., oxygen consumption in the resting

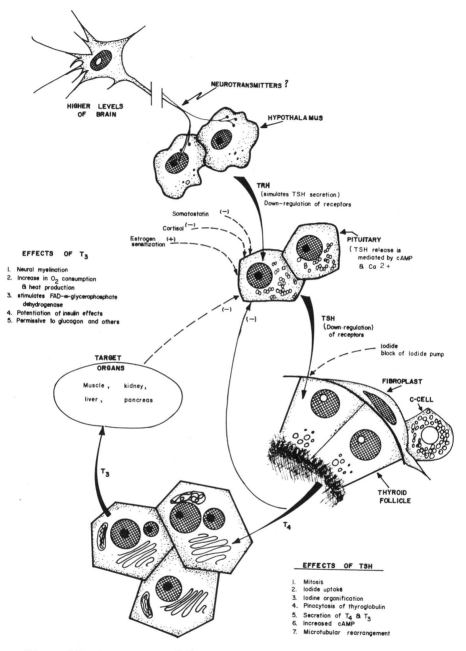

Figure 5.7 A summary of Chapter 5.

state. The mechanism is incompletely understood, but it does increase the concentration of one enzyme, glyceryl-1-phosphate dehydrogenase, an NADH shuttle enzyme. Mostly, T_3 appears to act as a permissive hormone allowing glucagon, epinephrine, STH, and others to perform their functions. Although it has no effect on the BMR of neural tissues, it is essential in neural myelinization of the newborn.

SUPPLEMENTAL BIBLIOGRAPHY

Ahren, B. Thyroid neuroendocrinology: Neural regulation of thyroid hormone secretion, *Endocr Rev 7*; 149–155, 1986.

Baird, A, P Mormede, S-Y Ying, WB Wehrenberg, N Ueno, N Ling, and R Guillemin. A nonmitogenic function of fibroblast growth factor: Regulation of thyrotropin and prolactin secretion. *Proc Natl Acad Sci USA 82*: 5545–5549, 1985.

Corda, D and LD Kohn. Thyrotropin upregulates α_1-adrenergic receptors in rat FRTL-5 thyroid cells. *Proc Natl Acad Sci USA 82*: 8677–8680, 1985.

Devisscher, M (ed). *The Thyroid Gland*. Raven Press, New York, 1980, 537 pp.

Engler, D and AG Burger. The deiodination of the iodothyronines and of their derivates in man. *Endocr Rev 5*: 151–184, 1984.

Fiddes, JC and K Talmadge. Structure, expression and evolution of the genes for the human glycoprotein hormones. *Recent Prog Horm Res 40*:43–74, 1984.

Gershengorn, MC. Thyrotropin-releasing hormone action: Mechanism of calcium-mediated stimution of prolactin secretion. *Recent Prog Horm Res 41*:607–646, 1985.

Grass, MD, B Shapiro, JH Thrall, JE Freitas, and WH Beierwaltes. The scintigraphic imaging of endocrine organs. *Endocr Rev 5*:221–281, 1984.

Ivarie, RD, JA Morris, and NL Eberhardt. Hormonal domains of response: Actions of glucocorticoid and thyroid hormones in regulating pleiotropic responses in cultured cells. *Recent Prog Horm Res 36*: 195–235, 1980.

Kourides, IA, JA Gurr, and O Wolf. The regulation and organization of thyroid stimulating hormone genes. *Recent Prog Horm Res 40*:79–117, 1984.

Larsen, PR, TE Dick, BP Markovits, MM Kaplan, and TG Gard. Inhibition of intrapituitary thyroxine to 3,5,3'-triiodothyronine conversion prevents the acute suppression of thyrotropin release by thyroxine in hypothyroid rats. *J. Clin Invest 64*:117–128, 1979.

Leblond, CP and G Bennett. Biogenesis of glycoproteins as shown by radioautography. *J Histochem Cytochem 27*:1185–1187, 1979.

Mercken, L, M-J Simons, S Swillens, M Massaer, and G Vassart. Primary structure of bovine thyroglobulin deduced from the sequence of its 8,431-base complementary DNA. *Nature 316*:647–651, 1985.

Mita, S, S Maeda, K Shimada, and S Araki. Cloning and sequence analysis of cDNA for human prealbumin. *Biochem Biophys Res Commun 124*:558–564, 1984.

Pierce, JG and RF Parsons. Glycoprotein hormones: Structure and function. *Annu Rev Biochem 50*:465–495, 1981.

Sundelin, J, H Melhus, S Das, U Eriksson, P Lind, L Tragardh, PA Peterson, and L Rask. The primary structure of rabbit and rat prealbumin and a comparison with the tertiary structure of human prealbumin. *J Biol Chem 260*:6481–6487, 1985.

Weintraub, BD, BS Stannard, JA Magner, C Ronin, T Tyalor, L Joshi, RB Constant, MM Menezes-Ferreira, P Petrick, and N Gesundheit. Glycosylation and posttranslational processing of thyroid-stimulating hormone: Clinical implications. *Recent Prog Horm Res 41*:577–603, 1985.

Yavin, E, Z Yavin, MD Schneider, and LD Kohn. Monoclonal antibodies to the thyrotropin receptor: Implications for receptor structure and the action of autoantibodies in Graves disease. *Proc Natl Acad Sci USA 78*:3180–3184, 1981.

6

Salt and Water Metabolism

Introduction   155
Vasopressin   156
Renin–Angiotensin–Aldosterone   159
    Renin   159
    Angiotensin II   162
    Aldosterone   163
Atrial Natriuretic Hormone   165
Regulation of Salt and Water Intake   168
Regulation of Salt and Water Output   171
Regulation of Hormone Secretion   174
    Antidiuretic hormone secretion   174
    Renin release   176
    Aldosterone 177
Receptors   178
    Angiotensin receptors   178
    Steroid receptors   179
    Atrial natriuretic hormone receptors   184
Clinical aspects   184
    Vasopressin–antidiuretic hormone   184
    Renin–angiotensin–aldosterone   186
    Atrial natriuretic hormone   188
Summary   188
Supplemental Bibliography   190

INTRODUCTION

Osmotic pressure is proportional to the number of ions and molecules of various types present in a stipulated volume of solvent, here, water. The units used are usually milliosmols per kilogram of water (mOsm/kg). In a "closed" system, such as a mammalian body, osmotic pressure may be varied by changes in the numerator, the denominator, or both of this ratio. Regulation occurs by adjustments in intake and renal output of salt and water. (In this discussion, I will ignore other routes of loss, such as sweat, tears, stools, menstrual discharge, and bleeding.)

The osmolarity of body fluids, as measured in the plasma compartment, is the most tightly regulated bodily variable. The osmotic threshold for vasopressin (VP) (often called antidiuretic hormone or ADH) release is 287.3 mOsm/kg. On the other hand, maximum diuresis occurs under a water load at a plasma osmolality of 281.7 mOsm/kg. Thus, a range of only 5.6 mOsm/kg or 2% is needed to swing from full diuresis to the initiation of antidiuresis.

The regulation of salt and water intake and their renal excretion is highly complex, and some aspects are controversial. There are, of course, both neural and humoral components, as well as tissue factors. The dominant hormones are VP–ADH, angiotensin II, aldosterone, and atrial natriuretic hormone, but a number of others modulate renal responses. An appreciation of the endocrine regulatory factors is difficult unless one has a conceptual grasp of the entire subject. Therefore, nonendocrine regulation is presented in sufficient detail so that the reader may have some understanding of the role of endocrine regulation.

VASOPRESSIN

Vasopressin (VP), oxytocin (OT), and vasotocin are so interrelated that I must discuss them here as a group even though, functionally, oxytocin belongs in Chapter 8 on reproduction. Figure 6.1 shows that seven of nine amino acid residues are common to these three polypeptides! Although their biological activities do vary quantitatively, qualitatively they overlap. For the same reasons, there can probably be no completely specific radioimmunoassay (RIA) for these peptides.

In Chapter 2 we spoke of the importance of the portal circulation delivering hypothalamic hormones to the adenohypophysis. Oxytocin and VP are different; they are true neurohormones, synthesized within nerve cell bodies of the paraventricular and supraoptic regions of the hypothalamus, and transported intraxonally to the neurohypophysis, where they are stored separately in granules.

The initial gene product for each is a higher–molecular-weight glycopeptide that upon specific cleavage yields equimolar amounts of hormone, a neural transport polypeptide called a neurophysin (NP) (Fig. 6.2) and an unidentified fragment. The fact

```
                                  1               5               9
ArginineVP/ADH            H₂N.cys.tyr.phe.gln.asn.cys.pro.arg.gly.NH₂
                               |_____|

Oxytocin                  H₂N.cys.tyr.ile.gln.asn.cys.pro.leu.gly.NH₂
  (milk-letdown factor)        |_____|

Vasotocin                 H₂N.cys.tyr.phe.gln.asn.cys.pro.val.gly.NH₂
  (amphibia)                   |_____|
```

Figure 6.1 Structures of hypophyseal neurohormones: VP, arginine vasopressin–antidiuretic hormone; OT, oxytocin or milk let-down factor; VT, amphibian vasotocin. Lysine-8 vasopressin occurs in pigs and hippopotami instead of arginine vasopressin.

```
                                 10          20          30          40
                                  !           |           |           |
(MSEL) Bovine-II      AMSDLELRQCLPCGPGGKGR CFGPSICCGDELGCFVGTAG
(MSEL) Porcine-III
(MSEL) Porcine-I

(MSEL) Rat-II         T   M
(VLDV) Bovine-I       VL    DV  T
(VLDV) Rat-I          AL    DM  K

                                 50          60          70          80
                                  |           |           |           |
       Bovine-II      ALRCQEENYLPSPCQSGQKP CGSGGRCAAAGICCNDESCV
       Porcine-III
       Porcine-I
       Bovine-I                                            SPDG H

                                 90     95
                                  VI     I
       Bovine-II      TEPECREGIGFPRRV.OH
       Porcine-III            AS L  A.OH
       Porcine-I             AS L.OH
       Bovine-I         ED A DPEAA SL.OH
```

Figure 6.2 Amino acid sequences of neurophysins. (See Appendix C for single-letter amino acid abbreviations.) The complete sequence of bovine neurophysin II is shown, and only the substitutions listed for the others. MSEL and VLDV denote amino acid residues at positions 2, 3, 6, and 7 (*Source*: from Breslow, 1979, with permission).

that interspecies variation for a given neurophysin is less than intraspecies variation between neurophysins leads to the conclusion that gene duplication early in mammalian evolution is responsible for the different structural classes of neurophysins.

No classification of neurophysins is completely satisfactory. One method notes that structural differences frequently occur at residues 2, 3, 6, and 7, producing the MSEL and VLDV classes (using the single letter code for amino acid residues in bovine-II and bovine-I neurophysins, respectively). Figure 6.2 shows some deviations from this pattern. Functionally, the MSEL group is compartmentalized with VP (bovine-II, porcine-I and -III, and human) and the VLDV group with OT (bovine-I and human). Again, the fit is imperfect because rat-II neurophysin (MSEL group) is associated with oxytocin and rat-I neurophysin (VLDL group) with VP.

There is also duplication of the same sequence within a single polypeptide chain (Fig. 6.3) with residues 12 to 31 showing a high degree of homology with residues 60 to 77 (with omission of Gly-17 and Lys-18); all replacements are conservative. The disulfide pairings and conformation of the duplicated segments are not firmly established.

After cleavage of the gene product, the hormone (VP or OT) remains bound to the appropriate NP by *noncovalent* bonds. There are two bonding sites on each NP, one being much stronger than the other. The K_a of the stronger site in 10^5 to 10^6 M^{-1} at 25°C under standard salt conditions. The weaker site is adjacent to Tyr-49 as

```
                        12          20          30
                        |           |           |
        Bovine-II       PCGPGGKGRCFGPSICCGDE
        Bovine-I

        Bovine-II               S  ()    AAAG    N
        Bovine-I                S  ()    AAAG    SPD
                        |                |       |
                        60               70      75
```

Figure 6.3 Internal duplication in bovine neurophysins omitting Gly 17 and Lys 18 (*Source*: from Breslow, 1979, with permission).

indicated by nitration and spin-label studies. The location of the stronger site is not established.

The principal site can bind OT, VP, or small peptide analogues of the NH_2-terminus of the hormones; this site is unaffected by nitration of Tyr-49. Most (two-thirds) of the free energy of bonding is attributable to the NH_2-terminal tripeptide. Interaction with NP requires a salt bridge (ion-pair) on residue 1, an aromatic ring on residue 2, and a bulky, hydrophobic side chain (*sec*-butyl or phenyl) on residue 3.

Neurophysins readily dimerize, and hormone affinity is said to be higher in this state. In the granule, the molar concentrations of NPs and hormones are equal and very high, leading to the assumption that dimerization is important and that even the weaker bonding site is at least partially occupied.

In retrospect, vasopressin is inaptly named because, compared with angiotensin II, it has rather weak pressor activity. Only in VP-producing tumors does it contribute significantly to the regulation of blood pressure.

RENIN–ANGIOTENSIN–ALDOSTERONE

Renin

Renin is a renal peptidase (EC 3.4.99.19) that is secreted from cells mainly within the portion of the renal afferent arteriole that is adjacent to an early segment of the distal convoluted tubule. (Do not confuse rennin and renin.) The juxtaglomerular apparatus includes both the renin-producing segment of the afferent arteriole and the macula densa. Renal renin is a protein of about 40 kDa.

Two aspects of renin chemistry produced confusion until recently. Unlike other prohormones, most (90%) of the circulating renin is prorenin (57 kDa), an inactive form of renin, and 10% is active renin (48 kDa). Furthermore, whereas circulating active renin appears to originate exclusively from the kidney, plasma prorenin has both renal and extrarenal sources. Put differently, active, circulating renin cannot be derived from plasma prorenin but must be secreted from the kidney. This leaves unresolved the reason for circulating prorenin to have ten times the concentration of circulating active renin and the nature of the precursor of active renin.

Prorenin is present in the plasma of anephric subjects, occasionally in quite high concentrations, indicating nonrenal sources. Immunoreactive renin is present in brain, salivary glands, and vascular smooth muscle. Prorenin is synthesized in the chorionic cells of the placenta, and it accumulates in the amniotic fluid to concentrations that are 2 orders of magnitude greater than that observed in normal plasma. This increase is reflected in the maternal plasma that increases as much as tenfold during the first 4 weeks of pregnancy.

Nucleotide sequencing of renin cDNA indicates that preprorenin contains 406 amino acid residues (37 kDa) including a presegment of 20 and a prosegment of 46 residues, located at the NH_2-terminus (Fig. 6.4). An antibody raised against a synthetic tetradecapeptide, residues 28 to 40 of prorenin, bound inactive renins from both human kidney and human plasma, but it did not bind active renin. These results were independently confirmed using a different portion of the prosegment. Thus, both renal and circulating inactive renin contain the prosegment, and renal inactive renin is probably prorenin, the precursor of renin.

Activation of prorenin produces a reninlike product. The two basic methods used are cryoactivation and acid activation; although they appear different, the two methods involve similar enzymatic processes. Sealey and coworkers (1979) have proposed a cascade mechanism (Fig. 6.5) containing Hageman factor (factor XII) and plasma kallikrein. Both are serine proteases acting optimally at alkaline pH. Both are normally present in plasma as inactive precursors, as are inhibitors of both enzymes that prevent accumulation of the active forms. Dialysis at pH 3.3 destroys the inhibitors; dialysis back to pH 7.4 produces an active preparation. Cryoactivation, which occurs at pH 7.4, requires refrigerator

---

Figure 6.4 Nucleotide and corresponding deduced amino acid sequence of human renal preprorenin. The mature polypeptide begins at the leucine residue labeled (1) with the positive numbers in braces referring to amino acid positions within mature renin. The single and double arrowheads indicate the probable ends of the leader and pro sequences, respectively. The two active-site aspartic acid residues, potential *N*-glycosylation sites, and the AATAAA sequence within the 3' untranslated region are underlined (*Source*: from Imai et al., 1983, with permission).

```
                                    -42 AACCTCAGTGGATCTCAGAGAGAGCCCCAGACTGAGGGAAGC   -1

  1  ATG GAT GGA TGG AGA AGG ATG CCT CGC TGG GGA CTG CTG CTG CTG CTC TGG GGC TCC TGT   60
     Met Asp Gly Trp Arg Arg Met Pro Arg Trp Gly Leu Leu Leu Leu Leu Trp Gly Ser Cys
                          {-60}         10              {-50}              20
      1
 61  ACC TTT GGT CTC CCG ACA GAC ACC ACC ACC TTT AAA CGG ATC TTC CTC AAG AGA ATG CCC   120
     Thr Phe Gly Leu Pro Thr Asp Thr Thr Thr Phe Lys Arg Ile Phe Leu Lys Arg Met Pro
                          {-40}         30              {-30}              40
121  TCA ATC CGA GAA AGC CTG AAG GAA CGA GGT GTG GAC ATG GCC AGG CTT GGT CCC GAG TGG   180
     Ser Ile Arg Glu Ser Leu Lys Glu Arg Gly Val Asp Met Ala Arg Leu Gly Pro Glu Trp
                          {-20}         50              {-10}              60
181  AGC CAA CCC ATG AAG AGG CTG ACA CTT GGC AAC ACC ACC TCC TCC GTG ATC CTC ACC AAC   240
     Ser Gln Pro Met Lys Arg Leu Thr Leu Gly Asn Thr Thr Ser Ser Val Ile Leu Thr Asn
                       {-1}{1}        70              {10}               80
241  TAC ATG GAC ACC TAT GGC GAG ATT GGC ATC GGC ACC CCA CCC CAG ACC TTC AAA   300
     Tyr Met Asp Thr Gln Tyr Tyr Gly Glu Ile Gly Ile Gly Thr Pro Pro Gln Thr Phe Lys
                          {20}         90              {30}              100
301  GTC GTC TTT GAC ACT GGT TCG TCC AAT GTT TGG GTG CCC TCC TCC AAG TGC AGC CGT CTC   360
     Val Val Phe Asp Thr Gly Ser Ser Asn Val Trp Val Pro Ser Ser Lys Cys Ser Arg Leu
                          {40}        110              {50}              120
361  TAC ACT GCC TGT GTG TAT CAC AAG CTC TTC GAT GCT TCG GAT TCC TCC AGC TAC AAG CAC   420
     Tyr Thr Ala Cys Val Tyr His Lys Leu Phe Asp Ala Ser Asp Ser Ser Ser Tyr Lys His
                          {60}        130              {70}              140
421  AAT GGA ACA GAA CTC ACC CTC CGC TAT TCA ACA GGG ACA GTC AGT GGC TTT CTC AGC CAG   480
     Asn Gly Thr Glu Leu Thr Leu Arg Tyr Ser Thr Gly Thr Val Ser Gly Phe Leu Ser Gln
                          {80}        150              {90}              160
481  GAC ATC ATC ACC GTG GGT GGA ATC ACG GTG ACA CAG ATG TTT GGA GAG GTC ACG GAG ATG   540
     Asp Ile Ile Thr Val Gly Gly Ile Thr Val Thr Gln Met Phe Gly Glu Val Thr Glu Met
                          {100}       170              {110}             180
541  CCC GCC TTA CCC TTC ATG CTG GCC GAG TTT GAT GGG GTT GTG GGC ATG GGC TTC ATT GAA   600
     Pro Ala Leu Pro Phe Met Leu Ala Glu Phe Asp Gly Val Val Gly Met Gly Phe Ile Glu
                          {120}       190              {130}             200
601  CAG GCC ATT GGC AGG GTC ACC CCT ATC TTC GAC AAC ATC ATC TCC CAA GGG GTG CTA AAA   660
     Gln Ala Ile Gly Arg Val Thr Pro Ile Phe Asp Asn Ile Ile Ser Gln Gly Val Leu Lys
                          {140}       210              {150}             220
661  GAG GAC GTC TTC TCT TTC TAC TAC AAC AGA GAT TCC GAG AAT TCC CAA TCG CTG GGA GGA   720
     Glu Asp Val Phe Ser Phe Tyr Tyr Asn Arg Asp Ser Glu Asn Ser Gln Ser Leu Gly Gly
                          {160}       230              {170}             240
721  CAG ATT GTG CTG GGA GGC AGC GAC CCC CAG CAT TAC GAA GGG AAT TTC CAC TAT ATC AAC   780
     Gln Ile Val Leu Gly Gly Ser Asp Pro Gln His Tyr Glu Gly Asn Phe His Tyr Ile Asn
                          {180}       250              {190}             260
781  CTC ATC AAG ACT GGT GTC TGG CAG ATT CAA ATG AAG GGG GTG TCT GTG GGG TCA TCC ACC   840
     Leu Ile Lys Thr Gly Val Trp Gln Ile Gln Met Lys Gly Val Ser Val Gly Ser Ser Thr
                          {200}       270              {210}             280
841  TTG CTC TGT GAA GAC GGC TGC CTG GCA TTG GTA GAC ACC GGT GCA TCC TAC ATC TCA GGT   900
     Leu Leu Cys Glu Asp Gly Cys Leu Ala Leu Val Asp Thr Gly Ala Ser Tyr Ile Ser Gly
                          {220}       290              {230}             300
901  TCT ACC AGC TCC ATA GAG AAG CTC ATG GAG GCC TTG GGA GCC AAG AAG AGG CTG TTT GAT   960
     Ser Thr Ser Ser Ile Glu Lys Leu Met Glu Ala Leu Gly Ala Lys Lys Arg Leu Phe Asp
                          {240}       310              {250}             320
961  TAT GTC GTG AAG TGT AAC GAG GGC CCT ACA CTC CCC GAC ATC TCT TTC CAC CTG GGA GGC  1020
     Tyr Val Val Lys Cys Asn Glu Gly Pro Thr Leu Pro Asp Ile Ser Phe His Leu Gly Gly
                          {260}       330              {270}             340
1021 AAA GAA TAC ACG CTC ACC AGC GCG GAC TAT GTA TTT CAG GAA TCC TAC AGT AGT AAA AAG  1080
     Lys Glu Tyr Thr Leu Thr Ser Ala Asp Tyr Val Phe Gln Glu Ser Tyr Ser Ser Lys Lys
                          {280}       350              {290}             360
1081 CTG TGC ACA CTG GCC ATC CAC GCC ATG GAT ATC CCG CCA CCC ACT GGA CCC ACC TGG GCC  1140
     Leu Cys Thr Leu Ala Ile His Ala Met Asp Ile Pro Pro Pro Thr Gly Pro Thr Trp Ala
                          {300}       370              {310}             380
1141 CTG GGG GCC ACC TTC ATC CGA AAG TTC TAC ACA GAG TTT GAT CGG CGT AAC AAC CGC ATT  1200
     Leu Gly Ala Thr Phe Ile Arg Lys Phe Tyr Thr Glu Phe Asp Arg Arg Asn Asn Arg Ile
                          {320}       390              {330}             400
1201 GGC TTC GCC TTG GCC CGC TGAGGCCCTCTGCCACCCAGGCAGGCCCTGCCTTCAGCCCTGGCCCAGAGCTGGA  1273
     Gly Phe Ala Leu Ala Arg
                          {340}406
1274 ACACTCTCTGAGATGCCCCTCTGCCTGGGCTTATGCCCTCAGATGGAGACATTGGATGTGGAGCTCCTGCTGGATGCGT  1352

1353 GCCCTGACCCCTGCACCAGCCCTTCCCTGCTTTGAGGACAAAGAGAATAAAGACTTCATGTTCAC
```

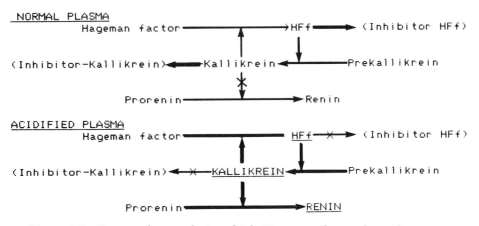

Figure 6.5 Proposed cascade in which Hageman factor-dependent activation of prorenin occurs in acidified plasma. Heavy arrows indicate predominant pathways: HFf, Hageman factor fragments (*Source*: from Sealey, Atlas, Laragh, Silverberg, and Kaplan, 1979, with permission).

storage for up to 40 days (no reaction occurs in the solid state). The low temperature affects the inhibitors more than the enzymatic reactions of the cascade.

These nonphysiologic procedures have more practical than theoretical interest. It is technically easier to do an assay of plasma renin activity (PRA) than a RIA for angiotensin or aldosterone. Because PRA is limiting, it is the assay commonly done. The assay is easy, but note the pitfalls! Acidification or refrigeration (or both) are commonly used methods of preservation. How many erroneous results for PRA must have been naively reported over the years!

Angiotensin II

The substrate for renin is angiotensinogen, a hepatic α_2-globulin (66–110 kDa); cleavage of a leucine-leucine bond produces a decapeptide, angiotensin I (Fig. 6.6). The K_m for the reaction is 1200 ng/ml; at plasma concentrations of 800–1800 ng/ml in normal human subjects, the reaction rate is dependent upon the concentrations of both substrate and enzyme. The concentration of substrate is increased by administration of glucocorticoids, estrogens, angiotensin II, bilateral nephrectomy, or hypoxia, and is decreased by liver disease or adrenal insufficiency.

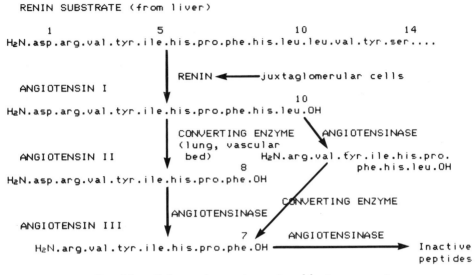

Figure 6.6 Peptides of the renin–angiotensin–aldosterone system.

Converting enzyme (kininase II), a calcium-dependent dipep-
tidase, cleaves a histidylleucine from the COOH-terminus of
angiotensin I to form the octapeptide angiotensin II (see Fig. 6.6),
the most potent pressor substance made in the mammalian body.
This ubiquitous enzyme with an enormous capacity for converting angiotensin I to II also inactivates vasodepressor kinins, such
as bradykinin.

Angiotensin II is degraded by both plasma and tissue peptidases. Angiotensin III (des-Asp-1-angiotensin II) is the only fragment with major biological activity.

Aldosterone

Besides its pressor activity, angiotensin II (and III) controls the
rate-limiting step in the synthesis of aldosterone from cholesterol
in the subcapsular zona glomerulosa of the adrenal cortex (Fig.
6.7). The major control point is presumably the mitochondral conversion of cholesterol to pregnenolone. Potassium and ACTH are
also potent stimulators of this step. In humans, increments in
plasma aldosterone are detectable following increments in

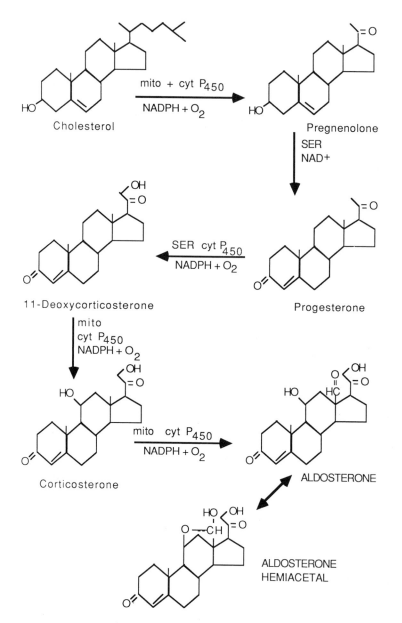

Figure 6.7 Synthesis of aldosterone from cholesterol in the zona glomerulosa of the adrenal cortex. The first step is rate-limiting.

plasma potassium as small as 0.1 mEq/ml. In fact, in the salt-depleted state, the renin–angiotensin system and potassium may be equally important in the short-term regulation of plasma aldosterone. Salt depletion increases the sensitivity of the zona glomerulosa to angiotensin II or III, which are both equipotent, and to ACTH.

Several other modulators of aldosterone synthesis exist. Atrial natriuretic hormone is discussed just below. Aldosterone-stimulating factor (ASF) is a pituitary glycopeptide of 26.0 kDa; a 4 kDa fragment is biologically active. It stimulates aldosterone secretion by a non–cAMP-dependent mechanism. Plasma ASF increases with dietary sodium intake; it is not suppressible with dexamethasone, and it is elevated in idiopathic hyperaldosteronism. Aldosterone secretion is also under maximum tonic dopaminergic inhibition. Dopaminergic suppression of angiotensin II-induced aldosterone secretion is directly related to sodium balance. Furthermore, dopamine suppresses posture-induced aldosterone responses, independently of known mechanisms.

Aside from the first step of side-chain cleavage of cholesterol to pregnenolone, which is regulated by a number of hormones, steroidogenesis follows a similar pathway in all tissues and organs making steroids. Mixed-function oxidases requiring NADPH, cytochrome P_{450}, and molecular oxygen are involved at three steps of hydroxylation, and an alcohol dehydrogenase–isomerase oxidizes ring A to the 4-en-3-one structure characteristic of all steroid hormones except the estrogens. In addition, there is the characteristic shuttle of the sterol–steroid from mitochondria to smooth endoplasmic reticulum back to the mitochondria. The reason(s) for this compartmentalization, which usually provides control points, is not known. Aldosterone exists as a mixture of 18-oxo compound and its hemiacetal.

ATRIAL NATRIURETIC HORMONE

The presence of dense perinuclear granules in atrial, but not ventricular, cardiocytes of mammals has been known since 1956. In the 1970s, the granules were shown to contain glycoprotein. The crucial experiment (1980) that stimulated an enormous amount of research was the intravenous administration of an extract of rat atria into normal rats which produced a very rapid, short, and massive diuresis and natriuresis. In a period of 4 years, the peptide responsible has been isolated, sequenced, and synthesized; the cDNA and the gene itself for both rat and human atrial natriuretic hormone (ANH) have been cloned and sequenced, and a rather impressive amount of physiological and pathophysiological information acquired. As the discussion will reveal, there is still no concensus in several areas.

This peptide has several names: cardionatrin, atriopeptin, and most commonly, atrial natriuretic factor. I call it a hormone because it has all the properties required of a hormone.

Chemically, there appears to be no consensus on the number of amino acid residues that should be included in the structure of ANH. This arises partly because of degradative artifacts that have been isolated and partly because, to some extent, the number of residues—up to a point—is not critical to the bioactivity of ANH. The gene, as usual, codes for a preproANH having 151 (human) or 152 (rat) amino acid residues with a signal peptide comprising 25 (human) or 24 (rat) amino acids (Fig. 6.8). A number of COOH-terminal ANH peptides have been isolated from human and rat atria, varying in size from 20 to 35 amino acid residues. It is not clear which of these peptides represents ANH. This may be an academic question because most are both biologically active and degradative artifacts.

Two questions need immediate answers. What is the circulating form of the hormone and what is the effect of amino acid deletion on function? The latter question is particularly critical because the basic dipeptide, Arg-101 and Arg-102, is a potential processing site. The latter question is easier to approach because all the synthetic peptides are available. Using a variety of bioassays, removal of NH_2-terminal amino acids produces only minor changes in bioactivity until the integrity of the Cys-SS-Cys loop is compromised. On the other hand, bioactivity is acutely sensitive to any deletion from the COOH-terminus, except the COOH-terminal tyrosine. The major circulating form of the hormone appears to be the ANH-Ser-99 to Tyr-126 form, but this has not been confirmed.

The method of denoting peptides in this area is cumbersome, i.e., naming the first and last amino acids in the sequence. Needleman and Greenwald have suggested simply denoting the

```
                 R  MET.GLY.SER.PHE.SER.ILE.....THR.LYS.GLY.PHE.PHE.LEU.
       SIGNAL    H  SER                   THR.THR.   VAL.SER.LEU.LEU

   PEPTIDE                                                 -1
                 R  PHE.LEU.ALA.PHE.TRP.LEU.PRO.GLY.HIS.ILE.GLY.ALA.
                 H              GLN        LEU     GLN.THR.ARG

                    +1                                10
              i  R  ASN.PRO.VAL.TYR.SER.ALA.VAL.SER.ASN.THR.ASP.LEU.MET.ASP.
              i  H          MET        ASN            ALA
              i
              i  R  PHE.LYS.ASN.LEU.LEU.ASP.HIS.LEU.GLU.GLU.LYS.MET.PRO.VAL.
              i  H                                               LEU.
   C          i
   O          i            30
   N     P    i  R  GLU.ASP.GLU.VAL.MET.PRO.PRO.GLN.ALA.LEU.SER.GLU.GLN.THR.
   N     E    i  H          VAL            VAL               PRO.ASN.
   E     P    i
   C     T    i                          50
   T     I    i  R  ASP.GLU.ALA.GLY.ALA.ALA.LEU.SER.SER.LEU.SER.GLU.VAL.PRO.
   I     D    i  H  GLU                   PRO     PRO
   N     E    i
   G          i                                               70
              i  R  PRO.TRP.THR.GLY.GLU.VAL.ASN.PRO.SER.GLN.ARG.ASP.GLY.GLY.
              i  H                      SER      ALA
              i
              i  R  ALA.LEU.GLY.ARG.GLY.PRO.TRP.ASP.PRO.SER.ASP.ARG.SER.ALA.
              i  H                                SER
              i
              i            90          93
              i  R  LEU.LEU.LYS.SER.LYS.LEU.ARG.ALA.LEU.
              i  H


                    94                  101               105
              i  R  LEU.ALA.GLY.PRO.ARG.SER.LEU.ARG.ARG.SER.SER.CYS.
              i  H      THR.ALA                              i
              i                                              i
              i            110                               i
   ANH        i  R  PHE.GLY.GLY.ARG.ILE.ASP.ARG.ILE.GLY.ALA.GLN.  i
              i  H                  MET                       i
              i                   _____i
              i                   i              126
              i  R  SER.GLY.LEU.GLY.CYS.ASN.SER.PHE.ARG.TYR.ARG.ARG.COOH
              i  H                                           .COOH
                          121
```

Figure 6.8 Comparison of the amino acid sequences of human and rat prepro-ANH. The circulating form of ANH is said to be the COOH-terminal 28 amino-acid fragment (*Source*: Cantin and Genest, 1985, with permission).

number of residues contained in the peptide with the understanding that the COOH-terminus is intact. Thus, ANH Ser-99 to Tyr-126 becomes simply ANH-28.

ProANH is atypical in one respect. Most prohormones are converted to the mature form of the hormone during their residence in the granules. This does not happen with proANH. Where cleavage and activation occur is not known.

The native and synthetic hormones exert identical effects, possibly through particulate guanylate cyclase stimulation and adenylate cyclase inhibition, on the kidney, blood vessels, adrenal cortex, and pituitary. These will be discussed in the appropriate sections.

REGULATION OF SALT AND WATER INTAKE

Water is the most abundant molecule in the body, constituting 60% of body weight, with intracellular and extracellular (interstitial fluid and plasma) water accounting for two-thirds and one-third of the total, respectively. Osmotic equilibrium exists between these two compartments. The osmotic content of the intracellular fluid is fixed by the mixture of negatively charged, indiffusible protein and positively charged ions inside the cell. Therefore, osmotic equilibrium can be achieved only by movement of water (and electrolytes) between the two compartments.

As examples, if one drinks water, extracellular fluid osmolality must drop, and water must then enter the cells to maintain osmotic equilibrium. On the other hand, if one becomes dehydrated, extracellular fluid osmolality increases, and water must leave the cells to maintain osmotic equilibrium (Fig. 6.9). As a consequence, cells everywhere shrink (intracellular fluid volume decreases), including groups of cells, identified as osmoreceptors, in the lateral preoptic area of the hypothalamus. These cells then send out signals that we interpret as thirst.

There are two ways in which a decrease in extracellular fluid volume can induce drinking. Baroreceptors, or stretch receptors, are located in the low-pressure side of the circulation in the left and right atria, vena cava, and pulmonary vein. These receptors fire at the end of diastole in response to the phase of maximum distension. A reduction in blood volume and, hence, a reduction in the rate of venous return reduces the rate of firing of these

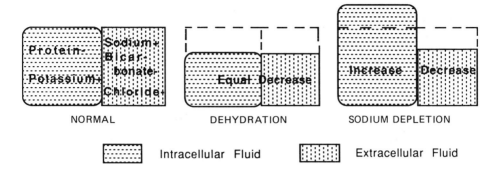

NORMAL   DEHYDRATION   SODIUM DEPLETION

Intracellular Fluid   Extracellular Fluid

Figure 6.9 Fluid movement during dehydration and sodium depletion. Although the composition of intracellular (ICF) and extracellular (ECF) fluid is different, the osmolalities are identical. Because ICF osmotic content is fixed, equilibrium is achieved by water movement between the two compartments. With water depletion, both compartments diminish equally; with sodium depletion, the ICF compartment increases, whereas that of the ECF decreases (*Source*: from Ramsay and Ganong, 1980, with permission).

receptors. This information relayed to the CNS induces drinking and correction of the deficit in extracellular fluid (ECF) volume.

If the decrease in ECF volume is severe enough, another mechanism is activated. A decrease in arterial blood pressure will cause an increase in firing of the sympathetic nerves that innervate the juxtaglomerular cells of the kidneys, thereby activating the renin–angiotensin system. Angiotensin II cannot pass the blood–brain barrier, but there are said to be receptors in the circumventricular organs, which include the subfornical organ, the median eminence, and the area postrema (Fig. 6.10). Evidence that angiotensin is involved in the drinking reflex includes experiments in dogs in which excessive drinking of water correlated with high concentrations of angiotensin II in the plasma. This response was abolished by the competitive angiotensin inhibitor, saralasin, or by nephrectomy. Thus, angiotensin II, which is more commonly associated with electrolyte regulation, also plays a part in correcting the deficit in ECF volume. The dual role played by angiotensin II ensures that the expansion of the ECF volume will not produce hypoosmolality, a condition which, by decreasing ADH secretion, would be counterproductive.

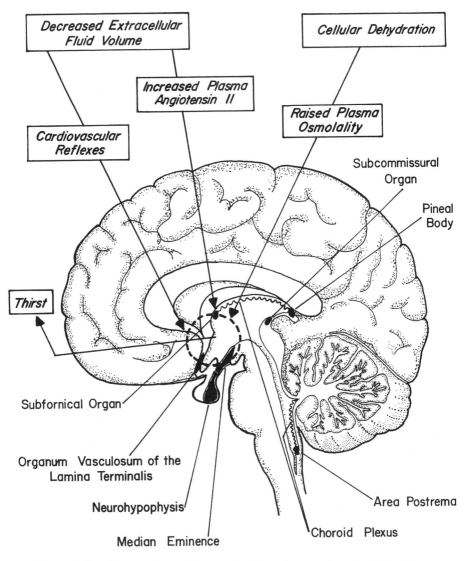

Figure 6.10 Interaction of hypovolemic and osmotic stimuli in the central nervous system. The ECF depletion provokes cardiovascular reflex mechanisms and synthesis of angiotensin II which interacts with specific receptors on the subfornical organ, thereby stimulating thirst and drinking. Intracellular dehydration also acts within the CNS to stimulate thirst and vasopressin secretion (*Source*: from Ramsey and Ganong, 1980, with permission).

The control of salt intake is located in the brain, but the stimulus comes from the taste buds detecting a low concentration of sodium in the saliva. In a salt-depleted state, this occurs by the mechanism described above, i.e., osmoreceptors sense a decrease in ECF volume and increase the production of renin, angiotensin II, and aldosterone. Aldosterone promotes reabsorption of sodium by the salivary glands, and the taste buds, detecting the decrease, signal the CNS. The same response is seen in sodium deprivation or administration of aldosterone in a situation of sodium balance. Paradoxically, addisonian patients (absence of functional adrenals) and adrenalectomized animals have an increased appetite for salt; the mechanism is not known.

REGULATION OF SALT AND WATER OUTPUT

Normally functioning kidneys ultrafilter the entire plasma volume in less than an hour. Obviously the kidneys must take heroic measures to prevent the daily loss of over 100 L of water and accompanying electrolytes. The mechanisms by which this is done are complex and are still incompletely understood. The basic unit is the nephron which accepts ultrafiltrate from the glomerulus. It can be divided, both on the basis of structure and of function, into several segments (Fig. 6.11). Electrolytes are secreted into the ultrafiltrate in certain segments, whereas others are reabsorbed elsewhere. Finally, as the nephrons anastomose into collecting tubules and then into collecting ducts, over 99% of the water is reabsorbed.

With the need to regulate Ca^{2+}, PO_4^{-3}, Na^+, K^+, and water excretion, it is not unexpected that a number of hormones have the kidney as a target organ, namely, parathyroid hormone (PTH), VP-ADH, catecholamines, steroid hormones, ANH, and possibly calcitonin. All but steroids and ANH act through adenylate cyclase. In addition, the kallikrein–kinin system and prostaglandins have effects.

Since 1975, microtechniques have enabled the measurement of hormone-dependent adenylate cyclase in isolated segments of the kidney tubule from mice, rats, rabbits, and humans. The results were sometimes surprising and are leading to investigations still underway to understand the significance of the new findings. A summary of these is presented omitting species variation.

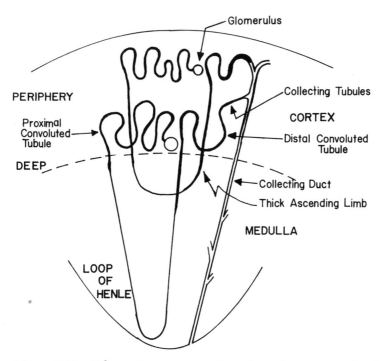

Figure 6.11   Schematic representation of renal structure showing outer cortical (peripheral) and inner cortical (deep) nephrons and major subdivisions of nephrons.

The proximal tubule (pars convoluta, pars recta) contains only two types of receptors. The presence of PTH receptors was expected because of the well known inhibitory effect of PTH on phosphate and fluid reabsorption. The presence of α-adrenergic receptors is inferred from (1) suppression of PTH-induced cAMP accumulation by norepinephrine (0.5 μM), which is reversed by phentolamine, an α-blocker, and (2) increased proximal fluid reabsorption by norepinephrine (0.1 μM), which is blocked by phentolamine.

The descending portion of the thin limb of the loop of Henle is apparently devoid of hormonal receptors, but surprisingly, ADH receptors are present in the ascending portion, and ADH may increase solute movement. The physiological relevance of this observation is not known.

The thick ascending limb (straight distal tubule) is separated into medullary and cortical portions. The two portions (1) are surrounded by extracellular environments of different ionic strengths, (2) have somewhat different cellular ultrastructure, and (3) exhibit different hormonal requirements (Table 6.1). Note that AVP–ADH has no detectable receptors in the human but has many in the medullary portion in mice and rats. Vasopressin stimulates chloride efflux in these animals. On the other hand, PTH receptors are usually in the cortical portion, which is reflected in stimulated calcium (and magnesium) transport (uptake) in that portion in response to PTH.

There is very little information available on hormone-dependent adenylate cyclase activity in the distal convoluted tubule.

The collecting tubules contain preponderantly receptors to ADH (Table 6.2), and it is here that most of the water in the glomerular filtrate is reabsorbed. The major effect of aldosterone on sodium reabsorption also occurs here.

A similar evaluation of the mechanism of action of ANH, which produces a rapid and transient natriuresis and diuresis

Table 6.1 Hormone-Sensitive Adenylate Cyclase in Renal Thick Ascending Limbs

Species	Nephron portion	PTH	sCT	AVP	Glgn	Isopr
Rabbit	Medullary	0	+ + +	(+ +)	+	0
	cortical	+ +	+	+	NT	0
Rat	Medullary	0	+ +	+ + + +	+ + + +	0
	cortical	+ + + +	+ + + +	+ +	+ + +	+ +
Mouse	Medullary	0	0	+ + +	NT	0
	cortical	+ + + +	+	+ +	NT	+
Human	Medullary	+ +	+ +	0	NT	NT
	cortical	+ +	+ +	0	NT	NT

Abbreviations used: PTH, 1-34 synthetic fragment of bPTH; sCT, synthetic salmon calcitonin; Glgn, porcine glucagon; Isopr, isoproterenol; 0, no effect; NT, not tested.

Source: from Morel, Imbert-Teboul, and Charbardes, 1981, with permission.

Table 6.2 Hormone-Sensitve Adenylate Cyclase in Renal Collecting Tubules

Species	Nephron portion	PTH	sCT	AVP	Glgn	Isopr
Rabbit	Medullary	0	0	+ + + +	0	+
	cortical	0	0	+ + + +	0	+ +
Rat	Medullary	0	0	+ + + +	+ +	0
	cortical	(+)	+ + +	+ + + +	+ +	+ +
Mouse	Medullary	0	0	+ + + +	NT	0
	cortical	0	+	+ + + +	NT	+ +
Human	Medullary	NT	0	+ + + +	NT	NT
	cortical	0	(+)	+ + + +	NT	NT

Abbreviations used: See Table 6.1.

and a modest kaliuresis, is now underway. Radiolabeled ANH-26 binds to canine renal membranes from glomeruli, thick ascending limbs, and collecting ducts, but not to proximal tubules; the dissociation constants are ca. 0.1 nM, typical of receptors. Also, cGMP and cAMP were measured in canine membrane preparations after addition of ANH-26. Cyclic GMP increased 30-fold in 1 min in glomerular membranes with much more modest (1.5- to 2.5-fold) changes occurring in membranes from the thick loop of Henle and from collecting ducts. Proximal tubular membranes showed no response. The response in the glomerular membranes was traced to the particulate guanylate cyclase. On the other hand, adenylate cyclase activity was inhibited in the same tissues.

REGULATION OF HORMONE SECRETION

Antidiuretic Hormone Secretion

There are three mechanisms controlling the secretion of ADH from the neurohpohysis in response to changes in plasma osmolality, blood volume, or blood pressure. Verney in 1947 proposed that osmoreceptors in or near the supraoptic nucleus respond to cellular dehydration by causing the release of ADH; the mechanism is not known. Bie (1980) has criticized the lack of critical evaluation of Verney's proposal, but the fact that it has endured for nearly 40 years attests to its basic validity. The response of reduced renal output (urine flow) coupled with increased drinking ensures rapid restoration of intracellular volume.

A decrease in extracellular fluid (blood) volume reduces the tonic inhibitory impulses from atrial and pulmonary baroreceptors which, through the CNS, stimulates ADH release and water drinking; again, the dual action ensures a rapid correction.

The most potent releasing stimulus for ADH is the hypotension following hemorrhage which is detected by aortic and carotid baroreceptors. This stimulus will override inhibitory influences, raising ADH plasma levels to as much as 1000 μU/ml. Such levels cause vasoconstriction as well as renal conservation of water.

Table 6.3 lists a large number of additional factors that may influence ADH release. Note that most of them have an obvious CNS and a hypothalamic effect, befitting the neural origin of VP–ADH and neural control of its release.

Table 6.3 Factors other than Plasma Osmolality, Blood Volume, and Blood Pressure Influencing ADH Secretion

Increased ADH secretion	Decreased ADH secretion
Emotional stress	Hypnotic suggestion
Pain	Psychologic conditioning
Vomiting	Inhalation of CO_2
Cholinergic stimulation	Atropine stimulation
β-Adrenergic stimulation	α-Adrenergic stimulation
Nicotine	Ethanol
Morphine	Diphenylhydantoin
Barbiturates	Reserpine
Vincristine	Chlorpromazine
Cyclophosphamide	
Clofibrate	
Chlorpropamide	
Tricyclic antidepressants (some)	
Anticonvulsants (some)	

Renin Release

Major control of renin secretion occurs by two independent mechanisms: a renal baroreceptor and the macula densa. There are baro- or stretch receptors within the afferent arteriole, and renin secretion increases in response to decreased stretch. Hemorrhage and suprarenal aortic constriction are potent stimuli (in the non-filtering kidney).

The contribution of the macula densa is more difficult to demonstrate. Renal arterial infusion of sodium chloride or potassium chloride inhibits renin secretion in the filtering, but not the nonfiltering, kidney. Although volume expansion partially ex-plains this result, a more complete answer must include chloride transport in the ascending limb of the loop of Henle. When chloride reaches the macula densa, it inhibits renin secretion. Diuretics that inhibit chloride transport, e.g., furosemide or ethacrynic acid, stimulate renin release, even if volume contraction is prevented.

Several other factors modulate renin release (Table 6.4). There is a CNS component that appears to be mediated by β-adrenergic receptors. There may also be some α-adrenergic control. Angioten-sin II directly inhibits release of renin. Indomethacin and other in-hibitors of prostaglandin synthesis reduce the release of renin in the basal state and in response to a low-sodium diet, diuretics, upright posture, hemorrhage, aortic constriction, and potassium depletion. These effects are in accord with the hypothesis that pro-staglandins mediate the stimulatory action of the renal barorecep-tor, the macula densa, and possibly, the sympathetic nervous system on renin release.

Table 6.4   Factors Influencing Renin Secretion

Increasing renin	Decreasing renin
Hemorrhage	Inhibitors of prostaglandin synthesis
Hypotension	High chloride concentration
sitting or standing up	
suprarenal aortic constriction	
renal artery stenosis	
Low sodium diet	High Angiotensin II concentration
Hypokalemia	
β-Adrenergic stimulation	

Aldosterone

The regulation of aldosterone secretion is exceedingly complex. Not only is there an interplay among the principal regulators—renin–angiotensin II, ACTH, and K^+—but these interactions are somehow modulated by the newer cast of actors that include ANH, ASF, and dopamine. Obviously, the mechanisms by which the latter modulate the former is unknown.

The binding of angiotensin II to its receptors on the zona glomerulosa cells induces at least two changes: an increase in the *rate* of calcium influx across the membrane and an activation of the specific phospholipase C that catalyzes the hydrolysis of phosphatidylinositol 4,5-bisphosphate. The latter leads to the rapid generation (within 15 sec) of inositol 1,4,5-triphosphate (IP_3) and diacylglycerol, each with a messenger function. The IP_3 induces the release of 10,000 to 20,000 nmol of calcium per liter from the endoplasmic reticulum, driving the intracellular free Ca^{2+} from 200 to 250 nM to 600 to 800 nM within 1 to 2 min, and a net efflux of calcium from the cell occurs. This rise is transient (3 to 5 min) because the pool of calcium in the endoplasmic reticulum is rapidly depleted, and most of the released calcium is pumped out of the cell. The transient rise is sufficient, however, to activate a variety of calmodulin-dependent enzymes.

In the meantime, angiotensin II has been activating the C-kinase system more slowly. The transient rise in calcium concentration and the increase in diacylglycerol content of the plasma membrane convert C-kinase from its Ca^{2+}-insensitive to its Ca^{2+}-sensitive, membrane-associated form. In this form, the activity of the enzyme is controlled by the rate of calcium influx across the plasma membrane. (As noted before, angiotensin II causes a rapid and sustained increase in the rate of calcium influx.) The C-kinase then phosphorylates a different set of proteins. The extent of C-kinase activity depends upon two factors: the amount of activated C-kinase bound to the plasma membrane and the rate of calcium cycling across this membrane.

Potassium and ACTH also stimulate aldosterone production. Each increases the rate of calcium influx into the cells, but neither stimulates phosphatidylinositol turnover. Instead, each activates adenylate cyclase, but by different mechanisms. The mechanism for potassium probably involves the Ca^{2+}–calmodulin-dependent activation of adenylate cyclase. Corticotropin produces its effects by combining with two types of receptors: one coupled to a calcium channel and the other to adenylate cyclase. Although separate, they are interrelated in that the increase in calcium influx sensitizes the adenylate cyclase. The major difference between the actions of potassium and ACTH lies in the relative magnitude of the two effects: potassium has a large effect on the calcium influx rate and a small effect on cAMP production, whereas ACTH has the opposite effects.

RECEPTORS

Angiotensin Receptors

Angiotensin II has demonstrated plasma membrane receptors in the aorta, uterus, and adrenal cortex, whereas only the adrenal cortex has demonstrated receptors for angiotensin III. In smooth muscle, angiotensin-receptor interaction induces changes in membrane permeability to ions, an increase in cytosolic unbound calcium concentration leading to contraction of actomyosin. In other target tissues, essentially nothing is known beyond the interaction other than that involvement of cyclic nucleotides is unlikely.

The binding data itself is scanty and not too consistent. The dissociation constants cover a range of more than 1 order of magnitude and overlap those of the low-affinity sites (Table 6.5). The latter, which are also observed with many other peptide hormones, may not be related to hormonal effects. The evidence for separate, distinct angiotensin III receptors is fragmentary, somewhat dated, and based mainly on differential competition with various angiotensin analogues. The angiotensin II receptor has been solubilized after photoaffinity labeling. Whether obtained from canine adrenal cortex or from uterine myometrium, a dimeric angiotensin complex (126 kDa) was identified by gel filtration and sucrose density gradient centrifugation. Analysis by SDS-PAGE resolved the dimer into a single species,(66.5 kDa) indicating two subunits of similar (or identical) molecular weight.

The binding of iodoangiotensin II is highly correlated with steroid production by collagenase-dispersed rat adrenal glomerulosa cells with significant increases in aldosterone and

Table 6.5 Binding Values for Angiotensin II Receptors

	K_d(nM)	
Target tissue	High-affinity site	Low-affinity site
Aorta		
rabbit		
plasma membranes	6	—
solubilized material	20	—
guinea pig		
plasma membranes	22–47	—
Uterus		
rat		
plasma membranes	8–20	—
Adrenal		
bovine cortex		
particulate fraction	2	83
	2	17–100
plasma membranes	4	—
zona glumerulosa cells	29	—
	3–5	25

Source: modified from Devynck and Meyer, 1978.

corticosterone production produced by 30 pM angiotensin II. This same preparation, incidentally, was also highly sensitive to ACTH, responding to a 3 pM concentration. Moreover, angiotensin II exerts a trophic action on the zona glomerulosa, inducing the formation of its own receptors and increasing steroidogenic capacity. This action contributes to the increased sensitivity and enhanced aldosterone response during sodium deficiency.

Steroid Receptors

The kidney has receptors for every class of steroid except progesterone which, nevertheless, competes with aldosterone, dexamethasone, and corticosterone for their renal receptors (Table 6.6). The corticosteroid receptors are subdivided into three types based primarily on differential affinities for various steroids. Thus, type 1, or aldosterone receptors, follow the order aldosterone

Table 6.6 Renal Corticoid Receptors

| | Mineralocorticoid | | | Glucocorticoid | | | |
| | Type I aldosterone | | | Type II dexamethasone/triamcinolone | | | Type III corticosterone |
	Rat	Rabbit	Human	Rat	Rabbit	Cattle	Rat
K_d(nM)	0.5–3	3.0–3.7	0.5	4–5	3.3	3	3
N_{max} (fmol/mg protein)	17–22	15	4	160–246	160	210	900

Source: from Fanestil and Park, 1981, with permission.

> deoxycorticosterone (DOC) > corticosterone > progesterone
> dexamethasone; type II, or glucocorticoid receptors follow the
order dexamethasone or triamcinolone > corticosterone > DOC
> aldosterone > cortisol > progesterone > estradiol >
dihydrotestosterone; and type III, or corticosterone receptors,
follow the order corticosterone > cortisol > DOC > progesterone > aldosterone > dexamethasone.

Aldosterone binds to two classes of receptors. The higher-
affinity site (type I) has a K_d of 0.5–3.7 nM and binds 4–22 fmol/mg
protein, whereas the lower-affinity site (type II) has a K_d of 25–60
nM and binds about 700 fmol/mg protein. It is obvious that
aldosterone at 1-nM concentration will bind almost exclusively to
type I sites.

All these receptors (see Table 6.6) are typical steroid receptors. In the absence of hormone, they are said to reside in the
cytoplasm (but see p. 22), and in the presence of hormone, the
steroid–receptor complex attaches to a genome and promotes
transcription and translation of specific proteins (Table 6.7). This
process characteristically has a lag period of 1–2 h before new
protein can be detected, and inhibitors of RNA and protein synthesis can abort the response. In addition, spironolactone, a potent aldosterone antagonist, can bind to cytoplasmic receptors
but fails to activate them, thus sequestering the receptor pool in
an inactive form.

Aldosterone stimulates the absorption of sodium from, and
the secretion of potassium, hydrogen (protons), and ammonium
ions into, the renal ultrafiltrate. Because inhibitors of RNA and
protein synthesis can block the sodium response to aldosterone,
but not the other responses, it is obvious that aldosterone must
be acting through two (or more) mechanisms. Most investigators
have concentrated on the mechanisms of sodium reabsorption.

Mention should be made of the toad bladder system, a widely
used paradigm for mammalian sodium transport; aldosterone
has *no* effect on potassium transport in this system. Two very
practical advantages explain its popularity; (1) it occurs as a very
thin membranous sheet appropriate for mounting between two
chambers, and (2) the extent of sodium transport from the
mucosal to the serosal side is directly proportional to the "short-
circuit current," i.e., the amount of current that must be applied
to nullify the potential difference across the membrane produced

Table 6.7 Aldosterone-Induced Changes in Enzyme Activity

Enzyme	Tissue	Change (%)		Aldosterone dosage	Dosage time
		Incr	Decr		
Carbonic	Mouse kidney	60		2 μg/d	3 day
anhydrase	Rat kidney		50	0.05 μg/100 g	4 hr
Na⁺K⁺-ATPase	Rat kidney	28		5 μg/100 g × 6	24 hr
	Medulla	12		100 μg/d	6 day
	Rat kidney	15		20 μg/100 g	3 hr
	Toad bladder	None		1000 nM	2.5 hr
cAMP phospho-diesterase	Toad bladder		20	200 nM	24 hr
Phosphoprotein phosphatase	Toad bladder	+		>20 nM	10 hr
FAD synthetase	Rat kidney	20		2 μg/100 g	2 hr
	Rat kidney		17	5 μg/d × 2	3 day
	Rat kidney	14		1.5 μg/100 g	3.5 hr
Citrate	Rat kidney	20		2 μg/100 g	4 hr
synthase	Rat kidney	12		0.8 μg/100 g	3 hr
	Rat kidney	25		0.8 μg/100 g	3 hr

Source: from Fanestil and Park, 1981, with permission.

by sodium migration. The simplicity and purity of this system explain the concentration given to it by nephrologists, and consequently their lack of attention to the mechanism of action of aldosterone on potassium and proton transport.

In sodium transport, sodium must cross two barriers: passive transit through the mucosal membrane driven by an electrochemical gradient, followed by active extrusion of sodium through the basolateral serosal membrane by a sodium pump, the requisite energy for the latter step being supplied by hydrolysis of ATP. This two-barrier model implies that aldosterone-induced protein(s) (AIPs) may play three distinct, but not necessarily independent roles: (1) facilitation of passive sodium transit across the mucosal membrane (the permease theory), (2) augmentation of the energy supply, and (3) increased sodium pump activity by either activating existing pumps or by increasing the number of pumps (the sodium pump theory).

The evidence for these three possibilities is considered in reverse order. A sodium pump is always equated with Na^+–K^+ ATPase activity, which must be increased by mineralocorticoids in proportion to the effect on sodium transport. There is some circumstantial evidence supporting this hypothesis (ouabain, hyperbaric oxygen, and phospholipid turnover), but the results do have alternative explanations. Direct experiments are negative. Aldosterone does not augment renal Na^+–K^+ ATPase activity in adrenalectomized rats at *physiologic* concentrations. Neither is it effective in the toad bladder in increasing the K_m of the enzyme for ATP and only marginally effective on the number of enzyme sites. Thus, there is no convincing evidence supporting the sodium pump theory.

There is suggestive evidence supporting increased energy production as a mediator of aldosterone action. Citrate synthase activity is moderately increased in 3 hr by moderate amounts of aldosterone (0.8 μg/100 g body weight) and FAD synthesis is similarly increased by somewhat larger amounts (see Table 6.7). The increase in renal citrate synthase activity is accompanied by a 55% increase in incorporation of methionine into the immunoprecipitated enzyme.

Increases in both types of mRNA [polyA(+)RNA and polyA(−)RNA], but not tRNA nor rRNA, are a requirement for the expression of aldosterone action; formation of the former can be detected 30 to 60 min after hormone addition. Actinomycin D inhibits the formation of both forms of mRNA and abolishes the sodium response to aldosterone (toad bladder). 3'-Deoxyadenosine (cordycepin), which inhibits only polyA(+)RNA formation, produces only a 50 to 60% inhibition of the physiologic response, indicating that the polyA(−)RNA pathway is also important. In contrast, 3'-deoxycytidine, which inhibits rRNA but not mRNA synthesis, does not impair the early response to mineralocorticoids.

Aldosterone also induces the synthesis of specific proteins from radioactively labeled amino acids. One of these may be citrate synthase. If so, increased activity of this enzyme would increase the concentration of NADH (at the expense of NAD^+) by increasing the activity of the tricarboxylic acid (TCA) cycle (assuming a demand for energy) and thus provide increased amounts of ATP.

There is also suggestive evidence supporting the permease theory. Aldosterone treatment increases membrane phospholipid fatty acid synthesis as well as their elongation and desaturation (toad bladder). Both the physiologic response to mineralocorticoids and the hormone-induced changes in membrane lipid metabolism are prevented by prior treatment of the tissue with 2-methyl-2-[p-(1,2,3,4-tetrahydro-1-naphthyl)phenoxy]propionic acid, an inhibitor of acetyl-CoA carboxylase. Inhibitors of RNA and protein synthesis also block both responses.

Atrial Natriuretic Hormone Receptors

Localization studies using ^{125}I-labeled ANH indicate that receptors are to be found in brain, especially in the circumventricular organs, the adrenocortical zona glomerulosa, and the vascular endothelial and smooth muscle cells. By the affinity-labeling technique, three polypeptides of ca. 60, 70, and 120 kDa have been isolated. The ratios of these three peptides varied with the tissues examined (adrenal, aorta, kidney), suggesting that there may be at least two different receptors.

CLINICAL ASPECTS

Vasopressin–Antidiuretic Hormone

Antidiuretic hormone secretion responds sharply to changes in osmolality of the plasma. Below 287 mOsm/kg, there is only a basal secretion (1–2 ng/ml of serum), whereas above 295–300 mOsm/kg, ADH levels are elevated fivefold, and maximal retention of water in the renal ultrafiltrate occurs. Thus, a change of less than 5% in osmotic pressure produces a 500% change in ADH secretion.

Hypovasopressinemia, diabetes insipidus, is a disease in which the most frequent complaint is one of polyuria, of such frequent voiding that it interferes with sleep. Typically, 5–10 L of a dilute urine free of sugar are excreted daily. The origin of the disease may be neurogenic, associated with cranial surgery or irradiation; nephrogenic, owing to defective or a lack of renal receptors for ADH; or psychogenic, resulting from compulsive drinking of water.

Replacement therapy in neurogenic diabetes insipidus usually uses the vasopressin agonist, 1-desamino-8-D-arginine vasopressin intranasally. These two changes in the structure of vasopressin have increased the antidiuretic/pressor potency ratio by a factor of 2000 and tripled the duration of action to 6 to 20 hr. Oxytocic activity is also depressed so that this drug can be used safely in pregnant women. A dosage of 2.5–15 μg twice daily usually provides good control.

Hypervasopressinemia is often the result of a tumor. As many as 40% of patients with pulmonary carcinomas and a smaller fraction of patients with other carcinomas have ectopic production of ADH. Central neurological disorders resulting from skull fractures, meningitis, or encephalitis may also cause inappropriately large ADH secretion.

Measurement of ADH by RIA in plasma and urine in relation to plasma osmolality during hydration or dehydration tests will establish the diagnosis of diabetes insipidus. The use of certain drugs can then locate the defect which may involve decreased synthesis, inadequate release, or renal resistance to the action of ADH (nephrogenic diabetes insipidus). Chlorpropamide is a sulfonylurea compound that stimulates release of ADH and potentiates its renal action. Clofibrate, a hypolipidemic drug, has only the former action.

A simpler and less expensive approach to diagnosis is the measurement of urine osmolality and plasma osmolality or sodium concentration. An example of this is shown in Figure 6.12.

1. Patients of the type shown in the graph on the left have no releasable AVP and administration of chlorpropamide or clofibrate is ineffective in initiating antidiuresis. Administration of AVP or 1-desamino-8-D-arginine vasopressin is effective.
2. Patients of the type demonstrated in the graph in the middle are excreting hypotonic urine on random fluid intake despite high plasma osmolality; upon dehydration sufficient to produce hypovolemia, the urine becomes hypertonic and polyuria ceases. Clofibrate raises urine osmolality. These results indicate a loss of response to an osmotic stimulus and retention of response to a volume stimulus.
3. Another group of patients (the graph on the right) demonstrates an abnormally high-set osmoreceptor. They respond, but they require higher plasma osmolality to do so. Clofibrate treatment produces hypertonic urine and prompt antidiuresis.

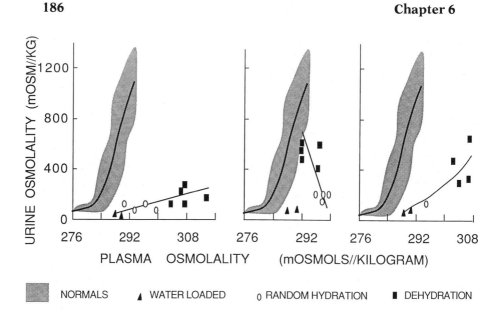

Figure 6.12 Use of urine and plasma osmolality in the diagnosis and treatment of diabetes insipidus. As plasma osmolality increases, urine osmolality also increases as shown by the curve and range of values obtained from normal subjects. This relationship is disturbed to various degrees in patients with diabetes insipidus. The patients in the first group have no releasable ADH; they must treated with replacement therapy. In the middle graph, we see patients who are able to respond to a volume stimulus but not to an osmotic stimulus; they can be treated with clofibrate or chlorpropamide. The right-hand graph shows less-sensitive response, i.e., the patients have a high set point; they respond to clofibrate (*Source*: modified from Moses, 1980, with permission).

Renin–Angiotensin–Aldosterone

Hypertension is so common in the United States that it is a public health problem. There is no widely accepted definition of hypertension: the World Health Organization uses 160/95 mmHg, whereas others use values as low as 140/90, excluding people over 65 years of age. Irrespective of the definition, uncorrected hypertension is a serious disease, leading, in time, to such cardiovascular diseases as acute myocardial infarction, aneurysms of the aorta, cerebrovascular accidents (stroke), and renal failure.

These are largely preventable or, at least, minimizable by a change in life-style, abstaining from smoking, and adopting a sensible regimen of diet and exercise, as well as taking antihypertensive drugs.

There are several clinical categories of hypertension: essential, juvenile, malignant, idiopathic, renovascular (Goldblatt), and others. As usual in endocrinology, research has not yet revealed the mechanism causing the disease in some categories, whereas in others two (or more) different biochemical defects requiring differing therapeutic approaches have been demonstrated.

Research has concentrated on exploring the renin–angiotensin–aldosterone axis. This system, as explained previously, has two ways of controlling blood pressure. Angiotensin II directly causes arterial vasoconstriction and indirectly, through aldosterone, causes sodium retention and volume expansion (Figure 6.13). Both mechanisms increase blood pressure. Although, normally, both are dependent upon renin, pathologically the renin–angiotensin vasoconstriction response may be more or less completely divorced from the aldosterone–volume expansion response. Thus, one may postulate four types of response.

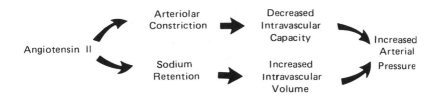

Figure 6.13 Renin–angiotensin hypertension. Hormonal and vascular responses to angiotensin that lead to alterations in blood pressure. Angiotensin II acts directly to produce arteriolar constriction and indirectly through aldosterone to produce sodium retention. Increasing osmotic pressure stimulates ADH secretion and increased water reabsorption, leading to an increased intravascular volume. Both responses, direct and indirect, lead to hypertension if carried too far (*Source*: from McKenna, TJ. Aldosterone secretion under physiological and pathological conditions. In K Fotherby and SB Pal (eds), *Hormones in Normal and Abnormal Human Tissues*, Vol 2, Berlin,Walter deGruyter & Co., 1981, p. 339, with permission).

1. Inappropriately high renin–angiotensin
2. Inappropriately high aldosterone
3. A combination of (1) and (2)
4. A different mechanism, i.e., neither (1) or (2) are elevated

In practice, all four types of response have been identified.

The key to identification of the type of response is specific pharmacological drugs. Saralasin (1-Sar-8-Ala-angiotensin) blocks the action of angiotensin II, whereas teprotide (pyroGlu-Trp-Pro-Arg-Pro-Glu-Ile-Pro-Pro) blocks its formation by inhibition of converting enzyme.

Atrial Natriuretic Hormone

It is too early for clinical applications of ANH agonists and antagonists to be available. The potential for treatment of certain cardiovascular and renal diseases ensures that ANH-based drugs are being actively investigated. The half-life of ANH in the plasma is about 3 min so hence, longer-lived analogues will be required for most applications.

Because ANH has direct effects on the glomerulus, it may be useful in maintaining diuresis when tubular diuretics have lost their effectiveness. Because ANH produces a diuresis and natriuresis without a marked kaliuresis, it has a clear advantage over conventional diuretics. Moreover, the fact that it can increase the glomerular filtration rate in animals with severe renal insufficiency suggests that it might be useful in reducing the frequency of dialysis of renal insufficient patients. Also, the therapeutic index of nephrotoxic drugs might be improved by concurrent administration of ANH agonists.

SUMMARY

The body's salt and water status is the balance of input and output. The major hormones involved are arginine vasopressin, angiotensin II, aldosterone, ACTH, and probably the newly discovered hormone, atrial natriuretic hormone.

Drinking can be induced in two ways. Baroreceptors located on the low-pressure side of the circulation fire at the end of diastole in response to the phase of maximum distension. A reduction in blood volume (extracellular fluid) reduces the rate of firing of these receptors. This information relayed to the CNS induces drinking and correction of the deficit in ECF volume. If the deficit is severe, sympathetic nerves will innervate the renal juxtaglomerular cells, thereby activating the renin–angiotensin system. Angiotensin II binding to its receptors in the circumventricular organs of the brain will also induce drinking.

The stimulus for the salt appetite comes from the taste buds. When aldosterone acting on the salivary glands causes an increased reabsorption of sodium from the saliva, the chemical change is detected by the taste buds.

Regulation of salt and water output is much more complex and is still incompletely understood. Even though the excretion of electrolytes and water cannot be physiologically divorced, let us consider them one at a time. Atrial natriuretic hormone is the only hormone that is said to increase renal blood flow and the rate of glomerular filtration, thereby increasing the potential urinary flow. Vasopressin–antidiuretic hormone acts mainly on the renal collecting ducts in humans promoting the reabsorption of water. Urine flow is the balance of these two forces. The ANH is released by all those factors leading to blood volume expansion and increased atrial pressure, such as high-salt diets and immersion in water. Vasopressin–antidiuretic hormone is released by factors leading to blood volume contraction, such as sweating, vomiting, or hemorrhage, as well as by pain, stress, and a number of drugs. Thus, the balance between these two will drive the fluid compartments back toward normality.

Electrolyte regulation is controlled by aldosterone (Na^+, K^+, H^+), ANH, (primarily Na^+, also K^+) and parathyroid hormone (Ca^{2+}, PO_4^{3-}). Aldosterone promotes Na^+ reabsorption from and secretion of K^+ and H^+ into the renal ultrafiltrate. Because the renin–angiotensin–aldosterone cascade is driven by blood volume contraction, the drinking induced by angiotensin must be accompanied by an appropriate retention of sodium to maintain the appropriate osmolality of the ECF. The counterregulatory hormone is again ANH. Not only does it promote the elimination of water, but also sodium, thus maintaining the appropriate osmolality of the ECF. Potassium, primarily an intracellular electrolyte, is released following tissue damage. It is one of the primary stimulants of aldosterone synthesis and release, thereby creating the condition for its own elimination.

Vasopressin–antidiuretic hormone is a nonapeptide containing a cyclic hexapeptide with a disulfide bridge. It is synthesized in the supraoptic nucleus of the hypothalamus as a single gene product along with its transport protein, neurophysin, and stored in the neurohypophysis. There it is hydrolyzed enzymatically into three products ready for secretion. Secretion is stimulated by hemorrhage, vomiting, emotional stress, pain, cholinergic and β-adrenergic stimulation, and a large number of drugs. Secretion is suppressed by ethanol imbibition, α-adrenergic stimulation, and a few drugs. Vasopressin is closely related to oxytocin, a specific smooth-muscle contractant.

Aldosterone is the product of a cascade that starts with the renal enzyme renin which is released by hypovolemia. It cleaves a fragment, angiotensin I, from a plasma globulin. A second hydrolysis by another enzyme produces angiotensin II, the most potent vasoconstrictor made and a hormone in its own right. One of its hormonal actions is the stimulation of aldosterone synthesis through the calcium–phosphotidylinositol second messenger. Aldosterone acts on renal receptors to promote Na^+ reabsorption and K^+, H^+, and NH_4^+ excretion.

Atrial natriuretic hormone is a newly discovered hormone. Although the gene product is large, the circulating form is a 28-amino acid peptide that promotes diuresis and natriuresis and, to a lesser extent, kaliuresis. Its release from atrial cardiocytes is prompted by hypervolemia and hypertension.

SUPPLEMENTAL BIBLIOGRAPHY

Aldosterone

Carey, RM and S Sen. Recent progress in the control of aldosterone secretion. *Recent Prog Horm Res 42*:251–289, 1986.

Edelman, JS. Mechanism of action of aldosterone: Energetic and permeability factors. *J. Endocrinol 81*:49P–53P, 1979.

Fanestil, DD and CS Park. Steroid hormones and the kidney. *Annu Rev Physiol 43*:637–649, 1981.

Morris, DJ. The metabolism and mechanism of action of aldosterone. *Endocr Rev 2*:234–247, 1981.

Rossier, BC. Role of RNA in the action of aldosterone on Na^+ transport. *J Membr Biol 40*:187–197, 1978.

Scott, WN, IM Reich, and DBP Goodman. Inhibition of fatty acid synthesis prevents the incorporation of aldosterone-induced proteins into membranes. *J Biol Chem 254*:4957–4959, 1979.

Angiotensin

Capponi, AM and KJ Catt. Solubilization and characterization of adrenal and uterine angiotensin II receptors after photoaffinity labeling. *J Biol Chem 255*:12,081–12,086, 1980.
Catt, KJ, G Aguilera, A Capponi, K Fujita, A Schirar, and J Fakunding. Angiotensin II receptors and aldosterone secretion. *J Endocrinol 81*:37P–48P, 1979.
Devynck, M-A and P Meyer. Angiotensin receptors. *Biochem Pharmacol 27*:1–5, 1978.
Simpson, RU, CP Companile, and TL Goodfriend. Specific inhibition of receptors for angiotensin II and angiotensin III in adrenal glomerulosa. *Biochem Pharmacol 29*:927–933, 1980.

ADH/VP

Bie, P. Osmoreceptors, vasopressin, and control of renal water excretion. *Physiol Rev 60*:961–1048, 1980.
Breslow, E. Chemistry and biology of the neurophysins. *Annu Rev Biochem 48*:251–274, 1979.
Handler, JS and J Orlott. Antidiuretic hormone. *Annu Rev Physiol 43*: 611–624, 1981.
Moses, MA. Diabetes insipidus and ADH regulation. In *Neuroendocrinology* (DT Krieger and JC Hughes, eds). Sinauer Associates, Sunderland, Mass, 1980, pp 141–148.
Robinson, AG. Neurophysins and their physiologic significance. In *Neuroendocrinology* (DT Krieger and JC Hughes, eds). Sinauer Associates, Sunderland, Mass, 1980, pp 149–155.
Russell, JT, MJ Brownstein, and H Gainer. Trypsin liberates an arginine vasopressinlike peptide and neurophysin from a M_r 20,000 putative common precursor. *Proc Natl Acad Sci USA 76*:6086–6090, 1979.

ANH

Atlas, SA. Atrial natriuretic factor: A new hormone of cardiac origin. *Recent Prog Horm Res 42*:207–243, 1986.
Cantin, M and J Genest. The heart and the atrial natriuretic factor. *Endocr Rev 6*:107–127, 1985.
Elliott, ME and TL Goodfriend. Inhibition of aldosterone synthesis by atrial natriuretic factor. *Fed Proc 45*:2376–2381, 1986.

Gellai, M, DE Allen, and R Beeuwkes, III. Contrasting views on the action of atrial peptides: Lessons from studies of conscious animals. *Fed Proc 45*:2387–2391, 1986.

Maack, T, MJF Carmargo, HD Kleinert, JH Laragh, and P Atlas. Atrial natriuretic factor: Structure and functional properties. *Kidney Int 27*:607–615, 1985.

Needleman, P and JE Greenwald. Atriopeptin: A cardiac hormone intimately involved in fluid, electrolyte and blood-pressure homeostasis. *New Engl J Med 314*:828–834, 1986.

Pegram, BL, NC Trippodo, T Natsume, MB Kardon, ED Frohlich, FE Cole, and AA MacPhee. Hemodynamic effects of atrial natriuretic hormone. *Fed Proc 45*:2382–2386, 1986.

Schwartz, D NC Katsube, and P Needleman. Atriopeptins in fluid and electrolyte homeostasis. *Fed Proc 45*:2361–2365, 1986.

Vandlen, RL, KE Arcuri, L Hupe, ME Keegan, and MA Napier. Molecular characteristics of receptors for atrial natriuretic factor. *Fed Proc 45*:2366–2370, 1986.

Winquist, RJ. Possible mechanisms underlying the vasorelaxant response to atrial natriuretic factor. *Fed Proc 45*:2371–1275, 1986.

Miscellaneous

Agus, ZS, A Wasserstein, and S Goldfarb. PTH, calcitonin, cyclic nucleotides and the kidney. *Annu Rev Physiol 43*:583–595, 1981.

Insel, PA and MD Snavely. Catecholamines and the kidney: Receptors and renal function. *Annu Rev Physiol 43*:625–636, 1981.

Jorgensen, PL. Sodium and potassium ion pump in kidney tubule. *Physiol Rev 60*:864–917, 1980.

Kinsella, J and B Sacktor. Thyroid hormones increase Na^+-H^+ exchange in renal brush border membranes. *Proc Natl Acad Sci USA 82*:3606–3610, 1985.

MacKnight, ADC, DR DiBona, and A Leaf. Sodium transport across toad urinary bladder: A model "tight" epithelium. *Physiol Rev 60*:615–715, 1980.

Morel, F, M Imbert-Teboul, and D Chabardes. Distribution of hormone-dependent adenylate cyclase in the nephron and its physiological significance. *Annu Rev Physiol 43*:569–581, 1981.

Nasjletti, A and KU Malik. The renal kallikrein–kinin and prostaglandin systems interaction. *Annu Rev Physiol 43*:597–609, 1981.

Ramsay, DJ and WF Ganong. CNS regulation of salt and water intake. In *Neuroendocrinology* (DT Krieger and JC Hughes, eds). Sinauer Associates, Sunderland, Mass, 1980, pp 59–65.

Wright, FS and G Giebisch. Renal potassium transport:Contributions of individual nephron segments and populations. *Am J Physiol 235*:F515–F527, 1978.

Renin

Atlas, SA, P Christofalo, T Hesson, JE Sealey, and LC Fritz. Immunological evidence that inactive renin is prorenin. *Biochem Biophys Res Commun 132*:1038–1045, 1985.

Bouhnik, J, JA Fehrentz, FX Galen, G Evin, B Castro, J Menard, and P Corvol. Immunologic identification of both plasma and human renal inactive renin as prorenin. *J Clin Endocrinol Metab 60*:399–401, 1985.

Imai, T, H Miyazaki, S Hirose, H Hori, T Hayashi, R Kageyama, H Ohkubo, S Nakanishi, and K Murakami. Cloning and sequence analysis of cDNA for human renin precursor. *Proc Natl Acad Sci USA 80*:7405–7409, 1983.

Kotchen, TA and GP Guthrie, Jr. Renin–angiotensin–aldosterone and hypertension. *Endocr Rev 1*:78–99, 1980.

Sealey, JE, SA Atlas, and JH Laragh. Prorenin and other large molecular weight forms of renin. *Endocr Rev 1*:365–391, 1980.

Sealey, JE, SA Atlas, JH Laragh, M Silverberg, and AP Kaplan. Initiation of plasma prorenin activation by Hageman factor-dependent conversion of plasma prekallikrein to kallikrein. *Proc Natl Acad Sci USA 76*:5914–5919, 1979.

7

Metabolism of Calcium and Phosphorus

Calcium   196
Bone and Teeth   197
    Basic histology and biochemistry   197
    Mineralization   201
    Nonhormonal factors influencing calcium homeostasis   204
Hormones Influencing Calcium Homeostasis   205
    Parathyroid hormone   205
    1α,25-dihydroxycholecalciferol 207
    Calcitonin   209
    Function   211
Clinical Aspects   214
    Tests   214
    Metabolic bone disease   214
    Hypercalcemia   217
    Hypocalcemia   218
Summary   219
Supplemental Bibliography   221

The plasma concentration of ionized calcium is extremely well regulated, for serious deviations have unwanted consequences including death. As a result, serum phosphate is also well regulated because the solubility product with calcium is a constant.

There are two hormones, parathyroid hormone and 1,25-dihydrocholecalciferol, intimately associated with the regulation of the plasma concentration of calcium and phosphate through intestinal absorption, renal excretion, and osseous mobilization. In addition, there are a number of environmental factors as well as other hormones that modulate the actions of the dominant duo. Lactation, in particular, places unusual demands on this system, and the body responds in kind.

CALCIUM

Calcium in the body may, with some rationality, be divided into three pools or compartments: plasma or serum, cellular, and skeletal (Table 7.1). In the plasma, a little more than one-half of the calcium is bound to either albumin or citrate; it is the unbound or ionic calcium that is physiologically active. Most of the cellular calcium resides in the endoplamic reticulum in an insoluble but readily mobilizable form. The major source of calcium is the skeleton, which acts as a calcium bank, receiving deposits in times of plenty (meal time) and returning them in lean times (between meals, starvation, pregnancy, lactation).

It is important to note that the pools are not equally accessible. In general, accessibility is a function of the ability to become soluble. A tiny fraction (ionic) is already soluble and instantly available. A larger fraction is present as amorphous $CaHPO_4$; this

Table 7.1   Pools of Body Calcium and Their Turnover

Compartment	Percentage of total	Concentration or amount
Serum		
protein-bound	40	1.8–2.2 mEq/L
citrate-bound	15	0.7–0.9
ionic	45	2.0–2.5
total	100	4.5–5.5 (0.5 g)
Cellular		
cytosol:basal		0.1 μOsm
cytosol:stimulated		10 μOsm
endoplasmic reticulum + mitochondria		500 × cytosol
total		12–14 g
Skeletal		
extracellular fluid (ECF)	0.1	1.5 g
intracellular fluid (ICF)	1	12–14 g
bone		1200–1400 g
Ca^{2+} turnover		
ECF (serum + skeletal)		40–50 ×/d
ICF		?
skeletal		3%/y

fraction is readily solubilized. The bulk of the calcium is present as crystalline hydroxyapatite, $Ca_{10}(OH)_2(PO_4)_6$; it took months to form this phase from amorphous $CaHPO_4$, and it is not readily available. Glimcher and coworkers (1981) recently concluded that changes in x-ray diffraction patterns with maturation of bone is not consistent with a two-phase mineral system, thus eliminating such precursors of hydroxyapatite as amorphous calcium phosphate, brushite, or any other distinct phase. Maturation is said to be "consistent with a general increase in the degree of crystal perfection of a calcium phosphate phase best described as a poorly crystalline hydroxyapatite" which lacks definition. Until such definition occurs, we use the term "amorphous" in a functional (rather than crystallographic) sense to designate a form that is more readily solubilized than crystalline hydroxyapatite. After all, the primary function of the skeleton is the maintenance of form and locomotion (see below for further discussion). The hormones involved in calcium homeostasis must respond to the most active pool and must, in turn, regulate that pool. Long-term imbalances will, of course, be reflected eventually in other pools.

BONE AND TEETH

Basic Histology and Biochemistry

Definitions

Comprehension of the literature on bone is difficult if one does not know the language. A few widely used terms are offered here to initiate the novice. An histology book is indispensable to a more complete understanding.

Compact or cortical bone: highly organized bone; the osteon is the basic unit with interstitial lamellae filling in the gaps between the osteons.
Endochondral bone: newly calcified bone, which is less structured than compact or cortical bone.
Howship's lacunae: osteocytes buried in the bone.
Osteitis fibrosa: replacement of bone with fibrous connective tissue.

Osteochondral complex: classically known as endochondral bone.
Osteoid: a zone of nonmineralized matrix.
Osteon: the basic unit of highly organized bone.
Perilacunar bone: noncrystalline bone surrounding deep osteo-
  cytes.
Periosteum: a membrane surrounding bone.
Trabeculae: spiderlike bone threads, which are the units of mes-
  enchymal, membranous, cancellous, or spongy bone.

There are four cell types in bone: osteoprogenitor cells,
osteoblasts, osteoclasts, and osteocytes. The osteoprogenitor
cells may be divided into two types by electron microscopic examination: preosteoblasts contain rough endoplasmic reticulum,
a well-formed Golgi apparatus, and relatively few mitochondria,
whereas preosteoclasts contain numerous mitochondria and free
ribosomes.

Osteoblasts, Odontoblasts, Cementoblasts

Osteoblasts synthesize and secrete the protein and polysaccharide complexes that form the osteoid of skeletal tissues; odontoblasts and cementoblasts are basically the same cells located in
the dentin or cementum layers of teeth, respectively. The principal protein component is type I collagen (see general biochemistry texts for details). Bone collagen differs, however, from
other type I collagens in being less soluble and failing to swell in
mild acids at low ionic strength, an indication of very extensive
cross-linking.

Another protein secreted by osteoblasts and odontoblasts is
osteocalcin, an abundant protein found in the bone, dentin, and
plasma of all vertebrates. The tissue content of osteocalcin is
unusually low in human bone, 0.05–0.1 mg/g or about 5% of that
in the bones of most other vertebrates. Plasma levels are also low,
5–10 ng/ml versus 100–300 ng/ml.

The primary structure of osteocalcin (Fig. 7.1) shows the
presence of three residues of γ-carboxyglutamic acid (Gla), a
vitamin K-dependent, posttranslational modification of glutamyl
residues; all are located in the NH_2-terminal portion of the
molecule. This amino acid occurs in a number of calcium-binding
proteins, such as prothrombin and clotting factors VII, IX, and X.
There are three calcium-binding sites on bovine osteocalcin, with

```
                 5                10                        15
h   TYR.LEU.TYR.GLN.TRP.LEU.GLY.ALA.PRO.VAL.PRO.TYR.PRO.ASP.PRO.
m                                  HYP.ALA
b        ASP.HIS                  HYP.ALA
s              ALA.THR.ARG         GLY.ASP.LEU.THR        LEU.GLN.


                 20          |    25          |  30
h   LEU.GLA.PRO.ARG.ARG.GLA.VAL.CYS.GLA.LEU.ASN.PRO.ASP.CYS.ASP.
m             LYS
b             LYS
s         SER.LEU                             VAL.ALA


                 35              40              45
h   GLU.LEU.ALA.ASP.HIS.ILE.GLY.PHE.GLN.GLU.ALA.TYR.ARG.ARG.PHE.
m
b
s      MET          THR.ALA    ILE.VAL.ALA        ILE.ALA.TYR.


                 49
h   TYR.GLY.PRO.VAL
m
b
s         ILE.GLN.PHE
```

Figure 7.1 The primary structure of osteocalcin from humans (h), monkey (*Macaca fascicularis*; m), cattle (b), and swordfish (s): Gla, γ-carboxyglutamic acid; Hyp, hydroxyproline. Note that there are three Glas (at residues 17, 21, and 24) in a region that is highly conserved (residues 16 to 27).

an average dissociation constant of 2 to 3 mM, about the value of plasma free calcium. Binding to the calcium of hydroxyapatite is much stronger, being about 0.1 μM.

No systematic study of structure and function has been done. It is known, however, that Gla and an intact disulfide bond between the two cysteines at residues 23 and 29 are required for calcium-binding activity. The highly conserved sequences (see Fig. 7.1) indicate that much of the molecule may be essential for activity.

A rat osteosarcoma cell line (ROS 17/2) provides a useful model. This cell line secretes osteocalcin into the medium, but intracellularly there is a mixture of the 5.8-kDa osteocalcin isolated from bone (20%) and a 9.0-kDa component (80%). Addition of 1,25-

dihydroxycholecalciferol [1,25-(OH)₂CC] increases intracellular levels sixfold within 12 hr and medium concentrations similarly in 15 hr. Because there is a substantial basal rate of synthesis of osteocalcin, synthesis is modulated by, rather than dependent upon, 1,25-(OH)₂CC. The response of osteocalcin synthesis in serum-free medium is dose-dependent and saturable with a half-maximal response at 0.1 nM 1,25-(OH)₂CC concentration. The action of the latter appears to be exerted at the transcriptional level.

Osteocalcin is a potent inhibitor of the *rate* of hydroxyapatite formation in vitro. Because the amount of hydroxyapatite formed is not affected by osteocalcin, its effect is exclusively on the kinetics of mineral formation rather than on the thermodynamic endpoint. Naturally, the effectiveness of osteocalcin is dependent upon its concentration.

Still another protein found in the matrix of bone and dentin is osteonectin (32 kDa), which selectively binds free calcium, collagen, and hydroxyapatite, leading to the hypothesis that it may function in the nucleation of the mineral phase.

Osteocytes

Osteocytes originate from osteoblasts that are surrounded and trapped by the collagen they produce. Eventually, they become buried in bone (deep osteocytes), each in its own lacuna, and change their structural appearance. They maintain communication with other osteocytes and osteoblasts by means of canaliculi (200 nm diameter) from which microcanaliculi (50 nm diameter) radiate. Although they occupy only 7% of the bone volume, they provide an enormous surface area (35,000 mm²/mm³) for the mobilization of calcium. In addition, perilacunar bone has fewer, more loosely packed, less mineralized fibers, i.e., the mineral is more amorphous and more readily solubilized. These last two statements are particularly important for calcium homeostasis (see p. 211).

Surface osteocytes (resting osteoblasts) are thin, flattened cells forming an incomplete, leaky envelope over 80% of the bone surface, where neither formation nor resorption is occurring.

Osteoclasts

Osteoclasts are multinucleated giant cells that resorb bone. The analogous cell type for resorption of cartilage is the chondroclast.

They apparently are identical except for the accident of location. Osteoclasts work at sites of active bone remodeling. These take various forms, but the most general is the cortical remodeling unit, a microscopic cavity inside compact bone, with calcium mobilization by osteoclasts occurring at one end and calcium deposition taking place at the other. Another form occurs during orthodontal manipulation when calcium is resorbed from one surface and laid down at another during tooth movement through alveolar bone.

An analogous, but somewhat different, process occurs in teeth. During tooth development, ameloblasts in the developing enamel layer, odontoblasts in the dentin layer, and cementoblasts in the cementum layer perform similar functions to the osteoblasts. The ameloblasts, however, are different from the other cell types in that they secrete mostly noncollagenous proteins, which are still incompletely characterized. During the process of calcification, most of these proteins are resorbed so that mature enamel contains only 0.05 to 0.2% protein and no cells. Dentin and cementum are more comparable to skeletal bone. It is noteworthy that tooth layers contain no osteoclastlike cells. As a consequence, calcium is not mobilized from maternal teeth during pregnancy or lactation. The same cannot be said for the bone into which the teeth are set. This bone can be resorbed to the point where teeth loosen and fall out.

Mineralization

There appears to be no direct hormonal control of the mineralization process. Rather it is a free-running process depending upon the interaction of nucleation sites and the local concentration of Ca^{2+} and HPO_4^{2-} ions. The chemical nature of nucleation sites remains undefined; hypotheses must recognize the experimental fact that mineralization is first observed in the "holes" in the quarter-staggered array of collagen fibrils. Hypotheses, in general, wish to create a high, local concentration and *chemical activity* of calcium and phosphate ions, which could form the first fragments of a Ca–P solid phase. Covalent or coordinate bonding of mineral ions to the organic matrix would do this *provided* the chemical activity is not greatly diminished. An accumulation of anionic groups (carboxyl, phosphate, sulfate) would favor a high local concentration of calcium. On the other hand, strongly chelated calcium would not have outer-shell electrons available for further reaction with phosphate. This is especially true of osteocalcin which chelates calcium with a dissociation constant in the physiologic range of ionic calcium. Covalently bonded phosphate, on the other hand, would remain active toward ionic calcium or positively charged calcium–phosphate clusters.

Osteonectin may also function to increase the local concentration of ionic calcium.

There is considerably more evidence in favor of *O*-phosphoserine as a nucleation site.

1. The structural characteristics of most Ca–P solids are determined primarily by the phosphate groups in the unit cell rather than by the calcium ions, which can be replaced by other cations without altering the basic crystal structure.
2. There are many specific phosphokinases in the body.
3. The concentration of organic phosphate in bone collagen is three to ten times greater than that in soft tissue collagens; this difference disappears in calcified bone and dentin collagen.
4. *O*-Phosphoserine is present in bone and dentin collagen as well as in noncollagen peptides of the organic matrix.
5. Considerably more *O*-phosphoserine is present in noncollagen enamel peptides.

Direct experimental confirmation of this mass of circumstantial evidence is rare. An elegant autoradiographic study is that of Weinstein and Leblond. After injections of [³H]proline, [³H]serine, or ³³Pi into rats, all three compounds were taken up by odontoblasts and deposited within the predentin. Only the [³H]serine or ³³P were rapidly displaced to the mineralization front. The ³³P, which was associated with collagen fibrils only at the mineralization front, was extractable with an aqueous buffer, suggesting that it had been incorporated into a soluble phosphoprotein.

More recent experimental work has confirmed and extended these observations. Phosphoserine, phosphothreonine, and osteocalcin appear in calcifying or recently calcified tissue (Table 7.2), and the phosphoamino acids occur mostly on small, water-soluble peptides associated with collagen (Table 7.3). Although

Table 7.2　The Concentration of O-Phosphoserine [Ser(P)] and γ-Carboxy-glutamic Acid (Gla) in Bovine Epiphyseal Cartilage of Calves

Cartilage	Residues (10^5 aa)		Ca (wt %)	P (wt %)
	Ser (P)	Gla		
Uncalcified	3	0.6	0.2	0.3
Calcified:density				
1.4–1.5 g/cm	16	16	0.7	0.6
1.5–1.6	18	17	3.9	2.3
1.6–1.7	20	27	10.3	6.1
1.7–1.8	32	32	14.3	8.2
1.8–1.9	50	52	16.7	9.3
>1.9	52	65	20.4	11.2

Source: from Glimcher et al., *Calcif Tissue Int* 27:187–191, 1979.

Table 7.3　The Concentration of Three Amino Acids[a] in Native, Calcified Tissue and in EDTA-Extractable Protein from Steers

Tissue	Native			EDTA-extractible		
	Ser(P)	Thr(P)	Gla	Ser(P)	Thr(P)	Gla
Cementum	79	10	55	500	67	745
Dentin	1710	Trace	23	11400	Trace	240
Bone						
mandible	22	3	90			
tibia	37	4	74			
Enamel	1000	ND[b]	ND[b]			

[a]O-phosphoserine, O-phosphothreonine, and γ-carboxyglutamic acid.
[b]not detectable.
Source: from Glimcher et al. *Calcif Tissue Int* 28:83–86, 1979.

still not proved, it appears that both calcium-binding protein and phosphoprotein in close proximity to each other may be required for nucleation.

　　Once a Ca–P solid begins to form, continued growth presumably requires both Ca^{2+} and HPO_4^{2-} to be present locally at concentrations (activities) exceeding their solubility product. The product, amorphous $CaHPO_4$, then undergoes an indeterminate number of solid-phase transitions over a period of months until finally crystalline hydroxyapatite, $Ca_{10}(OH)_2(PO_4)_6$, is formed.

Nonhormonal Factors Influencing Calcium Homeostasis

Many factors, in addition to hormones, may influence calcium homeostasis (Table 7.4). Consideration of the relationships

$$H_2PO_4^- \leftrightarrow HPO_4^{2-} + H^+$$

which has a pK_a of 7.21 and

$$Ca_{10}(OH)_2(PO_4)_6 \leftrightarrow 10\ Ca^{2+} + 2\ OH^- + 6\ PO_4^{3-}$$

shows the acute sensitivity of Ca–P solid to pH. Acidity neutralizes the hydroxide ion of hydroxyapatite, thereby destroying the crystalline lattice; by mass action, it also forces the formation of $(H_2PO_4)^-$, thus favoring the formation of relatively soluble $Ca(H_2PO_4)_2$. Alkalosis has the opposite effect.

The concentration of phosphate in the extracellular fluid is also important. Increasing the HPO_4^{2-} concentration will favor the formation of Ca–P solid and inhibit bone resorption. The normal concentration of inorganic phosphate is 1.5 mEq/L of which 80% is HPO_4^{2-}.

Fluoride ions (F^-) work in a different way. They substitute well for hydroxide ion in the hydroxyapatite crystal. In fact,

Table 7.4 Nonhormonal Factors Influencing Ca–P Homeostasis

Increased resorption	Decreased resorption
Acidosis	Alkalosis
Bed rest	
Immobilization	
Weightlessness	
Low ECF phosphate	High ECF phosphate
Polyanions	Fluoride

fluoroapatite ($Ca_{10}F_2(Po_4)_6$) is a more stable crystal than hydroxyapatite with a higher pK_a, thus enabling fluoroapatite to withstand acidity better. Fluoride in the diet (drinking water) or repeated application of a concentrated fluoride solution to teeth produces a limited amount of substitution of fluoride for hydroxyl ions (0.2–0.3% vs. 3.8% fluoride with complete substitution). Yet even this small amount is sufficient to reduce dental caries.

Polyanions, such as heparin or chondroitin sulfate, may stimulate bone resorption. Presumably this occurs because the polyanions complex calcium, lowering its effective concentration (activity). By mass action, this promotes solubilization.

HORMONES INFLUENCING CALCIUM HOMEOSTASIS

There are two primary hormones involved in calcium homeostasis arising from different sources and acting on three tissues (Table 7.5). In addition, calcitonin plays a secondary role that is still poorly defined.

Parathyroid Hormone

Parathyroid hormone (PTH) is synthesized in the four parathyroid glands situated at the poles of the bilobed thyroid gland. Each gland is about the size of a pea (30 mg). The upper two are derived from the fourth branchial arch, whereas the lower who, like the thymus gland, originate from the third arch. The chief cells secrete PTH, but the function of the less-prominent oxyphil cells is unknown.

Table 7.5 The Primary Hormones Involved in Human Calcium Homeostasis

Hormone	Source	Target tissues	Effect on plasma Ca^{2+}
Calcitonin	Thyroid C cells	Bone	Decrease
Parathyroid hormone	Parathyroid	Bone, kidney	Increase
1,25-(OH)$_2$CC[a]	Kidney	Gut, bone (permissive)	Increase

[a]1,25-Dihydroxycholecalciferol.

The PTH gene, which is closely linked to the β-globin gene, is located on a short arm of chromosome 11 in humans, as are the genes for calcitonin, c-Harvey-ras I oncogene, IGF II, and insulin. It controls the synthesis of preproparathyroid hormone, a single-chain polypeptide containing 115 amino acid residues. Synthesis of mature hormone follows the usual format. The first cleavage removing the NH_2-terminal leader sequence of 25 amino acids occurs cotranslationally in rough endoplasmic reticulum. The second cleavage occurs in the Golgi complex with the removal of another six NH_2-terminal amino acid residues to produce mature PTH containing 84 amino acid residues. There is a high degree of homology among mammalian species.

The PTH gene from humans, cattle, and rats contains three exons and two introns or intervening sequences. The first intron, which contains 1600 to 3400 bp, separates the 5′-noncoding region from the rest of the molecule, whereas the second short intron (103 to 119 bp) separates the nucleotides coding for the prepro-sequences from those encoding mature PTH. The human and bovine genes contain two transcription start sites, whereas the rat gene has only one. The significance of this observation is not yet apparent.

Structure–function studies show that all the bioactivity is contained in PTH1–34 (Fig. 7.2). Deletion of COOH-terminal

```
              1                 5                    10
human      H₂Nser.val.ser.glu.ile.gln.leu.met.his.asn.leu.gly.lys.
porcine
bovine        ala                              phe

              15                20                   25
human      his.leu.asn.ser.met.gln.arg.val.glu.trp.leu.arg.lys.
porcine            ser      leu
bovine            ser

                   30                35
human      lys.leu.gln.asp.val.his.asn.phe.val.ala.leu.
porcine
bovine
```

Figure 7.2 Amino acid sequence of PTH1–37. Only differences of porcine and bovine from human PTH are noted. All the bioactivity resides in the first 34 residues.

amino acids gradually decreases activity until reaching PTH1–26 which is inert. In contrast, deletion at the NH_2-terminus produces a sharp drop-off in activity and creation of hormonal antagonists through their continued ability to bind to PTH receptors. Modification [norleucine-8,18-tyrosine-34-PTH(3–34)-amide] has produced a potent antagonist useful for in vitro work.

The secretion of PTH responds inversely to the concentration of ionic plasma calcium, but the mechanism is unknown. There are conflicting reports on the effects of extracellular calcium and 1,25-$(OH)_2$CC on PTH mRNA levels and on rates of PTH and pro-PTH synthesis.

Other secretagogues of PTH, such as epinephrine, iso-proterenol, dopamine, secretin, or prostaglandin E, or inhibitors of secretion, such as α-adrenergic agonists or prostaglandin $F_2\alpha$, are believed to act through adenylate cyclase because the cellular concentration of cAMP changes in parallel with changes in PTH secretion. Dibutyryl-cAMP and inhibitors of phosphodiesterase activity mimic the effects of hypocalcemia.

β-Adrenergic agonists *augment* the secretion of PTH induced by hypocalcemia, and they do this at normal physiologic levels. The effects of catecholamines on PTH secretion are additive to those of hypocalcemia, suggesting separate receptors. Moreover, propranolol inhibits only the epinephrine-induced response.

1α,25-Dihydroxycholecalciferol

The second hormone arises from an endogenous sterol in a three-step synthesis (Fig. 7.3). Ultraviolet light acts on the skin sterol, 7-dehydrocholesterol, an intermediate in the synthesis of cholesterol from lanosterol. The light energy is sufficient to break the C-9 to C-10 bond of the sterol, opening ring B and forming cholecalciferol (vitamin D_3). (A vitamin by definition is a *natural*, required dietary substance. The "vitamin D" in milk and other dairy products is derived from irradiation of a homologous plant sterol (ergosterol) which is added to improve the nutritional properties of the product. The additive undergoes all the reactions described in Fig. 7.3.) This highly insoluble compound is also stored in the skin and slowly moved to the liver where it is hydroxylated (O_2, NADPH, and cytochrome P_{450} required) at C-25 by a microsomal hydroxylase (K_m, 10^{-8} M) (see gonadal steroidogenesis

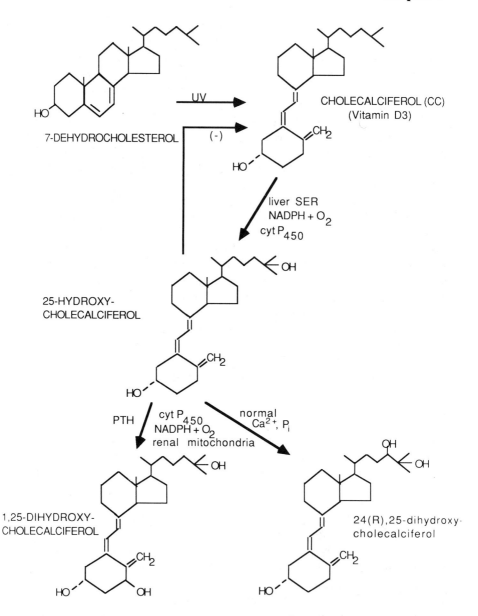

Figure 7.3 Synthesis of 1α,25-dihydroxycholecalciferol.

in Chap. 8 for a discussion of mixed-function monooxygenases). The reaction is regulated by product inhibition. 25-Hydroxycholecalciferol, the immediate precursor of the hormone, circulates at appreciable concentrations because of its binding to a plasma globulin.

The kidney contains two mitochondrial hydroxylases that work in an inverse relationship. When the plasma concentration of calcium is normal or high, the 24(R)-hydroxylase is active and 24(R),25-dihydroxycholecalciferol is made. At low calcium concentrations, PTH activates the 1α-hydroxylase, and the hormone, 1α,25-dihydroxycholecalciferol, is made, whereas synthesis of the 24(R)-isomer is strongly inhibited.

Calcitonin

Calcitonin is basically a neuropeptide secreted by certain cells migrating from the primitive nervous system and concentrating in certain organs. In the lizard, it is the lung; in birds, it is the ultimobranchial body; in the pigeon, the thyroid; and in mammals, the thyroid C cells and, perhaps, the thymus gland in humans. This wide distribution is reminiscent of gut hormones.

The calcitonin of seven species including the eel and salmon have been isolated and sequenced; five have been synthesized. All contain certain common structural features (Fig. 7.4). The NH_2-

```
            10          20          30
            |           |           |
h      CGNLSTCMLG TYTQDFNKFH TFPQTAIGVG AP.NH₂

rat                L           S

p       S      V S A WRNL N    R SGMGF VE T

b       S      V S A WK L NY   R SGMGF PE T

o       S      V S A WK L NY   RYSGMGF PE

sal     S      V   KLS ELH LQ  Y R NT S  T

eel     S      V   KLS ELH LQ  Y R DV A  T
```

Figure 7.4 Calcitonin sequences from seven species. Only differences from human calcitonin are noted.

terminal portion contains a seven-amino acid residue ring with Cys-1 and Cys-7 in a disulfide bridge; six of seven residues are invariant. These features are similar to those of vasopressin and oxytocin. The COOH-terminal amino acid is always prolinamide. There are two other invariant residues so that 9 of 32 are invariant. Naturally there is very extensive homology in the porcine–bovine–ovine group and in the eel–salmon group, but also in the rat–man group, which differ in only two residues.

From the diversity in sequences, one expects variable bioactivity. The variability found is, however, unexpected. Rat and human calcitonins differ by only two residues, but the former is four times more active (in the rat) whereas the nearly equipotent human and porcine hormones have 18 differences in their primary sequences. Work with many synthetic fragments and modifications leads to the conclusion that there is no single active site, most deletions or substitutions producing drastic reductions in activity.

Development of transplantable, calcitonin-producing rat medullary thyroid carcinomas has enabled the isolation of the mRNA and synthesis of the corresponding cDNA of calcitonin. Decoding of the cDNA sequence reveals preprocalcitonin to be a 127–amino acid polypeptide containing a 24–amino acid signal sequence, a 46–amino acid pro sequence, as well as a 17–amino acid COOH-terminal sequence. Calcitonin is flanked, as usual, by Lys-Arg and Gly-Lys-Lys-Arg peptides; the glycine in the latter leads to amidation of the COOH-terminal proline of calcitonin. The COOH-terminal peptide and calcitonin are liberated in equimolar amounts, although no biological function for the COOH-terminal peptide has been found. In addition, related products are found, called calcitonin–gene-related products, leading to the suggestion of alternative gene splicing. The former seems to predominate in thyroid medullary tissue and the latter in neural tissue.

The primary stimulus for secretion is hypercalcemia. The mechanism remains obscure because of the lack of a suitable purified calcitonin-secreting cell system. Calcitonin-secreting cell lines from medullary thyroid carcinomas have recently been established, but there is still no way to evaluate normal C cells. Recent results suggest at least two mechanisms for calcitonin secretion. One involves activation of adenylate cyclase by glucagon and isoproterenol, whereas the other, stimulated by K^+, Ca^{2+}, CCK, or pentagastrin, acts independently of cAMP.

Function

In general, one can view PTH and 1,25-dihydroxycholecalciferol as acting to raise hypocalcemic levels and calcitonin acting to lower hypercalcemic levels (see Table 7.5). Although the result is eucalcemia, each acts in a different way.

1α,25-Dihydroxycholecalciferol promotes calcium absorption by acting primarily like a steroid on the small intestine, i.e., it diffuses into the cell, binds to a cytosolic receptor, and is transported into the nucleus, where it presumably turns on a gene for synthesis of a cellular calcium transport protein. Protein synthesis inhibitors block the increase in calcium-45 transport, indicating involvement of a protein. Yet such a protein has not been found. A calcium-binding protein, previously assumed to be the putative protein, turned out to be synthesized too slowly to be responsible for the response seen.

Inorganic phosphate is also transported across the intestinal wall. Its mechanism of transport in the gut has been little studied.

The extent of PTH action is dependent upon its concentration. At low concentrations, it acts on the small amount of calcium in the extracellular fluid (see Table 7.1) that is turning over 40 to 50 times daily, causing increased urinary excretion of phosphate (phosphaturic effect) and enhanced tubular reabsorption of calcium. As noted earlier, it also activates the renal 1α-hydroxylase. At moderate or prolonged concentrations of PTH, it acts on amorphous Ca–P deposited in cells or in perilacunar bone. In high concentrations, PTH increases osteoclastic activity, thereby stimulating bone resorption; 1α,25-dihydroxycholecalciferol plays a permissive role in PTH action on bone.

There is no doubt that PTH (and calcitonin) binds to plasma membrane receptors and activates adenylate cyclase. Charbardes' group have measured adenylate cyclase activity on microdissected rabbit tubule preparations as a means of analyzing for hormone receptors (Fig. 7.5). There are discrete areas of receptors for PTH or calcitonin along the tubule and for vasopressin along the collecting duct. Cyclic cAMP-dependent protein kinase is located on the opposite side of the cell in the brush border microvilli. The concentration of cAMP at the luminal surface may explain the large urinary concentrations of cAMP when plasma levels of PTH are high. PTH also activates

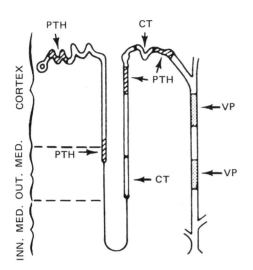

Figure 7.5 Schematic diagram depicting PTH and calcitonin (CT)-sensitive regions of the nephron of the rabbit: VP, vasopressin (*Source*: modified from Charbardes et al., 1978).

alkaline phosphatase, glucose-6-phosphate dehydrogenase, gluconeogenesis, and transport of sodium, phosphate, and calcium within the renal tubule. As yet there is no link between cAMP-dependent protein kinase and the end result of PTH action.

Less is known about bone, probably because of the difficulty in preparing reasonably pure cell populations. It is believed that cAMP causes release of lysosomal enzymes that induce bone resorption. However, cAMP also influences other cellular functions such as phosphorylation of microtubule assemblies, change in cell shape, and alterations in ion transport. It is interesting that colchicine and vinblastine, agents that interrupt microtubular function, inhibit bone resorption in vitro whereas ionophores that promote cellular calcium uptake induce bone resorption in vitro. The major functions promoted by cAMP and responsible physiologically for bone resorption remain unidentified.

Although the principal function of calcitonin is inhibition of bone resorption, the physiological importance of calcitonin has always been questioned. It is definitely not concerned with minute-to-minute regulation. Although one of its major functions may be the suppression of the postprandial rise in plasma calcium, the modern view emphasizes its role in restraining skeletal resorption during times of physiologic calcium stress, such as pregnancy or lactation.

The most extreme example of calcium stress is that of the lactating rat that transfers about 2.5 g of calcium, equivalent to 60% of its skeletal calcium, during the 21 days of lactation. Only 5 to 10% of the skeletal calcium is actually lost, however, the difference coming from the diet. In spite of the increased intake, serum calcium levels are about 10% lower than normal, producing elevated levels of PTH and 1,25-dihydroxycholecalciferol. The latter doubles the efficiency of intestinal absorption of calcium (from 17 to 33%) so that, combined with increased food intake, absorbed calcium increases from 40 to 250 mg daily. The increased PTH and 1,25-dihydroxycholecalciferol would normally produce a drastic mobilization of skeletal calcium, but the calcitonin levels have tripled and act to inhibit bone resorption. It is true that the elevated PTH will produce lowered urinary calcium excretion, but the conservation contributes minimally to the extraordinary demand.

The situation is somewhat different with women in whom the heaviest calcium drain comes during the last 2 months of gestation. During lactation, the loss of calcium in the milk is no greater than the urinary loss (ca. 100 mg/day). Nevertheless, calcitonin is elevated in pregnant and lactating women, especially if lactation is prolonged, and it is assumed that the same mechanisms are involved.

It has been said that there is no calcitonin-related disease aside from medullary carcinoma of the thyroid. Recently, it was noted that there is a marked sex difference in calcitonin response to an infusion of Ca^{2+}, with women having lower responses than men. Oral contraceptives or pregnancy bring their calcitonin response into the male range. There is also a marked age dependency with loss of response to calcium with advancing age in both sexes. It is now speculated that this progressive calcitonin deficiency contributes to the increased bone loss (osteoporosis) that occurs with age, especially in women.

Other hormones may have a profound influence on skeletal growth, although it is often difficult to separate effects on the organic matrix from those on mineralization. Somatotropin, acting through somatomedins, promotes osteoblastic function and linear growth. After the epiphyses close, there may be an increase in bone formation, particularly that of cortical bone.

Thyroid hormone is required for normal bone development in children. Skeletal growth is retarded in hypothyroidic and accelerated in hyperthyroidic children. In adult hyperthyroidism, however, decreased bone mass is associated with increased osteoclastic activity and a high rate of bone turnover. The molecular mechanisms are unknown.

High concentrations of glucocorticoids are, as a rule, catabolic, showing decreased DNA, RNA, and protein synthesis, as well as decreased sulfate incorporation into cartilage in vitro. In vivo, glucocorticoids produce secondary hyperparathyroidism by impairing intestinal absorption of calcium by means of an inhibition of proliferation of precursor cells.

In spite of the association of sex steroids with accelerated linear growth and epiphyseal closure at puberty, there is still no convincing evidence of a direct effect on bone collagen synthesis or bone resorption.

CLINICAL ASPECTS

Tests

Radioimmunoassay of PTH and 1,25-dihydroxycholecalciferol and measurement of serum and urinary calcium and phosphate are required.

Metabolic Bone Disease

Metabolic bone disease encompasses all conditions in which there are disruptions of the normal, orderly sequence of bone remodeling. There are some nonendocrine components as well as nondisease factors involved. It can occur as an identifiable abnormality of calcium metabolism or as an apparent derangement of osteoblastic or osteoclastic activity.

Osteoporosis is a major clinical problem, especially in geriatric practice. In osteoporosis, there is a deficiency in numbers of osteoblasts relative to osteoclasts, so that in bone remodeling, replacement does not keep pace with bone erosion. As a result, residual bone is normally calcified, but its mass is reduced. The lamellae are thin, and bone is brittle and easily fractured.

The leading factor in osteoporosis is aging (Table 7.6), the problem being particularly acute among postmenopausal women. Because estrogen production drops to male levels at the time of menopause, a cause-and-effect relationship has been postulated, and some clinicians even administer estrogens to postmenopausal women. There is, however, no solid evidence to support either the practice or the postulate. Even if one were to concede the efficacy of estrogen treatment, the possible side effects of estrogens (thromoembolism, hypertension, endometrial adenocarcinoma) make the wisdom of treating all Caucasian women to prevent symptomatic osteoporosis in a small minority (<10%) questionable.

Men also become osteoporotic, although less frequently. Estrogens have never been implicated. Hence, if one assumes a unitary cause, loss of estrogen is not involved in either sex. The recent observation that the calcitonin response to calcium infusion diminishes with age in both sexes may be important. Because osteoporosis develops over a period of years, any preventive treatment must be correspondingly prolonged.

There are well-established endocrine causes of bone loss which, if left unchecked, lead to osteoporosis at any age. Prolonged corticosteroid therapy or the hypercortisolemia of Cushing's syndrome (see Chap. 9) presumably produce a negative nitrogen balance and depletion of the organic matrix of bone.

Table 7.6 Factors in Osteoporosis[a]

Old age, especially in women
Cushing's syndrome
Corticosteroid therapy, prolonged
Immobilization, prolonged
Rheumatoid arthritis (partially owing to immobilization)
Paget's disease

[a]Frequently more than one factor may be operative.

In osteomalacia, a disease of *mature* bone, the mass of bone is normal, but new organic matrix fails to calcify from lack of 1,25-(OH)₂CC (Table 7.7). As a consequence, calcium and phosphate absorption from the intestine are impaired; hence, serum calcium concentrations tend to be low, leading to secondary hyperparathyroidism. This, in turn, stimulates osteoclastic activity and renal tubular reabsorption of filtered calcium while inhibiting tubular reabsorption of phosphate. Thus, the supply of mineral necessary for calcification is limited, and osteoid fails to calcify.

There are many causes of osteomalacia; those related to cholecalciferol metabolism (see Fig. 7.3) are summarized in Table 7.7. People who have insufficient exposure to sunlight (ultraviolet) *and* fail to ingest adequate amounts of milk fortified with the plant equivalent of cholecalciferol may have a deficiency of precursor of 1,25-(OH)₂CC. Those with chronic liver disease (cirrhosis) may have a deficiency of 25-hydroxylase, whereas those with chronic renal failure may fail to complete the synthesis of 1,25-(OH)₂CC. And finally, patients taking anticonvulsant drugs may induce hepatic enzymes responsible for the catabolism of cholecalciferol and its active metabolites. Each of these conditions will produce osteomalacia as will a deficiency of receptors for 1,25-(OH)₂CC.

Hypophosphatemia, or vitamin D-resistant ricketts, is a form of osteomalacia present in *growing* bone that is inherited as an X-linked dominant trait. The biochemical hallmarks of the disease are hypophosphatemia, eucalcemia, and elevated alkaline phosphatase levels. The defect is an impaired tubular reabsorption of

Table 7.7 Causes of a Deficiency of 1,25-Dihydroxycholecalciferol

Failure of epidermal synthesis of cholecalciferol (lack of exposure to UV)

Dietary deficiency of cholecalciferol (vitamin D₃)

Failure of cholecalciferol 25-hydroxylase (chronic hepatic disease)

Failure of 25-hydroxycholecalciferol 1α-hydroxylase (chronic renal failure)

Increased catabolism of cholecalciferol and its metabolites (induction of hepatic enzymes in patients taking anticonvulsants)

phosphate and impaired intestinal absorption of phosphate and calcium. It is not clear whether the defect in calcium absorption is primary or secondary.

Vitamin-D dependent ricketts, on the other hand, is a rare autosomal-recessive disorder that presents with evidence of vitamin D underactivity in the face of normal dietary intake and absorption of the vitamin. The basic defect is decreased (or absent) renal 1α-hydroxylase activity, leading to impaired intestinal absorption of calcium and phosphate. Consequently, serum calcium and phosphate concentrations are both suppressed, and alkaline phosphatase activity is elevated. Because of the enzymatic block, treatment with pharmacologic quantities of vitamin D or physiologic quantities of 1α-hydroxylated cholecalciferol is required.

Paget's disease is a localized disorder affecting one or a few bones that involve pain and deformity, a greatly increased rate of bone turnover, and bizarre architecture. Its etiology is unknown. Calcitonin is the treatment of choice because it markedly inhibits osteoclastic activity, suppresses pain, perhaps through stimulation of β-endorphin, and has only a few mild side effects (flushing, nausea, and urinary frequency) which decrease in frequency and severity with time.

Hypercalcemia

Some of the conditions producing hypercalcemia are shown in Table 7.8. Primary hyperparathyroidism is a relatively common condition, occurring in about 1:1500 adults (blood donors). It is twice as frequent in women as in men and is most often diagnosed

Table 7.8 Causes of Hypercalcemia

Endocrinopathies	Malignant disease
primary hyperparathyroidism	ectopic PTH production
hyperthyroidism	(lung, kidney)
Addison's disease	osseous metastases
pheochromocytoma	myelomatosis
Vitamin D intoxication	Milk–alkali syndrome
Immobilization	renal calcification

after 40 years of age. Usually (83%) the cause is a benign adenoma, rarely (3%) a carcinoma. In the remaining cases, there is hyperplasia of all four glands. Early on, there are often no clinical symptoms, the disease being detected during routine screening. A high PTH concentration by RIA in the presence of hypercalcemia is diagnostic. The source of PTH may be ectopic tumors, which are especially prevalent in lung and kidney tissue.

Multiple endocrine neoplasia syndromes are sufficiently common that they have been classified into type I (parathyroid hyperplasia with tumors of the pancreas or pituitary) and type II (parathyroid hyperplasia with medullary carcinoma of the thyroid or pheochromocytoma).

In 5 to 20% of patients with thyrotoxicosis, hypercalcemia will occur sporadically. The basis of this is not known, but there is much speculation. Osteoporosis is a well-recognized complication of thyrotoxicosis. Excess thyroid hormone may have a catabolic effect on bone, or it may stimulate the synthesis of adrenergic receptors, thereby increasing PTH secretion following β-adrenergic stimulation. Thus, the increased β-adrenergic activity of hyperthyroidism may blunt normal PTH suppression attending hypercalcemia.

Hypocalcemia

The causes of hypocalcemia are shown in Table 7.9. Urinary excretion of calcium amounts to about 100 mg daily which should, of course, be balanced by absorption of an equal amount from the gut. Absorption of polyvalent cations is, however, poor and variable.

Table 7.9 Causes of Hypocalcemia[a]

Hypoparathyroidism
Pseudohypoparathyroidism
Deficiency of 1,25-dihydroxycholecalciferol (chronic renal failure)
Inadequate dietary calcium
Malabsorption of calcium
Renal failure

[a]Assuming that systemic alkalosis does not exist.

Hence, the present RDA (recommended dietary allowance) for normal adults is 1 g for men or 1.2 g for women. Children and pregnant or lactating women require two to three times this amount. Intestinal malabsorption or failure of the kidney to reabsorb calcium both will produce a negative calcium balance.

Hypoparathyroidism is commonly produced by thyroid surgery, either by inadvertent removal of the parathyroid glands or by interference with their blood supply. Familial hypoparathyroidism, a rare disease, occurs in two forms. Type I is transmitted as a sex-linked, recessive disorder. Usually male children are mildly affected in the first year of life. Type II is attributed to either an autosomal-recessive gene or to an autosomal-dominant gene with variable penetrance. This form, which occurs in adults, is probably an autoimmune disease frequently associated with other endocrinopathies. Circulating antibodies directed against parathyroid, thyroid, adrenal, gonadal, and gastric mucosal cells are present in affected patients. Increased neuromuscular excitability is the most noticeable and potentially dangerous symptom. If the disease is long-standing, there may be epidermal abnormalities, such as dry skin, brittle nails, and chronic monilial infections. In children, the teeth may be discolored and hypoplastic.

Pseudohypoparathyroidism denotes a PTH-receptor disease. In these patients, there is resistance to PTH, i.e., there is hypocalcemia in the face of normal to elevated levels of PTH in the blood. The disease has been subclassified according to cAMP production. In type I pseudohypoparathyroidism, administration of exogenous PTH does not stimulate an increase in circulating or urinary cAMP, as it does in normal individuals. It is probably transmitted as a sex-linked dominant disorder. In type II disease, cAMP production does respond to exogenous PTH, but neither the phosphaturic nor the calcemic actions of the hormone are expressed. These two types represent blocks at different stages of receptor response. The former might be due to defective binding of PTH to its receptor, defective guanine-binding protein, or defective adenylate cyclase, whereas the latter is due to an undefined postreceptor event.

SUMMARY

The unbound calcium ion concentration in the plasma is very tightly regulated, a reflection of its importance in the physiology and biochemistry of the body. Phosphate ion concentration is less rigidly controlled, but it, in general, responds inversely to the calcium ion concentration. In response to a decrease in [Ca^{2+}], both PTH and, indirectly, 1,25-(OH)$_2$CC increase. The PTH acts on the kidney at very low concentrations to increase tubular reabsorption of calcium and to promote excretion of phosphate. It also activates renal 25-hydroxycholecalciferol 1α-hydroxylase, and the production of 1α,25-dihydroxycholecalciferol increases. This steroid hormone acts on the intestinal epithelium to promote absorption of calcium by inducing the synthesis of an unidentified calcium transport protein. Thus, in response to a small decrement in plasma calcium, PTH increases renal retention and the steroid hormone improves intestinal absorption, restoring calcium homeostasis.

If the calcium deficit is somewhat larger and somewhat more sustained, PTH can also draw on amorphous calcium phosphate pools in cells and in perilacunar bone. Only in aggravated deficits, does PTH, with the assistance of the steroid hormone, mobilize calcium from the hydroxyapatite of compact bone. (Because teeth have no analogue of the osteoclast, calcium cannot be withdrawn from dentin or enamel.) Aggravated deficits may occur as a result of a chronic deficit of dairy products or other dietary sources of calcium or because dietary sources are inadequate to compensate for the increased demands attending bone fracture, hemorrhage, pregnancy, or lactation.

Although calcitonin action opposes those of the two mentioned previously, its physiologic function is still ambiguous. Certainly it is not involved in minute-to-minute regulation of plasma calcium concentrations as are the other two. Current speculation has calcitonin responding to sustained calcium stresses, such as pregnancy or lactation, to suppress the otherwise devastating effect of PTH on the skeleton while allowing PTH to stimulate production of 1,25-(OH)$_2$CC and thereby intestinal absorption of calcium.

Even though this simple presentation can explain acute regulation of calcium in normal subjects and some pathologic manifestations, understanding at the molecular level is required for diagnosis and treatment of some diseases. Although progress is obviously being made, knowledge frequently stops short of an adequate explanation. For example, although we know the structure of preproparathyroid hormone and of the gene that encodes the sequence, we do not know what nor how the gene is turned on. We know very little about PTH receptors; they do activate adenylate cyclase. But then what?

Mineralization of the organic matrix of bone is crucial to vertebrate life. As far as we know, hormones play no direct part in it; perhaps that is why it is so slow. Some of the components that may play a role in producing high local concentrations of calcium and phosphate in mineralizing matrix are osteonectin, osteocalcin, and the phosphorylated hydroxyamino acids, serine and threonine. Physicochemical laws are believed to regulate nucleation, growth of the solid phase, and finally crystallization.

SUPPLEMENTAL BIBLIOGRAPHY

Parathyroid Hormone

Antonarakis, SE, et al. β-Globin locus is linked to the parathyroid hormone (PTH) locus and lies between the insulin and PTH loci in man. *Proc Natl Acad Sci USA 80*:6615–6619, 1983.

Brown, EM and GD Aurbach. Role of cyclic nucleotides in secretory mechanisms and actions of parathyroid hormone and calcitonin. *Vitam Horm 38*:206–256, 1980.

Goltzman, D, HPJ Bennett, M Koutsilieris, J Mitchell, SA Rabbani, and MF Rouleau. Studies of the multiple molecular forms of bioactive parathyroid hormone and parathyroid hormone-like substances. *Recent Prog Horm Res 42*:665–697, 1986.

Habener, JF, M Rosenblatt, and JT Potts, Jr. Parathyroid hormone: Biochemical aspects of biosynthesis, secretion, action and metabolism. *Physiol Rev 64*:985–1053, 1984.

Kronenberg, HM, T Igarashi, MW Freeman, T Okazaki, SJ Brand, KM Wiren, and JT Potts, Jr. Structure and expression of the human parathyroid hormone gene. *Recent Prog Horm Res 42*:641–661, 1986.

Vitamin D

Dame, MC, EA Pierce, and HF DeLuca. Identification of the porcine intestinal 1,25-dihydroxyvitamin D_3 receptor on sodium dodecyl sulfate/polyacrylamide gels by renaturation and immunoblotting. *Proc Natl Acad Sci USA 82*:7825–7829, 1985.

DeLuca, HF. Recent advances in the metabolism of vitamin D. *Annu Rev Physiol 43*:199–209, 1981.

Marx, SJ, UA Liberman, C Eil, GT Gamblin, DA DeGrange, and S Balsan. Hereditary resistance to 1,25-dihydroxyvitamin D. *Recent Prog Horm Res 40*:589–616, 1984.

Calcitonin

Amara, SG, DN David, MG Rosenfeld, BA Roos, and RM Evans. Characterization of rat calcitonin mRNA. *Proc Natl Acad Sci USA 77*:4444–4448, 1980.

Guttman, S. Chemistry and structure–activity relationship of natural and synthetic calcitonins. In *Calcitonin* (A Pecile, ed). Excerpta Medica, 1980, pp 11–24.

Lips, CJM, JA van der Donk, et al. The synthesis of calcitonin and β-endorphin by C-cell derived tumors; the possibility of a common precursor. In *Calcitonin* (A Pecile, ed). Excerpta Medica, 1980, pp 45–52.

MacIntyre, I and JC Stevenson. Calcitonin: A modern view of its physiological role and interrelation with other hormones. In *Calcitonin* (A Pecile, ed). Excerpta Medica, 1980, pp 11–24.

Munson, PL, SU Toverud, A Boass, and CW Cooper. Calcitonin: Role during lactation. In *Calcitonin* (A Pecile, ed). Excerpta Medica, 1980, 110–122.

Pecile, A, (ed). *Calcitonin 1984*. Excerpta Medica, 1985, 485 pp.

Miscellaneous

Glimcher, MJ, LC Bonar, MD Grynpas, WJ Landis, and AH Roufosse. Recent studies of bone mineral: Is the amorphous calcium phosphate theory valid? *J Cryst Growth 53*:100–119, 1981.

Godsall, JW, WJ Burtis, KL Insogna, AE Broadus, and AF Stewart. Nephrogenous cyclic AMP, adenylate cyclase-stimulating activity and the humoral hypercalcemia of malignancy. *Recent Prog Horm Res 42*:705–743, 1986.

Price, PA. Vitamin K-dependent formation of bone Gla protein (osteocalcin) and its function. *Vitam Horm 42*:65–108, 1985.

Raisz, LG and BE Kream. Hormonal control of skeletal growth. *Annu Rev Physiol 43*:225–238, 1981.

Toverud, SU and A Boass. Hormonal control of calcium metabolism in lactation. *Recent Prog Horm Res 37*:303–347, 1979.

8

Reproduction

The Gonadoliberin–Gonadotropin-Gonadal Steroid Hormone
System   224
    Regulation of menstrual cycles   224
    Regulation of male reproduction   254
    Melatonin   255
    Prolactin   257
Conception and Pregnancy   258
    Conception and implantation   258
    Placental hormones   259
    Ontogeny   267
    Parturition   273
    Lactation   279
Puberty   282
Steroid Receptors   285
    Activation–inactivation   287
    Transformation   288
    Translocation   291
    Nuclear binding   292
Clinical   293
    Amenorrhea   293
    Testicular disorders   300
    Precocious puberty   301
    Cancer   303
Summary   304
Supplemental Bibliography   310

It is difficult to present an orderly, rational account of reproduction from conception, to adulthood, to conception again, because explanation of any point in this cycle assumes knowledge of the rest. Even though conception is a logical starting point from a chronological viewpoint, relatively little is known about the biochemistry of the events in the fallopian tubes or during implantation and early embryonic development. A notable exception is the chick oviduct, a highly specialized organ. I have, therefore, elected to commence with a description of endocrine control of reproductive processes in adults, a much more thoroughly studied system.

THE GONADOLIBERIN–GONADOTROPIN–GONADAL STEROID HORMONE SYSTEM

Regulation of Menstrual Cycles

Gonadoliberin

Gonadoliberin or gonadotropin-releasing hormone (GnRH, also commonly and somewhat illogically called LHRH or LRH, implicitly denying its FSHRH properties) is a comparatively recent (1971) isolated and synthesized, hypothalamic, hypophysiotropic hormone. Like thyrotropin-releasing hormone (TRH), both the NH_2- and COOH-terminals are blocked.

1   5   10

pyroGlu-His-Trp-Ser-Tyr-Gly-Leu-Arg-Pro-GlyNH$_2$

The sequence Try-Gly-Leu-Arg-Pro may contain a β-turn. The strongest evidence for this is the increased potency (2.4×) of a conformationally constrained analogue of GnRH in which the α-carbon of glycine-6 is linked to the nitrogen of leucine-7 through an ethylene bridge. Another way to stabilize the β-turn is the substitution of a D-amino acid for glycine-6.

Gonadoliberin, like several small peptidic hormones, is synthesized as part of a larger peptide, have a 92-amino acid sequence consisting of a 23-amino acid signal peptide, GnRH, and a 56-amino acid peptide with prolactin release-inhibiting factor (PIF) properties. The two sequences that have hormonal activity are connected, as usual, by a basic dipeptide. This gene product is present in the human placenta and in the human and rat hypothalamus. Active immunization with synthetic peptides derived from the 56-amino acid sequence leads to greatly increased serum levels of prolactin in rabbits, indicating that PIF is important in the control of prolactin secretion. Thus, synthesis of this prohormone could ensure that secretion of gonadotropins and prolactin would be inversely related.

Gonadoliberin binds to plasma membranes. This can be shown visually by treatment of cultured gonadotrope cells with rhodamine-labeled GnRH or, indirectly, by binding experiments with fractionated cells. The Kd varies from about 10 nM for native hormone to 0.2 nM for GnRH analogues. The larger values may be inaccurate because of lack of attainment of equilibrium.

Internalization of GnRH receptors is not a prerequisite for secretion of gonadotropins. The fluorescent, rhodamine-labeled receptors are initially distributed over the cell surface, then aggregate into patches, and subsequently internalize (at 37°C) into endocytotic vesicles. The time course of internalization (10 min), however, makes it unlikely that release of gonadotropin requires internalization. Moreover, release of luteotropin (luteinizing hormone; LH) can be stimulated under conditions that preclude internalization.

Gonadoliberin probably does not act through an adenylate cyclase mechanism. Cholera toxin stimulates cAMP accumulation, but not LH release. Occupancy of the regulatory subunit of protein kinase does not change during incubation of cells with GnRH, and inhibitors of phosphodiesterase do not alter the dose-response curves for GnRH-stimulated release. Even for those few investigators whose work does show a cAMP response to GnRH, the cAMP response does not precede the release of LH. Thus, it is clear that the preponderance of evidence contravenes a cAMP mechanism.

On the other hand, there is considerable evidence supporting Ca^{2+} as the second messenger. Gonadoliberin does not stimulate gonadotropin release in the absence of extracellular Ca^{2+} nor in the presence of drugs that block Ca^{2+} entry. It is important to realize that incubation of cells in Ca^{2+}-free buffer will make the buffer about 0.2 mM in Ca^{2+} (the unbound Ca^{2+} concentration in serum is 1.0–1.3 mM), a sufficient amount to promote GnRH release.

The second criterion of Ca^{2+} as a second messenger is mobilization, either from intracelluar or extracellular sources. This is technically difficult to demonstrate. Measurement of $^{45}Ca^{2+}$ flux is not necessarily a measurement of *net* Ca^{2+} transport. Nevertheless, for what it is worth, GnRH specifically and *rapidly* (1.5 min) stimulates $^{45}Ca^{2+}$ flux preceding measurable LH release, and $^{45}Ca^{2+}$ flux and LH secretion can not be uncoupled.

The third criterion for Ca^{2+} as a second messenger is the dependence of LH release on cytosolic $[Ca^{2+}]$ independent of GnRH. Experimentally this has been demonstrated in three ways. The bacterial ionophores, A23187 and ionomycin, stimulate the release of LH in pituitary cultures in the presence of 1 mM Ca^{2+} in a dose- and time-dependent manner. Further, calcium-bearing liposomes insert themselves into the plasma membranes of pituitary cells and stimulate LH release; neither magnesium-bearing nor monovalent ion-containing liposomes will do this. And finally, veratridine, which activates the sodium channel of electrically excitable cells thus allowing calcium to enter upon depolarization, stimulates LH secretion in cultures. It should be noted, however, that action potentials have been demonstrated only in acidophilic cells of the pituitary.

With this background, you should expect the involvement of calmodulin, diacylglycerols (DAGs), inositol triphosphate, and protein kinase C. Understanding, however, has progressed unevenly. Gonadoliberin provokes the redistribution of calmodulin from the cytosolic fraction to the plasma membrane in the area of GnRH receptor patches. Furthermore, calmodulin inhibitors, such as some antipsychotics and the naphthalene sulfonamides, inhibit GnRH-stimulated LH release with the same potency series that they inhibit calmodulin. Indirect evidence implicates DAG, PI_3, and protein kinase C, but unexplained discrepancies remain.

Gonadoliberin and its analogues have a biphasic effect. Small amounts, especially if administered episodically (every 90 mins), induce a rise in GnRH receptors and promote the release and synthesis of gonadotropins by the gonadotropes of the adenohypophysis. When these same compounds are administered over an extended period, there is down-regulation of GnRH receptors, desensitization of the pituitary to GnRH, depletion of the releasable LH pool, and reduced secretion of LH. Direct interactions of GnRH analogues with Leydig cells or granulosa cells impair their steroidogenic responsiveness to LH or hCG. There is also a suggestion that 5α-steroid reductase and 3α-hydroxysteroid oxidoreductase activities are enhanced by this treatment, hence, 5α-androstane-$3\alpha,17\beta$-diol is formed in the testis at the expense of testosterone.

Native GnRH is susceptible to proteolytic digestion by endopeptidases between the Tyr-5 and Gly-6 and Gly-6 and Leu-7 bonds and by a carboxamide peptidase between the Pro-9 and GlyNH$_2$-10 bond. Placement of an ethylamide at Pro-9–desGly-10 (ProNH-CH$_2$-CH$_3$) and substitution of a D-amino acid at Gly-6 offers considerable protection against degradation and provides superagonist activity. Like other hypothalamic hormones, GnRH has a wide distribution in testis, corpus luteum, CNS, and gut. I am unaware of any extensive interspecies and interphyla comparisons, as yet.

Gonadotropins

Gonadotropins are luteotropin (luteinizing hormone; LH) and folliculotropin (follicle-stimulating hormone; FSH). Again, the names are more restrictive than the hormones, for they both act in males as well as in females. As mentioned in Chapter 5, they are both subunit proteins with α-subunits nearly identical with those of thyrotropin (TSH) and human chorionic gonadotropin (hCG). Specificity resides in the β-subunit which recognizes and binds to the appropriate receptor. No biological effect is seen, however, unless an α-subunit is also present. The LH receptors are subject to down-regulation; FSH receptors have not been as extensively investigated. Both hormones act through an adenylate cyclase mechanism.

Follicle-stimulating hormone, a 34 kDa glycoprotein containing 16% carbohydrate, might more appropriately be called gametotropin, for it acts on both types of gonads. In the ovary in the absence of progesterone, it stimulates the growth of granulosa cells in selected follicles; nothing is known about the process of selection. It also promotes the synthesis of the steroid aromatase enzyme in the granulosa cells as well as that of inhibin and of prolactin (PRL) receptors. In the testes, FSH acts on the Sertoli cells in the presence of testosterone (which requires LH for its synthesis) to promote spermatogenesis, as well as the synthesis of inhibin and of prolactin receptors.

Luteotropin, a 30 kDa glycoprotein containing 2% carbohydrate, stimulates theca interna cells of the ovary to produce androgen which is aromatized to estradiol in the granulosa cells, stimulates progesterone production by the corpus luteum, and causes ovulation 24 to 36 hr after a midcycle surge in all ovulatory cycles. It also increases lipoprotein, PRL, and β-adrenergic recptor formation; downregulates its own receptor, and increases the secretion of plasminogen activator, prostaglandins and relaxin (see p. 275), and mucopolysaccharides. A number of general cell functions, such as glycolysis, protein synthesis, and ornithine decarboxylase activity (synthesis of polyamines) are also increased in primary cultures of rat granulosa cells. In the testes, it stimulates testosterone production by the Leydig (interstitial) cells.

Although prolactin is not considered a gonadotropin, I introduce it here because of its numerous interactions with gonadotropins and steroidogenesis. It plays a definite, but still ill-defined, role in reproduction on both sexes. The most conclusive evidence of its involvement resides in a pathological condition of hyperprolactinemia produced by prolactin-secreting microadenomas of the pituitary. People with such condition may be infertile. Chemical suppression of PRL or surgical removal of the tumor restores plasma PRL levels to normal, and fertility frequently returns.

A glimpse of its functions was obtained from experiments using primary cultures of rat follicular granulosa cells in a defined medium. In this situation, PRL at physiologic concentrations induces the synthesis of LH receptors, stimulates pregnenolone and progesterone biosynthesis, inhibits aromatase activity and estrogen biosynthesis, and promotes the secretion of meiotic maturation inhibitor. In addition it plays a well-defined role in lactation (see p. 279).

Preprolactin was described in Chapter 1 (see Table 1.1), and the relationship of PRL to other members of the somatomammotropin family was discussed in Chapter 4. Human PRL is a 199–amino acid polypeptide containing two disulfide bridges: (Cys-58-SS-Cys-174; Cys-191-SS-Cys-199) homologous to those in STH, and a third that forms a small loop near the NH_2-terminus (Cys-4-SS-Cys-11).

Steroidogenesis

All steroid-producing tissue in the normal adult has the same embryologic origin and the same steroidogenic potential. During differentiation, most of the genomes for steroidogenic enzymes are expressed in both the adrenal cortex and the gonads, but certain ones are repressed to serve the local purpose. (All but the germ cells have a full complement of chromosomes and, one supposes, the potential for steroidogenesis everywhere. Recently, evidence in support of this has begun to accumulate. Stromal cells of adipose tissue from women convert androstenedione to estrone in the presence of glucocorticoid and other serum factors. Even though the specific activity of the aromatase is low, the amount of tissue in obesity can be enormous. Thus, the production of estrogen may contribute to the known relationship between obesity and endometrial carcinoma). As a result, the adrenal has little or no aromatase, and gonads no 11β-hydroxylase or 21-hydroxylase. Hence, it is obvious that all three steroidogenic tissues may produce androgens and estrogens, the amount varying greatly from one tissue to another. In certain tumors, however, derepression occurs, and abnormally large amounts of certain steroids may be secreted.

As is customary in biochemical reactions, the first committed step is often the rate-limiting step and the one that is controlled. In steroidogenesis, this is a side-chain cleavage (SCC) of cholesterol producing pregnenolone and isocaproaldehyde (Fig. 8.1). The hormone promoting SCC differs with the tissue:

Zona glomerulosa of adrenal cortex	Angiotensin II/III
Zona fasciculata/reticularis of adrenal cortex	ACTH
Growing ovarian follicle	LH
Testicular Leydig cells	LH
Corpus luteum	LH

The mechanism also differs because angiotensin receptors do not act through adenylate cyclase, whereas ACTH and LH definitely do.

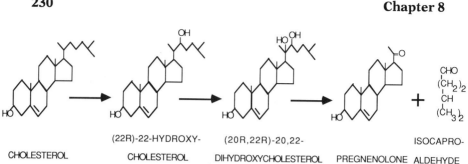

CHOLESTEROL   (22R)-22-HYDROXY-CHOLESTEROL   (20R,22R)-20,22-DIHYDROXYCHOLESTEROL   PREGNENOLONE   ISOCAPRO-ALDEHYDE

Figure 8.1 Side-chain cleavage (SCC), the rate-limiting step in steroidogenesis, is still incompletely understood. It is a mitochondrial reaction promoted by a different hormone in each tissue. The reaction requires a cytochrome P_{450}-containing enzyme, NADPH, and molecular oxygen.

Even though the mechanism of action of ACTH has been more thoroughly investigated than that of LH, it is generally felt that they are comparable. Some of the basic facts are summarized as follows:

1. Activation of cholesterol esterase to supply cholesterol to the mitochondria requires the synergistic action of ACTH or LH and γ_3-MSH (see also Chap. 9).
2. Reaction is very rapid. Corticosterone release from isolated cells can be detected in less than 1 min , in vivo in less than 3 min.
3. The SCC reaction is not blocked by inhibitors of protein synthesis at low concentrations, but it is at high concentrations; inhibitor may be added before or after stimulation with hormone.
4. Cyclic AMP (actually Bu$_2$cAMP) can replace ACTH or LH.
5. At very low doses of ACTH or LH, an increase in the level of cAMP bound to the regulatory subunit of protein kinase can be detected before a measurable increase in cytosolic cAMP.

The synthesis of all these facts leads to the current hypothesis outlined in Fig. 8.2. Through their receptors, ACTH and LH activate adenylate cyclase. Cyclic AMP, in turn, activates a protein kinase which promotes the phosphorylation of a labile protein that turns over very rapidly. The phosphorylated protein stimulates SCC in an undetermined manner. This model requires that the nonphosphorylated inactive form be present in excess.

The side-chain cleavage involves two consecutive hydroxylations at C-22 and C-20 and then scission of the C-20 to C-22 bond to liberate pregnenolone and isocaproaldehyde (see Fig. 8.1). The intermediates have been isolated, and kinetic and $^{18}O_2$ labeling experiments are consistent with this pathway. No further intermediates, such as 20, 22-epoxycholesterol, 20,22-dehydrocholesterol, or the 20,22-ketol, are involved. Lieberman cautions, however, that the hydroxylated cholesterols may be artifacts and that a concerted reaction in an enzyme complex may be the true mechanism of side-chain cleavage.

The steps in the conversion of pregnenolone to androgens and estrogens are well worked out (Fig. 8.3). The order of reactions is still controversial. Historically, the Δ^4-pathway (pregnenolone → progesterone) was described first; later, evidence accumulated that 17-hydroxypregnenolone (the Δ^5-pathway) forms more readily than progesterone except in the corpus luteum.

Figure 8.3 looks more complex than it really is. In spite of the 15 arrows shown, there are only six reactions involved (Table 8.1).

1. The conversion of a 5-en-3β-ol steroid to a 4-en-3-one structure typical of most steroid hormones requires two enzymes. The 3β-hydroxysteroid dehydrogenase uses any C-21 or C-19 steroid with the requisite ring A and B structure. The preferred proton acceptor is NAD^+; $NADP^+$ can substitute, but

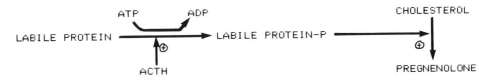

Figure 8.2 A model to explain hormone (ACTH) promotion of SCC. The labile protein is a small polypeptide (20 amino acid residues) with a blocked NH_2-terminus (*Source*: Pederson and Brownie, private communication).

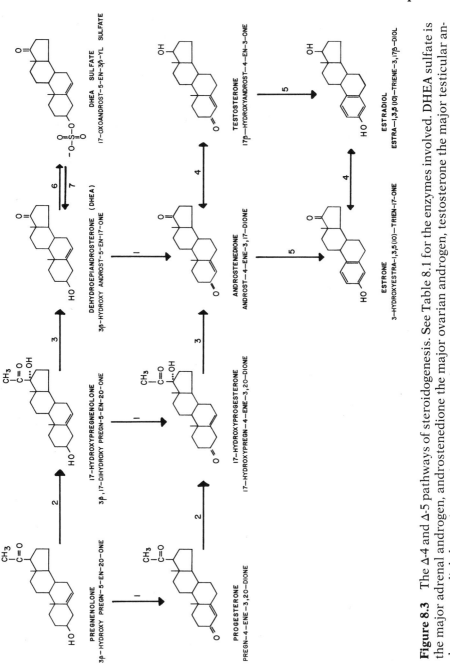

Figure 8.3 The Δ-4 and Δ-5 pathways of steroidogenesis. See Table 8.1 for the enzymes involved. DHEA sulfate is the major adrenal androgen, androstenedione the major ovarian androgen, testosterone the major testicular androgen, estradiol the major ovarian estrogen, and progesterone the major corpus luteal hormone.

Table 8.1 Properties of Steroidogenic Enzymes

Reaction No.[a]	Enzyme	Species	Organ	Location	Cofactor	K_m' (µM)
1	5-En-3β-ol dehydrogenase	Rabbit	Adrenal	SER[b]	NAD⁺	6
		Human	Placenta	SER	NAD(P)⁺	0.2[c]
2	17-Hydroxylase	Rabbit	Adrenal	SER	NADPH	0.4
3	C17–20 Lyase	Many	Testes	SER	NADPH	—
4	17β-Hydroxy-C18-steroid dehydrogenase	Human	Placenta	Cytosol	NAD(P)⁺	0.2[d]
	17β-Hydroxy-C19-steroid dehydrogenase	Guinea pig	Liver	SER	NAD⁺	80
			Cytosol	NADP⁺	200
5	Aromatase	Human	Placenta	SER	NADPH	—
6	Steroid alcohol sulfotransferase	Human	Adrenal	Cytosol	—	1

[a]See Figure 8.3.
[b]SER, smooth endoplasmic reticulum.
[c]K_m, 0.2 µM (pregnenolone); 0.04 µM (DHEA); 0.02 µM (NAD⁺).
[d]K_m, 13 µM (NAD⁺); 1 µM (NADP⁺); 0.2 µM (estradiol-17β).

less efficiently. The product, a 5-en-3-one steroid, is then isomerized by a Δ^5-Δ^4 isomerase. Although the two activities in mammalian tissues are separable, they have never been purified. (The two enzymes have been purified from the oddity, *Pseudomonas testosteroni*.) The dehydrogenase reaction is rate-limiting.

2. 17-Hydroxylase is a mixed-function oxidase (see later) that prefers pregnenolone over progesterone as a substrate. Note that in the rabbit adrenal gland the 17-hydroxylase sites will be 50% occupied at a pregnenoione concentration that will minimumly activate the 5-en-3β-hydroxysteroid dehydrogenase.

3. The C17-20 lyase converts 17-hydroxy-20-oxo-C-21 steroids to 17-oxo-C-19 steroids in the presence of cytochrome P_{450}, NADPH, and O_2. The reaction is not strictly analogous to the C20-22 lyase reaction which does not involve an α-ketol.

4. The 17-hydroxysteroid dehydrogenase is essential for full gonadal hormonal activity. The 17-oxo analogues (dehydroepiandrosterone, DHEA; androstenedione; estrone) have only about 20% of the bioactivity of the corresponding 17β-hydroxysteroids (testosterone, estradiol). Note that the 17α-epimers are inactive in most species. Three different enzymes have been isolated from mammmalian sources as well as 3(17β)-hydroxysteroid dehydrogenase from *P. testosteroni*. From guinea pig liver cytosol, two C-19 dehydrogenases, each with isozyme forms, have been isolated in pure form. One group has a dual coenzyme requirement and specificity for 5β-androstanes, whereas the second group exhibits specificities for $NADP^+$ and 5α-androstanes and 4-en-3-oxoandrostenes. The placental cytosolic enzyme is specific for C-18 steroids. The dual coenzyme requirement enables it to serve also as a transhydrogenase, although the physiological significance of this putative function is not clear. This is the only enzyme of this series available in gram quantities, and detailed structural studies are in progress.

5. The C-19 steroid aromatase is in reality another lyase, different from both the C17-20 and C20-22 lyases. C-10 is a quaternary carbon. Therefore, initially there are two consecutive hydroxylations at C-19. A third is sterically forbidden. Instead, three cleavages occur in concerted fashion between C-10 and C-19, C-1 and H-1β, and C-2 and H-2β, eliminating the C-19 carbon with the H-1β proton as formaldehyde. The C-2 proton enolizes irreversibly, producing a change in conformation of ring A that precludes reversal.

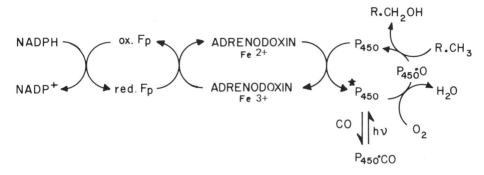

Figure 8.4 Schematic representation of the pathway of electron transport for mitochondrial hydroxylation reactions: Fp, flavoprotein; P_{450}, cytochrome p_{450} (* denotes reduced form); R, substrate.

6. Much DHEA is secreted from the adrenal as a sulfate. Even though some is synthesized directly from cholesterol sulfate, the major pathway involves sulfation of DHEA, 3'-phosphoadenosine-5'-phosphosulfate being the donor of the sulfate group. The DHEA sulfotransferase is a dimer (68 KDa) of two identical subunits having a rather broad specificity for steroid alcohols that have a 5-en-3β-ol or a fully reduced ring A structure.
7. Steroid sulfatases are believed to be ubiquitous. The enzyme from mammalian sources has not been studied extensively.

All hydroxylases are mixed-function monooxygenases requiring a cytochrome P_{450}-containing enzyme, NADPH, and oxygen. On the basis of one or two well-studied systems, it is now believed that all hydroxylases are actually enzyme systems. The best studied is the mitochondrial 11β-hydroxylase system, the components of which have been isolated in pure form. They are an FAD-containing flavoprotein, a nonheme iron protein called adrenodoxin, and a protoporphyrin hemoprotein called cytochrome P_{450} (Fig. 8.4). Cytochrome P_{450} normally absorbs light at 420 nm, but upon inactivation with CO, it absorbs at 450 nm; irradiation with light at 450 nm reverses the inactivation. The reaction of substrate with P_{450} changes the spin state of the ferrous iron in the cytochrome. This can be detected by low-temperature NMR or by spectroscopy in the visible region.

The cytochrome P_{450}s of the smooth endoplasmic reticulum have not been studied as thoroughly. Electron transport is different in that a different flavoprotein that reduces cytochrome c directly is the primary electron transfer agent and a phospholipid facilitates transfer to microsomal cytochrome P_{450}.

Although Figure 8.3 gives one a general idea of what steroids may be produced, Table 8.2 places them on a quantitative basis. Notice that there are no qualitative differences between the sexes, only quantitative ones. Notice, too, that there are no sex differences in the adrenal androgens, DHEA, and its sulfate. Control of their secretion resides in corticotropin-releasing hormone (CRH) and corticotropin (ACTH). These so-called weak androgens are believed to be responsible for stimulation of libido in women.

Biologically, testosterone is the dominant circulating gonadal steroid in men. Women also have some; most of it (57%) is produced by "peripheral" (a deliberately vague term that obscures our ignorance and really means nonsteroidogenic tissue in the classic sense) conversion of androstenedione to testosterone, androstenedione, in turn, being produced in small amounts by the adrenals and ovaries.

Testosterone is not, however, the most potent androgen. In certain tissues, a δ^4-5α-reductase:NADPH enzyme converts testosterone to 5α-dihydrotestosterone (Fig. 8.5). In the rat prostate, this androgen is five times more potent than testosterone. Dihydrotestosterone mediates prostatic growth, growth of facial hair, recession of temporal hairline, and acne, whereas testosterone increases muscle mass, voice changes, and male psychosexual orientation (Table 8.3).

Estradiol is the dominant gonadal hormone in women. Note that estrogens are much more potent on a mass basis than most other steroid hormones so that daily production of a few hundred micrograms suffices. It is barely detectable in the plasma of men, children, and postmenopausal women. Its synthesis, at least in rat, rabbit, and cattle ovaries, is thought to involve a cooperative arrangement between theca interna and granulosa cells whereby LH stimulates the production of androstenedione in the thecal cells. This diffuses across the lamina basalis (basement membrane) and is aromatized in the granulosa cells to estrone and reduced there by 17-hydroxysteroid dehydrogenase to estradiol. Estradiol and androstenedione both leave the ovaries in the venous drainage. Aromatase activity is mainly stimulated by FSH (Fig. 8.6). The applicability of this two-cell, two-gonadotropin model to primates remains unsubstantiated.

Table 8.2 Daily Steroidogenesis in the Normal Adult Human

Steroid	Plasma concentration (µg/L)		Secretion (mg)		Production (mg)	
	Male	Female	Male	Female	Male	Female
DHEA	2–8	2–8	15–50	5–11		23–35
DHEA sulfate	1–20	1–25		10–18		11–19
Androstenedione	1–2	0.3–3	0.9	3.3	1.4[a]	3.3[a]
Testosterone	3–12	0.2–0.5	5–9	0.5–1.1	4–12[b]	0.9–3.7[b]
Estrone sulfate	0.4–0.5	0.8–0.9				
Estradiol	<0.04	0.03–0.5		0.1–0.5		
Progesterone	<0.5	0.5–15				

[a]Peripheral conversion from testosterone: male, 37%; female, 0.7%.
[b]Peripheral conversion from androstenedione: male, 1%; female, 57%.

Table 8.3   Biological Actions of Androgens

Action	Hormone
Stimulate development of spermatozoa (with FSH)	T
Stimulate development of male internal ducts (epididymus, vas deferens)	T
Stimulate development of male secondary reproductive organs: prostate (with PRL), seminal vesicles, scrotum, penis	DHT
Male secondary sex characteristics: increased facial hair, recession of temporal hairline, diamond-shaped pubic escutcheon, sebaceous gland hypertrophy (acne)	DHT
Stimulate growth of axillary hair, libido	DHEA
Hypertrophy of the larynx (voice deepening)	T
Anabolic effects (positive N balance): increase in size of kidney, heart, skeletal muscle, bone growth, epiphyseal closure	T
Moderate retention of sodium, potassium, water, and calcium	T
Behavioral effects: aggressiveness	T
Inhibit LH secretion	T

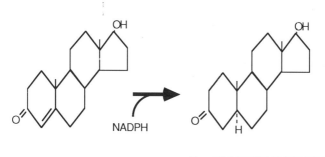

TESTOSTERONE   5 α -DIHYDROTESTOSTERONE

Figure 8.5   Reduction of testosterone to the more potent 5α-dihydro-testosterone by testosterone 5α-reductase.

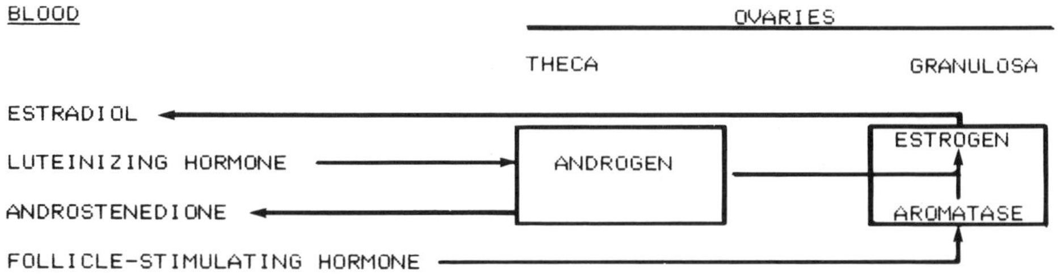

```
BLOOD                                              OVARIES
                                        THECA                    GRANULOSA

ESTRADIOL        ◄───────────────────────────────────────┐
                                         ┌──────────┐      ┌─────────────┐
LUTEINIZING  HORMONE  ─────────────────► │ ANDROGEN │  ──► │  ESTROGEN   │
                                         │          │      │             │
ANDROSTENEDIONE  ◄───────────────────────│          │      │  AROMATASE  │◄─┐
                                         └──────────┘      └─────────────┘  │
FOLLICLE-STIMULATING  HORMONE  ──────────────────────────────────────────┘
```

Figure 8.6 The two-cell, two-gonadotropin model of ovarian estrogen synthesis. It may not be applicable to primates.

The plasma concentration of progesterone in men, children, postmenopausal women, and women in the follicular phase of the menstrual cycle is also near the limit of detectability. It increases more than tenfold during the luteal phase.

The target tissues for these steroids, including the anterior pituitary, are mostly those associated with reproduction (Tables 8.3 to 8.5). Note that estradiol increases gonadotropin synthesis in the pituitary. Note also that testosterone is an anabolic hormone, increasing protein synthesis in selected tissues. Both gonadal hormones have a modest effect on mineral and water metabolism, and both affect epiphyseal closure during puberty. Dogma states that these tissues should have the appropriate receptors, and indeed, they have usually been demonstrated. Steroid receptors are discussed in detail later.

Estrogens have a number of *direct* effects on ovarian granulosa cells in primary culture which have been most extensively documented for the rat (Table 8.4). Probably the most notable are the formation of gap junctions, which may lead to a virtual syncytium, and the synergistic action with FSH in promoting the formation of LH, FSH, and estrogen receptors. It is conceivable that this could produce a positive feedback situation in the dominant follicle, leading to a preovulatory surge of LH and estradiol.

Table 8.4 Biological Actions of Estrogens

Development of female secondary sex characteristics

Initiate mitotic activity in uterus, especially the endometrium, and in vagina; both used for bioassay

Increase synthesis of FSH and LH in pituitary gonadotropes

Stimulus for ovulation (positive feedback)

Decrease LH and FSH secretion (negative feedback)

Cause salt and water retention

Stimulate ductal growth in breasts

Cause epiphyseal closure

Direct effects on rat ovarian follicular granulosa cells in primary culture
  proliferation (antiatretic action)
  increased coupling between granulosa cells through gap junctions
  increased FSH induction of antrum formation
  increased FSH-induced LH, FSH, and estrogen receptor content
  increased FSH-induced cAMP formation, aromatase activity, and pro-gesterone production

Table 8.5 Biological Actions of Progestins

Cause proliferation of uterine endometrium
Large amounts inhibit LH secretion
Decrease excitability of uterine myometrium
Development of lobules and alveoli in breasts primed with estrogens

Regulation

Regulation differs somewhat at the CNS level between primates and rodents. For years, Knobil and coworkers have studied the regulation of the menstrual cycle (28 days) in rhesus monkeys. Their model has three basic components. The arcuate nucleus in the hypothalamus, operating in its basic, unmodulated mode, generates a signal about once an hour, releasing a bolus of GnRH into the pituitary portal circulation. The gonadotropes respond by secreting FSH and LH in a pulsatile fashion. The ovary times the cycle, which is the sum of the duration of follicular development and of the life span of a corpus luteum (ca. 14 days).

In Knobil's most dramatic experiments, he infused 1 μg/min of GnRH for 6 min once an hour into female monkeys with hypothalmic lesions in the medial basal hypothalamus (no endogenous GnRH). In those monkeys that were ovariectomized (Fig. 8.7), administration of estradiol (starting on day 174), operating through a negative-feedback, produced the expected fall in plasma gonadotropins. But within 2 more days, the estrogen in *constant* supply produced a positive-feedback, and LH increased to a dramatic peak at 20 ng/ml. At that point, negative-feedback was reestablished, and LH dropped to low levels. Remember that a constant, pulsatile infusion of GnRH was continued throughout!

In the lesioned monkeys with intact ovaries, constant, pulsatile infusion of GnRH reestablishes normal, ovulatory, menstrual cycles. Thus, the ovary is the dominant *Zeitgeber* (metronome) for the monkey menstrual cycle, estradiol controls gonadotropin secretion by direct action on the pituitary, and the circhoral [approximately (*circa*) hourly (*hora*)] release of GnRH is a permissive, albeit obligatory, component of the control system.

An additional point concerning these experiments should be made for future use. The arcuate nucleus acting as a transducer of neuronal into endocrine signals translates frequency, the language of the nervous system, into hormone concentrations in the plasma, the language of the endocrine system. For example, as the frequency of pulsatile (6 min) injection of GnRH is increased from once in 3 hr to once an hour, the LH concentration

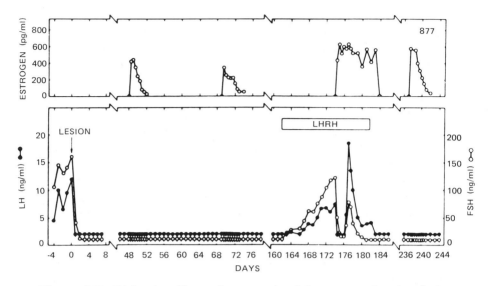

Figure 8.7 Biphasic effect of a sustained increment in circulating estrogen, produced by implantation of estradiol-containing Silastic capsules on day 174, on plasma luteinizing hormone (LH) and follicle-stimulating hormone (FSH) concentrations in a lesioned monkey given replacement gonadotropin-releasing hormone (GnRH) (1 μg/min for 6 min each hour). Estradiol benzoate given before or after the GnRH replacement regimen was ineffective (*Source*: from Y Nakai, TM Plant, DL Hess, EJ Keogh, and E Knobil. *Endocrinology 102*:1008, 1978, reproduced with permission).

in the plasma is increased twofold, whereas that of FSH is decreased twofold. Increased frequency beyond once an hour suppresses the release of both gonadotropins.

There is CNS input to the arcuate nucleus, of course, and the menstrual cycle can be modulated. Suckling completely inhibits it. Stressful situations may upset the cycle, but the mechanism is obscure. Puberty and menopause represent changes that will be discussed later.

At this point, we have sufficient background, at least from an endocrine viewpoint, to review the events of the menstrual cycle. Unless otherwise stated, this summary applies to monotocous (single ovulatory) species, primarily the primates including humans. Striking differences with polytocous species will be mentioned.

Selection of a follicle destined to ovulate is at least a two-step process. *Recruitment* is the process of selection of those few primordial follicles that will grow at the beginning of each cycle from among the thousands present at the beginning of reproductive life. *Selection* is the process whereby one (or occasionally more) follicle is chosen for maturation and ovulation; the fate of all others is atresia. *Asymmetrical ovarian function* is an inherent characteristic of monotocous species.

The process of recruitment is initiated by FSH. The scanty glomerulosa cells in the primordial follicle (Fig. 8.8) start to divide and differentiate and to make LH and PRL receptors and the steroid aromatase complex. These actions of FSH are mediated by activation of adenylate cyclase and cAMP-dependent protein kinase and can be mimicked by choleragen, forskolin (colforsin), and cAMP analogues. Agonists of GnRH inhibit these responses in a calcium-dependent manner and promote phosphoinositide turnover. Phorbol-12-myristate-13-acetate suppresses cAMP formation and the other responses to FSH as well as a rapid and marked decrease in protein kinase C activity, suggesting that the inhibitory actions of GnRH on granulosa cell maturation are mediated by protein kinase C.

The number of follicles recruited is roughly proportional to the exposure to gonadotropins (product of concentration and time) so that supraphysiologic exposure may produce superovulation (>1) (Fig. 8.9). The time span from recruitment to ovulation is inherent in the species as well as the individual, being 13 to 15 days in a "normal" 28-day cycle.

By day 7 of recruitment, two factors point to selection of a "dominant" follicle, even though one may not be visibly apparent

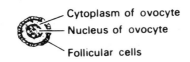

Primordial follicle

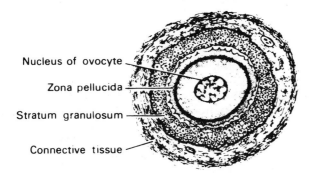

Early unilaminar primary follicle

Multilayered primary follicle

(a)

Figure 8.8   Various stages of folliculogenesis and corpus luteum formation (*Source*: from CR Martin, *Textbook of Endocrine Physiology*. Oxford University Press, New York. 1976, Chap. 21, with permission).

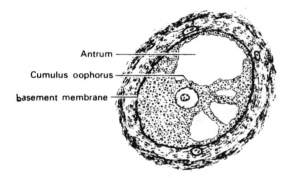

Theca interna
Stratum granulosum
Vesicles
Capillary
Theca externa

Early vesicular or secondary follicle.

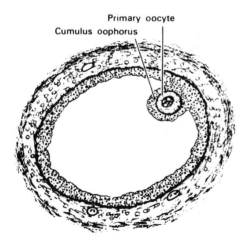

Antrum
Cumulus oophorus
basement membrane

Late secondary follicle.

Primary oocyte
Cumulus oophorus

Mature Graafian follicle

(b)

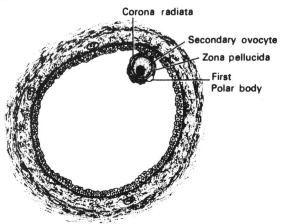

Corona radiata

Secondary ovocyte

Zona pellucida

First
Polar body

Follicle at time of ovulation

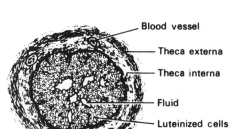

Follicle after ovulation

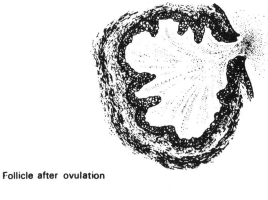

Blood vessel

Theca externa

Theca interna

Fluid

Luteinized cells

Corpus luteum

(c)

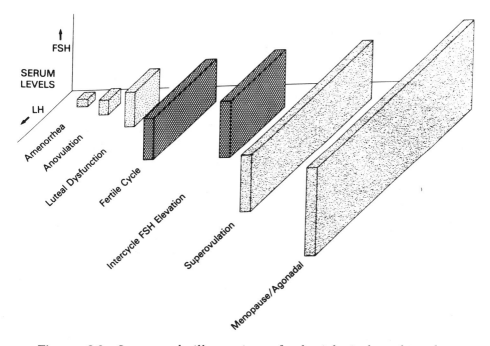

Figure 8.9 Conceptual illustration of physiological and pathophysiological states related to gonadotropin-dependent ovarian function, emphasizing a relative differential threshold to increasing LH and FSH secretion and their synergistic actions (*Source*: from diZerega and Hodgen, *Endocr Rev 2*:36, 1981, with permission).

at that time. Estradiol secretion is significantly higher in the ovary bearing the dominant follicle, and uptake of hCG by LH or hCG receptors on thecal cells surrounding the growing follicle is apparent by day 7. By day 10, the dominant follicle becomes visibly larger than the others.

By means not yet detected, the dominant follicle "rules the roost," suppressing its cohorts in *both* ovaries. Moreover, suppression appears to be irreversible. Removal of the dominant follicle does not allow another of the same cohort to assume that position. Rather, all are apparently already consigned to their atretic fate; a new dominant follicle will be selected from the recruitment of a new cohort of proliferating follicles. In monotocous species, the location of the dominant follicle alternates between the ovaries.

One regulator undoubtedly is folliculostatin or inhibin, apparently a family of peptides made by the granulosa cells and secreted into the circulation as well as into the follicular fluid. α-Inhibin-92 from human semen is easily fragmented into two fragments having 31 and 52 amino acid residues. A β-inhibin-94 that has a different amino acid composition has also been isolated, as has an inhibin from porcine follicular fluid that contains two chains held together by disulfide bonds. All selectively suppress FSH secretion from pituitary cells, with α-inhibin-92 being more potent than the smaller fragments.

Inhibin acts selectively on the gonadotropes of the pituitary to inhibit FSH secretion. Thus, by limiting the follicular FSH surge, the number of primordial follicles recruited may be limited. Inhibin concentration is higher in the follicular fluid of small follicles.

The follicular fluid also contains a large number of chemically uncharacterized activities. These include oocyte meiosis inhibitor and stimulator, luteinization inhibitor and stimulator, FSH receptor-binding inhibitor, and GnRH-like substances. These factors have not been isolated, they do not appear to be steroids (not charcoal-extractable), and they are presumed to be polypeptides.

Follicular fluid, of course, contains androgens and estrogens, the androgen/estrogen ratio being higher in atretic follicles.

In addition, a number of growth factors or hormones may be involved. Both insulin and EGF have receptors on granulosa cells; the affinity (K_d) of these receptors for their ligands is comparable with the concentration of hormone in serum; and these two hormones modulate the response of granulosa cells to the three major pituitary hormones. Gonadoliberin, FGF, SM-C/IGF-I, MSA, OGF (ovarian growth factor), and PGE_2 and $PGF_2\alpha$ have less well-defined, but definite, actions (see Hsueh et al., 1984, for details).

During pregnancy and lactation, cycles cease. This is not due to ovarian refractoriness, for the ovaries remain sensitive to exogenous gonadotropins as evidenced by recruitment. Rather, negative feedback reduces pituitary secretion of gonadotropins.

There are some striking species' differences in folliculogenesis. In polytocous species, initiation of follicular maturation commences at the previous midcycle LH–FSH surge, whereas in monotocous species it does not commence until the corpus luteum and its accompanying progesterone secretion have disappeared. By definition polytocous species possess ovarian symmetry, bicornuate uteri, and multiple dominant follicles. Unlike monotocous species, extinction of dominant follicles leads to their rapid replacement from among the cohort of growing antral follicles.

Folliculogenesis logically leads to ovulation. The initiating event is a surge in estradiol secretion, starting on day -1 or -2 of the cycle. Two time scales are widely used in reporting menstrual cycle data. The classic scale uses the commencement of menses as day 0. Since the discovery that LH causes ovulation and the advent of RIA, the day of the LH surge is taken as day 0 whenever this information is available; the days of the follicular phase are then numbered negatively. Even though the follicular phase lasts statistically for 14 days, individually it may last from 7 days to several weeks.

If the plasma estradiol maintains a critical concentration of about 150 pg/ml for 36 hr, it is followed by a large surge in plasma LH that triggers ovulation 24 hr later. Failure to initiate this series of events produces an anovulatory cycle. None of these events can be explained on a molecular basis.

After extrusion of the secondary ovocyte, now in the second meiotic division, into the abdominal cavity in the vicinity of the fimbriated opening of the oviduct (fallopian tube), the ovocyte is usually swept into the oviduct to start its journey to the uterus. These details are presented in the section on pregnancy. The emptied graafian follicle is rapidly converted into a corpus luteum. (Even though the name means "yellow body," only the corpora lutea of a few primates justify the name, all others being a brownish red.)

The corpus luteum is an independent, endocrine organ most noted for its transience. The duration of its existence is inherent in the species, but interspecies variation is extreme—from 1 to 2 days (rat) to 10 months (roe deer); in humans and monkeys, it is 14 days. The second common characteristic is its ability to secrete progesterone in large amounts—a hormone that changes the uterine endometrium from the proliferative phase (in response to estrogens) to the secretory phase in prepration for the possible implantation of an embryo (see p. 258). A possible relationship to viviparity breaks down when one realizes that in addition to mammals, the reptiles, amphibians, and fish, but not birds, produce corpora lutea; of these, only a few are viviparous.

Luteinization involves a marked enlargement of the granulosa cells, a great increase in the nucleus/cytoplasm ratio, a change from rough endoplasmic to smooth endoplasmic reticulum, a loss of most (and in some species all) of the cells, and extensive vascularization. There is a striking increase in progesterone secretion accompanied by a severe fall (or even loss in some species) in the capacity to synthesize estrogen and androgen, the latter being related to loss of thecal cells in the corpus luteum.

The relationship of progesterone production to trophic hormone stimulation is remarkably variable. In several species including rat, rabbit, hamster, sheep, pig, horse, cow, human, and monkey, granulosa cells maintained in culture luteinize spontaneously and secrete progesterone for several days in the absence of added luteotropins. In vivo, however, trophic hormones are required, at least during a portion of the life of the corpus luteum. For example, hypophysectomy or treatment of rats with LH antisera on day 8 of pregnancy produces abortion unless they are treated for 4 days with a progestin. Luteotropic agents include FSH, LH, PRL, or estrogens, depending upon the species (Table 8.6).

Prostaglandin $F_2\alpha$, ($PGF_2\alpha$) originating from the uterus, has been implicated in termination of luteal function in guinea pigs, pigs, cows, sheep, and perhaps rats; hysterectomy in these species prolongs the luteal life span. The mechanism is not well established, but it is known that there are $PGF_2\alpha$ receptors on the plasma membranes of luteal cells and that the decrease in progesterone secretion is more rapid than the decrease in LH receptors in the pseudopregnant rat, suggesting interference at a later step in progesterone synthesis.

The mechanism of luteolysis in primates is different because hysterectomy does not prolong the luteal life span. Also, there are

Table 8.6 Hormones Required for Luteal Function in Various Species

Species	Length of estrus or menstrual cycle(d)	Luteal life span (d)	Pituitary	Prolactin	LH	FSH	Estrogen
Rat	4–5	1–2	+	+	+	?	+
	(10–14)[a]		+	+	+	?	
Mouse	4	1–2	+	+	−	?	+
Hamster	4	1–2	−	−	−	−	+
	(8–10)		+	+	+	+	
Guinea pig	15–18	12–13	−?		−		
Pig	21	13–15	−	−	−	−	Luteotropic[b]
Sheep	21	13–14	+	+?	+	−	Luteotropic[b]
Cow	21	14–16	+		+		Luteotropic[b]
Rabbit	(17)		+				+
Woman	28	14	−	−	−[c]	−[c]	Luteolytic
Rhesus monkey	28	14	−	−	−[c]	−[c]	Luteolytic

[a]Numbers in parentheses represent length (days) of pseudopregnancy produced by sterile mating.

[b]Not a direct effect.

[c]Required in small amounts throughout the luteal phase for normal luteal life span. An abbreviated corpus luteum can be maintained in the absence of LH and FSH.

Source: reproduced from Channing et al., 1980, with permission.

no changes in luteal $PGF_{2\alpha}$ levels with age of the corpus luteum in women. Two hypotheses, not mutually exclusive, have been proposed. One is based on the established fact that estrogens are luteolytic in primates. The other postulates an LH receptor-binding inhibitor that increases in concentration as the corpus luteum ages.

In summary, events in the menstrual cycle of women are timed by the ovary, which has a preset follicular phase of about 14 days with considerable individual variation (1 to several weeks) and a preset luteal phase of 14 days with, normally, very little variation. Estradiol synthesized in the growing follicles modulates the sensitivity of the adenohypophyseal gonadotropes to GnRH, which is normally released from the hypothalamus in unvarying pulses occurring every 2 hr, day and night. For example, the maximum secretory capacity is 500, 2000, and 10,000 IU of LH every 4 hr in the early and late follicular phases and the day before the LH surge, respectively. Estradiol exceeding its critical concentration of 150 pg/ml for more than 36 hr produces an LH surge (day 0) and ovulation between days 1 and 2 as evidenced by a rise in basal body temperature (Fig. 8.10). The marked increase in progesterone during the luteal phase suggests that ovulation has occurred. Menses follow the decrease in plasma progesterone and estradiol, and the cycle restarts.

A different neural arrangement in the rat regulates the estrus cycle, which is either 4 or 5 days in length depending upon the individual. In female, but not male rats, there is a "cyclic" center in the preoptic–suprachiasmatic area that receives information from the internal and external environment and, in turn, modulates the "tonic" center which includes the arcuate nucleus and medial parts of the ventrochiasmatic area. The tonic center, which is present in both sexes, releases GnRH into the portal circulation.

Many factors affect the estrus cycle in animals. Pheromones are volatile compounds present in bodily excretions (urine, vaginal fluid, etc.) that are detected by the olfactory glands. The first estrus cycle in immature females can be advanced by male urinary pheromones (the male himself need not be present). A group of females cycling randomly will be synchronized by the introduction of pheromones. Even though a neural connection between the olfactory nerve and the cyclic center has not been established, it would be logical to postulate one.

Other examples are reflex ovulators, species (rabbit, cat) in which the LH surge is initiated by the neural stimulus of

---

Figure 8.10 Patterns of hormone secretion in a single menstrual cycle demonstrating the early rise in gonadotropin (FSH and LH). During the second half of the follicular phase, estrogens, androgens, and 17-hydroxyprogesterone begin to rise. Estradiol peaks 1 day before the LH surge (ovulatory cycle). The rise in progesterone during the luteal phase is followed by an increase in basal body temperature. In late luteal phase, steroids decline, presaging the onset of menses (*Source*: from Yen, 1980, with permission).

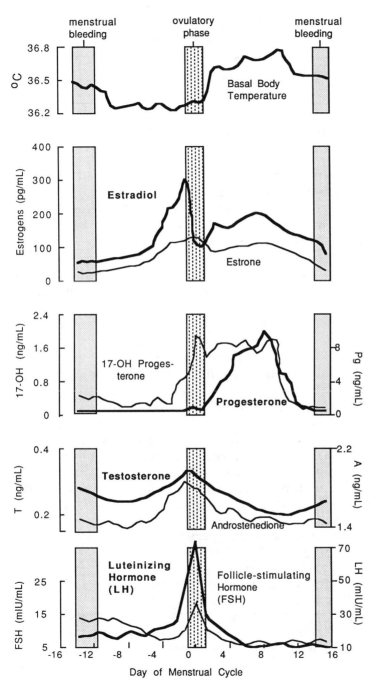

menstrual bleeding

ovulatory phase

menstrual bleeding

Basal Body Temperature

Estradiol

Estrone

17-OH Proges-terone

Progesterone

Testosterone

Androstenedione

Luteinizing Hormone (LH)

Follicle-stimulating Hormone (FSH)

Day of Menstrual Cycle

copulation, and seasonal breeders in which the reproductive cycle of both sexes is controlled by the light–dark cycle. Indeed, even nonseasonal breeders are affected somewhat by lighting which is the reason well-run animal facilities have the light–dark cycle regulated.

Regulation of Male Reproduction

Turning now to reproduction in the male, one finds many similarities and only one major difference, namely, gametogenesis is continuous in males rather than cyclic. The process from spermatogonia to spermatozoa requires 14 days in the rat and 72 days in men. In most species, it requires a temperature of 4°C lower than body temperature which is achieved by having scrotal testes. Testes that fail to descend before puberty remain infertile. In some seasonal breeders, the testes are normally abdominal (and infertile); they descend into the scrotum during the breeding season.

The bulk (95%) of the testes is composed of seminiferous tubules, the epithelium of which is composed of two cell types, the sex cells and the somatic Sertoli cells. The rest of the testicular volume contains interstitial or Leydig cells. The former are sensitive to 37°C temperature, the latter are not.

The Leydig cells, under the direct stimulation of LH and the indirect stimulation of PRL, manufacture mainly testosterone, but also some androstenedione and DHEA and its sulfate (see Fig. 8.3). Most of the steroids are secreted into the capillary blood stream, but some pass directly in high concentration into the neighboring seminiferous epithelium. In analogy with the follicle, there are also many FSH receptors in the seminiferous epithelium. These two hormones, FSH and testosterone, then act through the Sertoli cells on specific stages of spermatocyte development (there are 14 morphologically recognizable steps in gametogenesis in the rat) to promote differentiation.

The Sertoli cells manufacture folliculostatin (inhibin), which inhibits FSH secretion, whereas testosterone from the Leydig cells inhibits LH secretion. Even though the hypothalamus has high concentrations of aromatase, the fact that nonaromatizable androgens, such as dihydrotestosterone (DHT), can suppress LH indicates that androgen-to-estrogen conversion is not a prerequisite for the suppressive action of testosterone on the hypothalamus and pituitary. Moreover, estradiol and testosterone have opposing actions on the pattern of LH secretion in men, the former reducing the amplitude and increasing the frequency of spontaneous LH discharges and the latter increasing the amplitude and decreasing the frequency. Furthermore, the positive-feedback effect of estradiol is more difficult to demonstrate in normal men than in certain hypogonadal states.

In summary, the adult human brain has undergone sexual differentiation. The secretion of LH is regulated by a complex interaction of gonadal steroids and GnRH which differs in detail between men and women.

Testicular spermatozoa (sperm) are incapable of fertilizing mature ova until a maturing process called capacitation is completed. The principal site of capacitation is the epididymis, although in some species further capacitation occurs in the female reproductive tract. The biochemical mechanism of capacitation is not understood.

Melatonin

The pineal gland is the organ that responds to changing photoperiods by modulating the secretion of melatonin. The synthesis of melatonin bears considerable analogy to that of epinephrine (see Chap. 9). An amino acid, tryptophan, is hydroxylated and decarboxylated to produce the neurotransmitter, serotonin (Fig. 8.11). Only the pinealocytes have the capacity to produce serotonin. Much (30%) of it is stored, however, in the sympathetic nerve endings. Serotonin is then N-acetylated by acetyl-CoA, a step with no analogy in epinephrine synthesis, and O-methylated by hydroxyindole-O-methyl transferase (HIOMT) using S-adenosylmethionine (SAM) as cosubstrate during periods of darkness. It is unusual to see the last step in a synthesis the rate-limiting one. Melatonin concentration in the plasma from the confluens sinuum draining the pineal gland is about eight times higher than that in peripheral plasma.

Pinealectomy does not eliminate plasma melatonin, indicating other minor sources of synthesis. These include the retina, harderian gland, and intestine of the rat. Melatonin

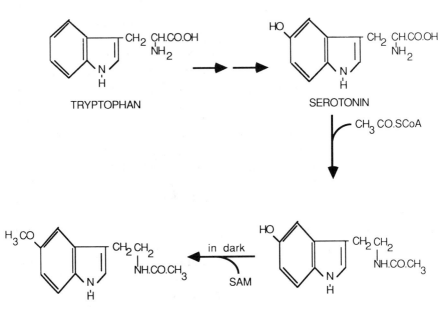

Figure 8.11 Synthesis of melatonin from tryptophan.

rapidly equilibrates with CSF to about 40% of plasma levels. About 60 to 70% of plasma melatonin is bound to albumin; none is bound in CSF.

Regulation of melatonin synthesis is a composite of neural and endocrine inputs. Environmental lighting, acting through the eye in adult mammals and, in part, directly on the pineal in lower vertebrates and birds, markedly suppresses HIOMT activity and melatonin synthesis. Any manipulation causing a major activation of the sympathetic nervous system (presumably through catecholamines) may override the inhibiting effect of light. The neuronal pathway for photosensory information is well defined in the rat at both ends and rather vaguely defined in the middle. In the absence of visual input, a circadian signal, probably arising from the suprachiasmatic nucleus, drives the circadian pineal melatonin rhythm in darkness.

Most of the hormones in the gonadal axis modulate the secretory activity of the pineal gland. Both FSH and LH probably act through the gonadal hormones because pineal receptors include only those for estradiol, testosterone, dihydrotestosterone, progesterone, and PRL. Progesterone decreases and the gonadal hormones increase melatonin syntheses and release, testosterone being aromatized to estradiol the same as it is in other areas of the brain. Prolactin increases HIOMT activity in castrated rats.

A biological function of melatonin is definitely established in seasonal breeders in which short photoperiods increase melatonin synthesis and suppress gonadal function to ensure that the young will be born only in the spring. The mechanisms by which this is accomplished are myriad; thus, it is dangerous to make generalizations. While melatonin treatment can affect STH, TSH, and ACTH release, the physiological significance of these experiments remains to be established.

Prolactin

The hypothalamus controls pituitary release of PRL through both a prolactostatin or prolactin release-inhibiting hormone, widely believed to be dopamine, but which might also be the prolactin release-inhibiting factor (PIF) cosynthesized with GnRH (discussed earlier), and a prolactin-releasing factor (see Table 2.1). Dopamine meets most of the requirements of a hormone: it is present in high (1–30 nM) concentration in rat adenohypophyseal portal blood, its concentration varies with various stimuli and it acts in vitro on isolated pituitary cells. There is, however, only one value for adenohypophyseal receptor binding (K_d, 35 nM). γ-Aminobutyric acid (GABA) is also a candidate as a PIF; its physiological significance has not been assessed. Prolactin also acts in a short-loop feedback to increase the release of dopamine and thereby limit its own release. Estradiol has antidopaminergic activity.

Throtropin-releasing hormone (TRH) and vasoactive intestinal peptide (VIP) are the only isolated hypothalamic peptides demonstrating direct prolactin-releasing action on the pituitary. There is a sleep-associated discharge of PRL occurring usually around 3:00 to 5:00 AM that is believed to have a serotoninergic origin.

Prolactin is another example of an "old" polypeptide that through evolution has changed its biological function. In fish, it primarily regulates salt and water metabolism, a function assumed by aldosterone in humans. In birds and lower mammals, it promotes maternal behavior, such as nest building. In all mammals it, in conjunction with several other hormones, is required for lactation (see p. 279).

The fact that the plasma PRL concentration in men is only a slightly less than that in women has led some to investigate its possible role in men. Indeed, PRL receptors are present in a number of tissues in the rat: prostate, adrenal, kidney, and testes in decreasing order of concentration. Oddly, the highest concentration of PRL receptors occurs in *female* rat liver! Production of anti-PRL antibody in intact mice, rats, or rabbits produces prostatic atrophy. Through its testicular receptors PRL modulates the level of testicular LH receptors. Are these two facts related? The biochemistry of this newest pituitary hormone is just starting to unfold.

CONCEPTION AND PREGNANCY

Conception and Implantation

Millions, or even hundreds of millions, of sperm in seminal fluid are deposited in the female reproductive tract with each ejaculation, another example of extreme redundancy to ensure attainment of a vital goal—perpetuation of the species. (Remember the ovarian counterpart.) In primates and many other mammals, ejaculation occurs in the vagina, and the cervix is the first barrier to the ascent of the sperm. During most of the menstrual cycle, the cervix is coated with a thick, impenetrable mucus. The preovulatory surge of estradiol makes the mucus thin and watery, as well as increasing vaginal secretions. Under these conditions, dozens of sperm traverse the cervix and the convoluted topography of the uterus and enter the fallopian tubes within a few (5–15) minutes of ejaculation. Sperm motility is a prerequisite for a successful transit of the cervix, but the distance covered in the uterus in such a short time dictates that in some way the sperm must be aided by the female reproductive tract.

Conception occurs in the fallopian tubes. Study of this process in mammals is difficult; the most widely used model is fertilization in echinoderms, such as sea urchins. Sperm recognize ova by virtue of receptors located on the vitelline layer (Figure 8.12). The acrosome of the sperm head carries a highly specific protein called bindin that interacts with the receptor. Hundreds of sperm can bind to one ovum. Polyspermy, a fatal condition that occurs if more than one sperm enters the egg, is normally prevented by a very rapid sequence of events initiated by the first sperm to penetrate the plasma membrane (Table 8.7). Within 1 or 2 sec, a membrane potential is created by the influx of sodium ions, producing a partial block. Within 20 sec, a cortical reaction is initiated. Cortical granules lying directly beneath the plasma membrane fuse with it and discharge their contents into the space between the plasma membrane and the overlying vitelline layer. By 60 sec, an impenetrable fertilization membrane is complete. The two nuclei fuse within a few minutes to produce a new individual with the proper number of chromosomes. The first cell division occurs about 100 min later.

Although this scenario occurs in seawater, mammalian conception and the first few cell divisions occur in the fluid of the fallopian tubes. This fluid is mainly a transudate of plasma, only the levels of amylase and lactate dehydrogenase being higher (two and ten times, respectively). Receptors for estradiol have been detected in the fallopian tube.

The developing embryo has progressed to a late morula stage by the time it is released into the uterus (about 3 days in humans). The trophoblastic cells of the blastocyst, the next developmental stage, attach to an implantation site on the uterine wall. From them arise the membranes (amnion and chorion) needed for nourishment of the conceptus and removal of metabolic wastes and for the secretion of pregnancy hormones (hCG, hCS). In the human, implantation occurs about 8 days after conception.

Placental Hormones

In spite of the fact that human chorionic gonadotropin (hCG) shares an α-subunit with TSH, FSH, and LH and has a β-subunit

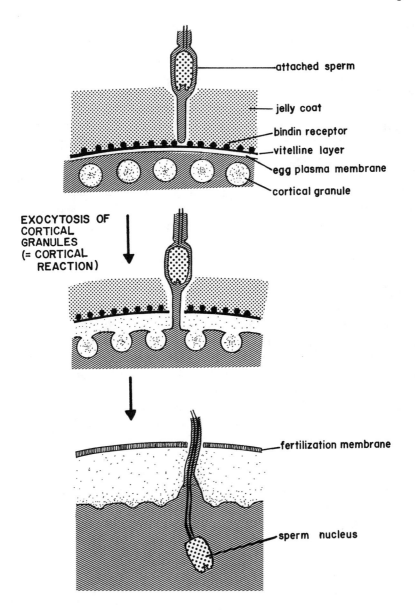

attached sperm

jelly coat

bindin receptor

vitelline layer

egg plasma membrane

cortical granule

**EXOCYTOSIS OF
CORTICAL
GRANULES
(= CORTICAL
REACTION)**

fertilization membrane

sperm nucleus

that is highly homologous with that of LH, it differs from the pituitary hormones in several interesting ways.

1. It is not stored in secretion granules, but is secreted as rapidly as it is made.
2. Concanavalin A stimulates the secretion of hCG and its β-subunit in a dose-dependent manner, but it inhibits the release of the pituitary hormones.
3. Human CG-like activity can be detected by immunological and receptor-binding techniques in nearly all normal autopsy tissues. Its physiological role, if any, in nonpregnant humans is unknown.

The α- and β-subunits of hCG are synthesized separately under the control of separate chromosomes. Synthesis is often unbalanced with production of the β-subunit being rate-limiting. Thus, normal placental extracts contain intact hCG and α-subunit, but not β-subunit, when analyzed by gel filtration and RIA. Mature α- and β-subunits pair in a second-order reaction into an inactive loose complex that slowly refolds in a first-order reaction into the active, stable dimer.

The structure of hCG is shown in Figures 8.13 and 8.15. The α-subunits of the four human glycoprotein hormones are nearly identical, consisting of 89 to 92 amino acids in the same sequence but differing considerably in the carbohydrate portion.

Figure 8.12 A schematic diagram showing the early events in fertilization of a sea urchin egg. Sperm pass through the jelly coat by dissolving holes in it with acrosomal digestive enzymes and bind to receptor sites (bindin) on the vitelline layer. Just below it are thousands of cortical granules that release their contents into the perivitelline space and promote the conversion of the vitelline membrane into an impermeable fertilization membrane, thus preventing polyspermy. These events occur very rapidly (see Table 8.6). [*Source*: modified from *Molecular Biology of the Cell* (B Alberts, D Bray, J Lewis, M Raff, K Roberts, and JD Watson). Garland Publishing, 1983, p. 807].

Table 8.7 Timetable of Events Following Fertilization of an Egg of the Sea Urchin (*Strongylocentrotus purpuratus*)

Time[a] (sec)	Event
2	Minor influx of Na^+; membrane potential change
8	Liberation of Ca^{2+} from intracellular depots
20	Cortical reaction: release of acid and major influx of Na^+
30	Conversion of NAD to NADP
38	Rise in oxygen consumption
60	Formation of fertilization membrane is completed
60–300	Increase in intracellular pH
375	Increase in protein synthesis
400	Activation of transport systems
1100	Fusion of egg and sperm nuclei
1300	Initiation of DNA synthesis
5500	First cell division

[a]Time is measured from the binding of sperm to receptor sites on the ovum.
Source: from Epel, 1977.

```
                     10
H₂N ala.pro.asp.val.gln.asp.cys.pro.glu.cys.thr.leu.gln.glu.asp.pro.phe.phe.ser.
    20                              30
gln.pro.gly.ala.pro.ile.leu.gln.cys.met.gly.cys.cys.phe.ser.arg.ala.tyr.pro.
    40                 50        52
thr.pro.leu.arg.ser.lys.lys.thr.met.leu.val.gln.lys.asn(CHO).val.thr.ser.glu
         60                         70
ser.thr.cys.cys.val.ala.lys.ser.tyr.asn.arg.val.met.gly.gly.phe.lys.
    78    80                         90
val.glu.asn(CHO).his.thr.ala.cys.his.cys.ser.thr.cys.thr.thr.his.lys.ser.OH
```

Figure 8.13 α-Subunit sequence of hCG, which is nearly identical to that of FSH, LH, and TSH. The structure of the carbohydrate (CHO) units is shown in Figure 8.15 (*Source:* from Hussa, 1980, with permission).

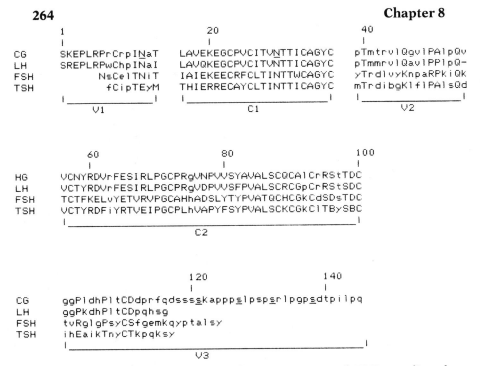

Figure 8.14 β-subunit sequences of CG, FSH, LH, and TSH are aligned for maximum correlation. Upper-case letters represent strongly conserved positions. Vl, V2, and V3 indicate variable regions of sequence homology while C1 and C2 indicate constant regions. Carbohydrate is attached at the underlined positions (see Fig. 8.15) (*Source*: from Hussa, 1980, with permission).

Although the β-subunits naturally differ enough to account for the unique immunological and biological activities of each, there is still extensive homology with two constant regions (Fig. 8.14). Luteotropin and hCG, which share biological activities, have an 80% homology in the first 115 residues. The sequence Cys-Ala-Gly-Tyr (residues 34 to 37 of hCG), found in all four β-subunits, is also present in serine proteases. This common sequence creates problems in producing immunological specificity.

Each subunit of hCG contains two asparagine-linked complex-type oligosaccharides. In addition, there are four simple oligosaccharides linked *O*-glycosidically to serine residues in the unique COOH-terminal sequence of hCG (Fig. 8.15).

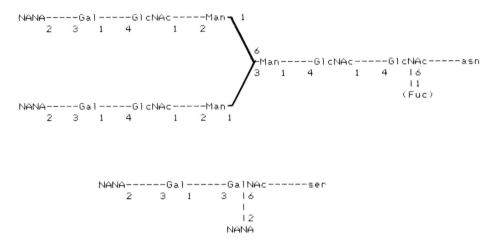

Figure 8.15 Structure of carbohydrate units of hCG. Top: *N*-glycosidic units attached to asparagine-52 and -78 of hCGα and -13 and -30 of hCGβ. L-Fucose is found in hCGβ only. Bottom: *O*-glycosidic units attached to serine-121, -127, -132, and -138 of hCGβ (*Source*: from Hussa, 1980, with permission).

The control of hCG secretion is not understood. Human chorionic gonadotropin is detectable in plasma within a few days of implantation. Indeed, it is the basis of the best test for pregnancy (an immunoassay for hCGβ). By the tenth week of pregnancy, the concentration of hCG in plasma is impressive; it then subsides to a high plateau. Some investigators have found a GnRH-like immunoreactivity in maternal serum, cord serum, and amniotic fluid. Natural or synthetic GnRH can stimulate the release of hCG, both in vivo and in vitro, in certain, but not all, choriocarcinoma cell lines.

A second pregnancy hormone is human chorionic somatomammotropin (hCS) (see Chap. 4), also called placental lactogen. The principal role of hCS may be its action as an insulin antagonist. It may also be responsible for the development of diabetic ketoacidosis in pregnant women who normally are not diabetic. Because the plasma concentration of hCS is proportional to the mass of the placenta, it is widely used as a test of placental function. The rate of secretion (1 g/day at term) is the greatest of any protein hormone in humans, accounting for 10% of all placental protein production at term. The regulation of hCS secretion, if any, is unknown.

Placental ACTH has never been isolated in pure form, but by virtue of selective RIAs and gel filtration, it is apparent that the placenta can make proopiomelanocortin, the precursor of ACTH, β-lipoprotein, β-endorphin, and α-MSH (see Chap. 9 for details). The relative proportions of these four peptides are more similar to those of an intermediate lobe of the pituitary than to those of an anterior lobe in which the major products are ACTH and β-lipoprotein. Corticotropin probably cannot cross the placental barrier.

Steroid hormone production by the fetoplacental unit is remarkable. In pregnant women at or near term, there is a daily production of 15–20 mg estradiol, 50–100 mg estriol, 250–600 mg progesterone, 1–2 mg aldosterone, and 3–8 mg deoxycorticosterone. Because the placenta lacks a 17-hydroxylase, the C-21 to C-19 conversion is impossible there; a cooperative effort with the fetus, however, circumvents this block.

The human placenta produces two principal steroid hormones, progesterone and estrogen; the latter is mostly estriol but also some estradiol and estrone are produced. The placenta does not become the dominant source until the eighth week of gestation. Before this time, hCG produced by the trophoblasts stimulates the corpus luteum to produce progesterone and estradiol.

Progesterone biosynthesis from low-density lipoprotein (LDL) cholesterol in the maternal plasma is autonomous, limited only by the number of LDL receptors on the surface of the trophoblasts. Neither the addition of hCG nor of anti-hCG antibody to cultured cells modifies the rate of secretion. De novo synthesis is low because of the low specific activity of hydroxymethylglutaryl (HMG)-CoA reductase, the rate-limiting enzyme in cholesterol biosynthesis. The cholesterol ester content of placental tissue is also low because progesterone inhibits acyl-CoA: cholesterol acyl transferase. Therefore, it is apparent that maternal LDL cholesterol is converted to pregnenolone and progesterone as rapidly as it is taken up by the trophoblasts. The principal roles of progesterone in pregnancy are its anesthetic effect on the uterine myometrium and suppression of lactation (see p. 279).

The capacity of the placental trophoblasts to convert androgens to estrogens is so great that the placental aromatase cannot be saturated, i.e., production of estrogen is solely dependent upon the supply of precursor C-19 steroids. The latter are supplied, principally as dehydroepiandrosterone (DHEA) sulfate, by both the maternal and fetal adrenals. The fetal liver and, to a lesser extent, the fetal adrenal gland extensively hydroxylate dehydroepiandrosterone sulfate, forming 16α-hydroxyDHEA sulfate. In the placenta, the sulfate conjugate is hydrolyzed and both DHEA and 16α-hydroxyDHEA aromatized to estradiol and estriol, respectively.

The fetal adrenal is quite different from the adult adrenal gland. The fetal gland consists of a small zona glomerulosa or definitive zone and a large inner fetal zone; the zona fasciculata and zone reticularis are missing, and the medulla consists merely of clumps of medullary cells. The definitive zone under the stimulation of ACTH produces the normal complement of steroid hormones, i.e., cortisol, deoxycorticosterone, corticosterone, and aldosterone. The fetal zone produces principally DHEA sulfate and smaller amounts of 16α-hydroxyDHEA sulfate. The relative importance of several alternate routes of synthesis (Fig. 8.16) is not known.

Ontogeny

Ontogeny, the development of a complex organism from a single cell, is a fascinating and incompletely understood subject. Here we shall follow only phenotypic sexual development. Central dogma states that sexual differentiation is a sequential, ordered, and relatively simple process (Figure 8.17).

Chromosomal sex refers to the sex chromosomes which are XY in males and XX in females. In the human there are also 22 pairs of autosomes, portions of which also contribute to sexual development. The two keys to understanding sexual development are as follows:

1. Male development occurs a few weeks earlier than does female (Fig. 8.18).
2. Feminine development is innate unless a positive signal for male development intervenes.

A short arm of the Y chromosome normally carries such a signal, a gene specifying a cell surface antigen termed the H–Y antigen. At 5 to 6 weeks of age, the embryonic gonads are indifferent, i.e., they appear identical in XX and XY fetuses and consist of three compartments: the primordial germ cells, the connective tissue of the genital ridge, and a covering layer of epithelium. Under

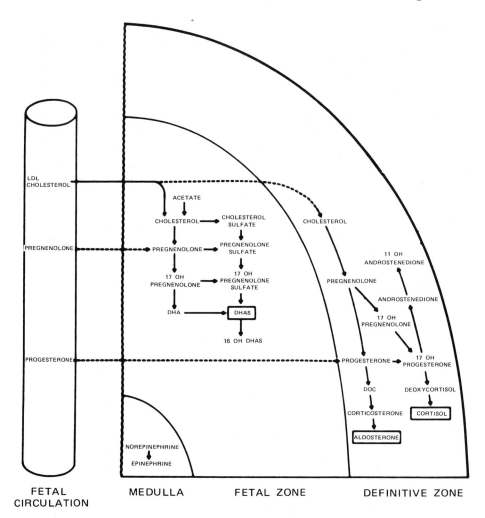

Figure 8.16 Schematic depiction of pathways of hormone formation in the human fetal adrenal gland. [Reproduced, with permission, from the Annual Review of Physiology *43*: 141,   1981 in an article by M. Seron-Ferre and RB Jaffe]

CHROMOSOMAL SEX -------> GONADAL SEX -------> PHENOTYPIC SEX

Figure 8.17 The Jost model for sexual differentiation.

the influence of the H–Y antigen, the germ cells of the potential testes line up to form spermatogenic cords, and shortly thereafter Leydig cells appear in the connective tissue. On the other hand, fetal ovaries develop at about the sixth week of gestation.

Regardless of sex, the embryo has two internal duct systems: wolffian and mullerian (Fig. 8.19). In the male, the wolffian ducts develop and the mullerian ducts disappear; in the female, the mullerian ducts develop, however the embryonic wolffian ducts

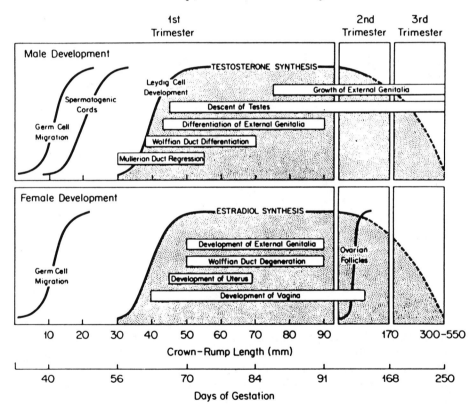

Figure 8.18 The temporal relationship during sexual differentiation in a human embryo (*Source*: from Wilson et al., 1981, with permission).

INDIFFERENT STAGE

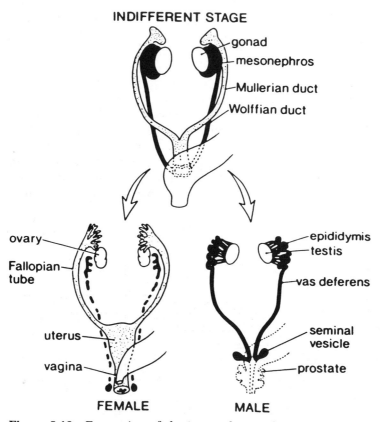

Figure 8.19 Formation of the internal genital tract in male and female embryos (*Source*: from Wilson et al., 1981, with permission).

do *not* disappear. The mechanism involves release of an antimullerian duct hormone, a 124 kDa glycoprotein dimer, by the testicular Sertoli cells that causes involution of the mullerian duct system. This hormone is not species-specific. Shortly thereafter, the Leydig cells stimulated by hCG commence secretion of testosterone, which causes virilization of the wolffian ducts. The upper portion forms the epididymis, the central portion develops a thick muscular coat to become the vas deferens, and the terminal portion becomes the ejaculatory duct and seminal vesicles. Simultaneously, the prostate gland arises from endodermal buds appearing in the lining of the primitive urethra. If no signals are received (female or an abnormality in a male), the mullerian ducts develop into the fallopian tubes, uterus, and upper portion of the vagina (see Fig. 8.19).

In contrast to the internal organs of reproduction, the external genitalia of both sexes arise from a common anlage (Fig. 8.20). The external genitalia of the female enlarge but undergo little change, whereas in the male, androgen prompts the genital folds to fuse and elongate to form the penis and urethra and the genital swellings to fuse to form the scrotum. Differentiation is largely completed by the end of the first trimester. In the latter part of gestation, two aspects of male development are completed: namely, descent of the testes (in some instances this may finish after birth) and accelerated growth of the genital tract. Thus, both antimullerian hormone and testosterone must be secreted by the testes at a critical period in utero for the proper sexual development of the male.

One further step is required in certain androgen target tissues to attain complete masculine development. In the anlage of the external genitalia, testosterone serves as a prohormone, being converted by a microsomal steroid 4-ene-5α-reductase to 5α-dihydrotestosterone. Failure to carry out this conversion produces male pseudohermaphrodites (XY males with a female phenotype). In the wolffian duct, however, synthesis of 5α-dihydrotestosterone does not occur until differentiation is completed.

One may ask, in view of the sensitivity of the developing fetus to steroid hormones, why the relatively enormous amounts of hormone being produced by the fetoplacental unit usually have so little effect. The answer lies in the conjugation (mainly sulfation) of most of the steroid produced; conjugates are biologically inactive.

Differentiation is a multifactorial process under complex genetic control. The Y chromosome is involved in testicular differentiation from the bipotential gonad through the action of the H–Y antigen. From human subjects in whom inherited deficiencies have occurred, it appears that the enzymes involved in testosterone and dihydrotestosterone biosynthesis are regulated

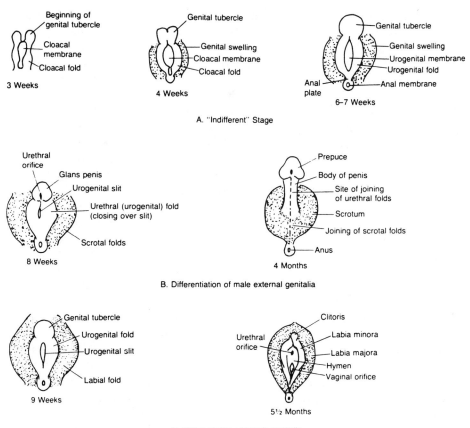

Figure 8.20 Formation of the external genitalia in male and female embryos (*Source*: from Wilson et al, 1981, with permission).

by autosomal genes. Inherited forms of antimullerian hormone deficiency (either synthesis or action) are transmitted as a recessive trait, either autosomally or X-linked. From linkage studies in *Tfm/y* mice, we know that genes (either structural or regulatory) located on the X chromosome control the cytoplasmic receptor at androgen-dependent target areas. Thus, normal male phenotypic development is regulated by gene loci on autosomes as well as on both X and Y chromosomes.

And finally, portions of the brain also undergo sexual differentiation. The evidence in humans is weak, but it does fit with exhaustive experiments with rats. The rat is unusual in that sexual differentiation of the CNS occurs during the first 4 days after birth. In most other species, including man, this event occurs in utero.

Again, the basic neural substrates of reproductive function are female, and functions recognized as typical of the male are the consequence of androgen-directed sexual differentiation. Control of *cyclic* gonadotropin secretion resides in the preoptic area of the hypothalamus (Fig. 8.21). Afferent nerve fibers proceed from this area to the region of the ventromedial hypothalamus which possesses *tonic* activity. The output of GnRH from the latter area is more or less constant (but episodic), unless the output of the cyclic center is superimposed on it. Testosterone, either endogenous or exogenous, in the first 4 days of life in the rat obliterates the cyclic center. At puberty, the recipient rat, if female, goes into constant estrus and has polycystic ovaries as a result of the constant high level of gonadotropin and estradiol secretion.

It is somewhat odd that CNS androgenization requires aromatization of testosterone to estradiol. Administration of estradiol to female rat pups, therefore, has the same masculinizing effect as testosterone. Because the ovaries of female rat pups actively secrete estradiol during the perinatal period, one must ask how they escape androgenization. The answer lies in the production of large amounts of α-fetoprotein by neonatal rats, a plasma protein that binds estrogens much more effectively than androgens.

Parturition

It is axiomatic that a quiescent uterus and a tightly contracted cervix are required throughout gestation, whereas a contracting uterus and dilated cervix are prerequisites for delivery. The role of many factors in parturition have been investigated: the role of the fetus and its pituitary–adrenal function; of progesterone,

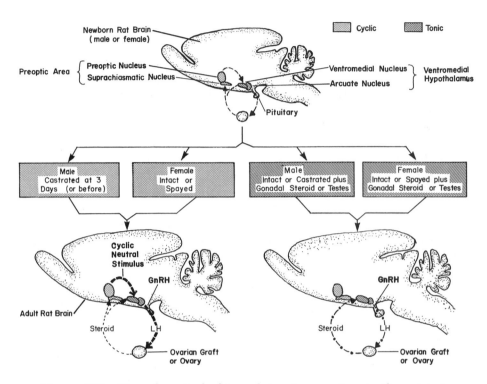

Figure 8.21 Neural control of gonadotropin secretion in the rat is inherently cyclic and remains so unless gonadal steroid (estrogen or androgen) is present during the neonatal period (center). Control of cyclic release (left) resides in the preoptic area of the hypothalamus. In the absence of input from this area to the ventromedial hypothalamus, secretion is tonic (*Source*: fom Gorski, 1980, with permission).

estrogen, relaxin, oxytocin; and of prostaglandins. Species variation, the lack of a dominant role by any one substance or, put differently, the complexity of interplay among some of these hormones, and the lack of adequate data have precluded the synthesis of tenable, integrative hypothesis of the control of parturition. The alternative, then, is the recitation of fragmentary bits of evidence which, for the moment, lead nowhere. Before starting, however, we should quickly review two subjects new to us.

Relaxin

Even though the effect of relaxin was discovered in 1926, little work was done on it until 1972. Now it is a respectable, putative hormone involved in the remodeling of collagen in the reproductive tract, making it potentially significant in ovulation, parturition, and sperm transport.

Relaxin is a chemically defined ovarian polypeptide in three species (pig, rat, and shark) (see Fig. 4.3) which resembles insulin (23% homology for pig and rat relaxins). Interestingly, shark relaxin, presumably little changed in 500 million years, resembles porcine insulin more than porcine relaxin does!

Analysis of rat relaxin cDNA has led to the structure of preprorelaxin. The surprising finding is the size of the connecting peptide (Fig. 8.22). In spite of the variation in size of the connecting peptides of relaxin, insulin, and IGF, the tertiary structure of the three prohormones must be very similar because the same disulfide bonds form, connecting opposite ends of the prohormone.

The corpus luteum of gestation is the only known prolific source of relaxin, although it has been detected in ovarian follicles and follicular fluid, placenta and decidua, prostate and seminal fluid, and perhaps, in the uterus.

The biological roles of relaxin may be divided into two classes: the acute effects, such as induction of quiescence in smooth muscle; and the more chronic effects, such as its role in collagen metabolism. Little will be said about the former except to speculate that relaxin may somehow alter the Ca^{2+} flux in smooth muscle.

The effect of relaxin on collagen metabolism has been extensively investigated. Indeed, the original bioassay is based on the observation that relaxin causes an elongation of the collagenous interpublic ligament and the separation of the pubic bones. This is essential to the safe delivery of the young in those species in which large, mature fetuses are born. In women, the pubic bones separate as much as 10 mm at term.

Relaxin has several effects. In the uterus, it produces quiescence, as noted earlier, and increased collagen and glycogen content. Myometrial receptors for relaxin have been characterized in the rat and the pig. Interrelationships with other

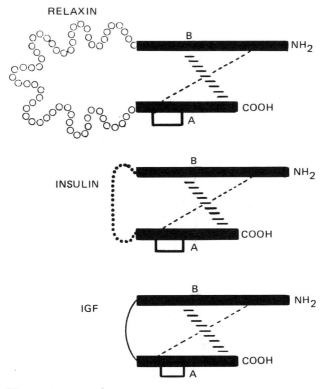

Figure 8.22 A diagrammatic representation of the prohormone structures of relaxin, insulin, and IGF. Note that the major differences lie in
the size of the connecting peptides. The A and B chains have considerable
species homology with three disulfide bonds located in nearly identical
positions (*Source*: from Bryant-Greenwood, 1982, with permission).

hormones are incompletely understood. In the cervix, relaxin
plays a major role, together with other hormones (estrogens, progesterone, and prostaglandins), in increasing collagen synthesis
(with no change in tensile strength) leading to increased disten-
sibility of the cervix at parturition in many mammals.

Prostaglandins

Some endocrinologists classify prostaglandins (PGs) as hormones, whereas others, citing the almost complete inactivation of PGEs and PGFs in one passage through the lungs, consider them as paracrine substances. In any event, the rate-limiting event in PG synthesis is the release of arachidonic acid (all cis-5,8,11,14-eicosatetraenoic acid) from the C-2 carbon of phospholipids by lysosomal phospholipase A_2. The control of this enzyme is still the subject of many investigations.

Arachidonic acid is oxidized in successive steps to form a series of substituted cyclic fatty acids (Fig. 8.23). The cyclooxygenase step (step 1) can be inhibited by a number of drugs, including aspirin and indomethacin. The products are lettered according to the ring structure, and the substituents on it are numbered according to the number of double bonds in the fatty acid. Each class has specific actions on smooth muscle, platelet aggregation, or renin release, some opposing the actions of others. Prostacyclin (PGI_2) and the thromboxanes (TxA_2 and TxB_2), the newest discoveries, are particularly potent compounds.

Parturition

In sheep, the fetus through the activity of its pituitary–adrenal axis determines the timing of its own birth. Corticotropin and cortisol rise sharply just before birth. (Maternal ACTH does not cross the placenta.) Fetal hypophysectomy prolongs pregnancy and is associated with a failure of fetal plasma cortisol to rise and of maternal plasma progesterone to drop. Infusion into the fetus of either ACTH or dexamethasone induces delivery of the hypophysectomized fetal lamb, concomitant with the normal fall in maternal plasma progesterone.

In primates, the pituitary–adrenal axis matures during the second half of gestation, but the production of cortisol appears to modulate (rather than initiate) the timing of delivery. Anencephalic infants, who have involuted adrenals, have a normal gestational length, although the spread of values is significantly greater than for normal infants.

In some species, progesterone maintains uterine quiscence through suppression of the spontaneous generation and propagation of action potentials. The myometrium is refractory to stimulation by oxytocin, $PGF_2\alpha$, or an extrinsic electrical field. These variables define the excitability of a contractile cell that characteristically rises with the onset of parturition. A decrease

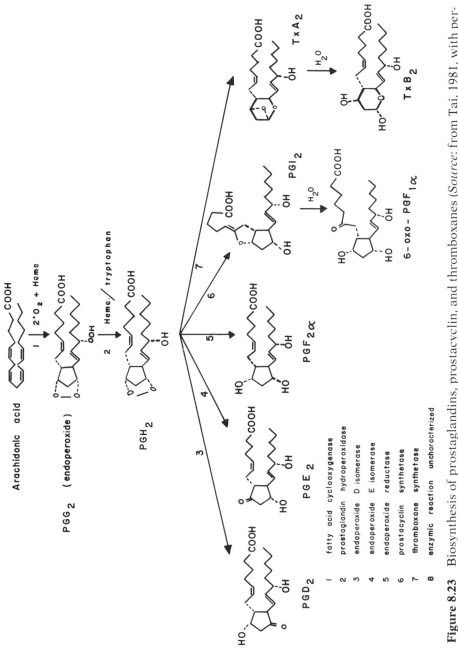

Figure 8.23 Biosynthesis of prostaglandins, prostacyclin, and thromboxanes (*Source*: from Tai, 1981, with permission).

in plasma progesterone concentration and withdrawal of the progesterone block precedes parturition in some species (e.g., rabbit). In primates, however, plasma progesterone may not decrease until delivery of the placenta.

During late pregnancy, estrogens may stimulate uterine contractility through protein synthesis, especially that of contractile protein, through an increase in the number of oxytocin receptors, and following progesterone in an increase in prostaglandin synthesis. In women with placental sulfatase deficiency and low estrogen production, pregnancy is prolonged. Moreover, the cervix is small and contracted. In one study, administration of estrogen stimulated uterine contractility but not labor. Currently, the evidence for the involvement of estrogen in human parturition is only suggestive.

Relaxin is involved in parturition in some species. In human pregnancy, however, plasma relaxin concentrations tend to be higher in early pregnancy than in the second and third trimesters. There is no peak at the time of delivery. Therefore, it does not seem likely that relaxin is actively involved. An increase in the number of relaxin receptors would be equivalent to an increase in relaxin concentration. This, however, has not been measured.

In spite of the widespread use of oxytocin (see Chap. 6) to initiate or augment labor, the role of oxytocin in initiation of parturition remains obscure. It may be that the role of oxytocin is to ensure uterine involution once the products of conception have been delivered.

Prostaglandin synthesis may represent a common final pathway responsive, in still poorly defined ways, to the steroid and polypeptide hormones discussed earlier. At the time of parturition, PGE and PGF increase in the amniotic fluid and uterine venous blood, and a metabolite, 13,14-dihydro-15-oxoPGF$_2\alpha$, increases in the peripheral blood. Drugs that inhibit PG synthesis prolong gestation, and PGs have been used for induction or augmentation of labor at term or for induction of midtrimester abortion. Control of PG synthesis reduces to control of phospholipase A$_2$ activity, and although the current thinking suggests that control centers mainly in the fetal membranes, there is no compelling evidence concerning the mechanism by which it occurs.

Lactation

Following birth, a successful outcome of pregnancy in many cultures depends upon lactation. The mammary gland is a complex organ requiring many hormones for its preparation and function. There are, moreover, marked species' variations. In organ culture, insulin and glucocorticoid are indispensable for maintaining viability, growth, and differentiation, and STH is required for maximum response; thyroid hormones play a permissive role. Various undefined epithelial growth factors may be important. In vivo, estrogens promote development of the duct system and perhaps, in conjunction with progesterone, the lobuloalveolar system as well. During pregnancy, further development occurs under the influence of prolonged elevated levels of estrogens, progestins, and prolactin. Adipose tissue is replaced by epithelial components, and milk synthesis is inhibited by progesterone.

The major milk proteins are casein and α-lactalbumin. Prolactin alone can stimulate the synthesis of these proteins by a poorly defined mechanism. The number of PRL receptors in the mammary gland increases dramatically ($20\times$) at the time of parturition and nursing. A portion of the increase may be due to a release of a progesterone block, whereas the rest may be explained by the increase in plasma PRL in response to suckling and by the self-induction of PRL receptors by PRL.

Although the mechanism of PRL action is not known, it is clear that cAMP is *not* an intermediate and that the stimulation of synthesis probably occurs at the transcriptional level. The intermediate steps are obscure. Prolactin binds to a plasma membrane receptor, and much of it is internalized and degraded. Whether or not this is a required step in its action is not known. Prostaglandins, which may be involved as PGB_2, PGE_2, or $PGF_2\alpha$, stimulate RNA synthesis in murine mammary gland explants in a PRL-like manner, and indomethacin blocks the stimulatory effect of PRL. Prostaglandins alone cannot, however, mimic the effect of PRL on casein synthesis; a combination of prostaglandins and polyamines (e.g., spermidine) is required. Mitoguazone [methylglyoxal bis(guanylhydrazone)], an inhibitor of polyamine synthesis, abolishes the stimulation of casein synthesis by PRL. Furthermore, PRL stimulates the synthesis of ornithine decarboxylase, an enzyme involved in polyamine biosynthesis (ornithine$\rightarrow$putrescine) in mammary gland organ cultures.

Protein phosphorylation may also be important in PRL action. Prolactin induces the synthesis of cAMP-dependent protein kinases (inhibited by actinomycin D or cycloheximide). Extensive phosphorylation of proteins in the plasma membrane, ribosomes, and nucleus occurs with lag periods of 8 to 24 hr after addition of PRL. Thus, as a working hypothesis, one might suggest that PRL stimulates RNA synthesis through the combined action of prostaglandins and polyamines. This leads to the formation of protein kinases that then activate many functional proteins and to gene expression by phosphorylation that, in turn, further stimulates RNA synthesis, including the mRNAs, for milk proteins.

The lactose synthetase system, which is unique to mammary glands, catalyzes the formation of lactose. It consists of two subunits, A and B, the former being the enzyme galactosyltransferase and the latter, the milk whey protein α-lactalbumin, the regulatory subunit. The concentration of the B-subunit increases dramatically at parturition because its synthesis, which is stimulated by a combination of PRL and T_3, is suppressed by progesterone.

Prolactin also has many other effects in the mammary gland. It increases the synthesis of lipoprotein lipase, thus allowing the gland to utilize triglycerides in chylomicrons. It, along or in combination with insulin and glucocorticoid, stimulates the synthesis of fatty acids, especially the short-chain (C_8 and C_{10}) fatty acids. This is important because the absorption of short-chain triglycerides is much simpler than that of long-chain triglycerides, and the newborn are lacking some of the enzymes required for absorption of the latter. The major ions in milk are Na^+, K^+, Ca^{2+}, and Cl^-. Even though PRL action on mammalian renal tubules is questioned, there is no doubt that PRL acts to make the concentration of Na^+ in milk low and that of K^+ high relative to plasma. Ouabain abolishes the effect of PRL.

A nursing infant cannot obtain milk from a full breast without the action of oxytocin, a response that is called "milk letdown." The stimulus of suckling initiates a neurogenic reflex transmitted through the spinal cord and midbrain to the hypothalamus, where it triggers the release of oxytocin from the neurohypophysis. The released hormone causes contraction of myoepithelial cells that encircle the mammary acini, thereby expelling the milk into the nipple. It takes about one-half-minute of suckling before an infant can obtain milk. The reflex can be inhibited by emotional stress and triggered by sexual excitement.

PUBERTY

At the time of delivery, the neonate leaves the nutritionally and hormonally rich environment of the placenta. As the effects of maternal, placental, and fetal hormones die away, the baby enters a quiescent period in which gonadotropins and gonadal hormones are barely detectable. At some time between 8 and 14 years, puberty arrives. What events reawaken the hypothalamoadenohypohyseal–gonadal system that functioned during fetal life and early infancy and then became dormant?

First, however, some general comments. There was a widespread trend toward earlier onset of puberty, earlier menarche, and greater height between 1850 and 1950, attributable in Western industrialized countries to improvement of socioeconomic conditions, nutrition, and general health. The average age of menarche decreased from 15.5 to 12.5 years and of voice changes from 18 to 12.5 years. Further decreases are unlikely.

In the United States population, adrenarche begins in 98.8% of the population at 8 to 13 (mean, 11) years of age for girls and 9 to 14 (mean, 11.6) years of age for boys. Completion of puberty requires 1.5 to 6 (mean, 4.2) and 2 to 4.5 (mean, 3.5) years for the two sexes, respectively. Tanner's classification is widely used to describe pubertal changes: pubic hair (PH 1–5), breast (B 1–5), and genital (G 1–5) development where 1 is zero or none and 5 is adult. The growth spurt associated with puberty is also staged: peripubertal "take-off," peak height velocity, and decrease at epiphyseal closure. The mean height difference of 10 cm between the adult sexes is largely due to a difference before take-off because boys grow an average of 28 cm and girls 25 cm during puberty. The latter reach peak height velocity before menarche.

All the components below the level of the CNS—the pituitary gland, gonads, and sex hormone target tissues—can be activated precociously by administration of the appropriate hormone. Therefore, they can, at most, play only a minor role in the suppression of the onset of puberty. On the other hand, certain CNS lesions, such as neoplasms involving the hypothalamus and nearby structures, can cause true precocious puberty including fertility. Thus, childhood can be regarded as an interval of functional GnRH insufficiency that is terminated by the reactivation of pulsatile GnRH secretion.

Two independent, temporally related processes are required for the initiation of sex steroid secretion. One process, adrenarche, involves the increase in adrenal androgen secretion that precedes by about 2 years the second event, gonadarche—the reactivation of the hypothalamic–pituitary gonadotropin-gonadal system. As Figure 8.24 shows, the normal temporal relationship is excluded in certain endocrinopathies so that one process may occur without the other, indicating (but not proving) the lack of interaction between the two.

Adrenarche is associated with the differentiation and growth of the zona reticularis of the adrenal cortex, with an increased secretion of dehydroepiandrosterone (DHEA) and its sulfate by the adrenal and with the growth of axillary or pubic hair. Cortisol secretion remains constant (based on total body surface area), thus removing ACTH from consideration as a postulated adrenal–androgen-stimulating hormone. Its trophic action is, however, essential.

Studies of growth in children with chronic adrenal insufficiency who are receiving adequate replacement therapy, with isolated gonadotropin deficiency or with hypergonadotropic hypogonadism indicate that adrenal androgens in physiologic concentrations are not necessary for the adolescent growth spurt, whereas the gonadal sex steroids are essential and act in concert with growth hormone, insulin, and triiodothyronine. (T_3).

The first sign of gonadarche is a sleep-associated increase in the episodic secretion of LH. As puberty progresses, the amplitude and frequency of the nocturnal pulses increase, later spreading to the day as well. The adult pattern of about 12 discrete bursts over a 24-hr period with no diurnal variation is attained in late puberty.

There are at least two mechanisms involved in the prepubertal restraint of gonadotropin secretion. One is a supersensitive negative-feedback, the other an intrinsic CNS inhibitory influence.

There are three lines of evidence supporting the concept of a supersensitive negative-feedback control of the hypothalamoadenohypophyseal–gonadal system. The secretion of small amounts of LH and FSH during childhood indicates that the system is operative, albeit at a low level. Second, the administration of *small* amounts of estrogen indicates that the prepubertal child is five to ten times more responsive than adults in suppressing gonadotropin secretion. Finally, agonadal

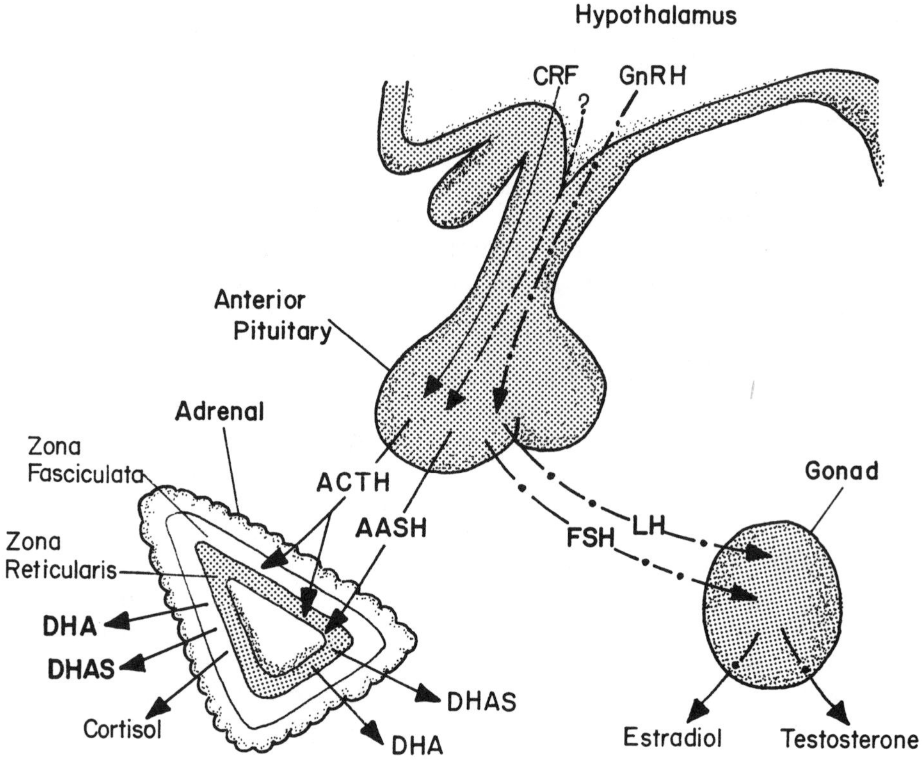

+	Premature Adrenarche	−
−	Primary Adrenal Insufficiency	+
−	Idiopathic Precocious Puberty (onset 6 years)	+
+	Idiopathic Precocious Puberty (onset 6 years)	+
+	Gonadal Dysgenesis Syndrome	−
+	Isolated Gonadotropin Deficiency	−
−	Constitutional Delayed Adolescence	−

Figure 8.24 Adrenarche and gonadarche are independent but temporally associated processes controled by different mechanisms: AASH, a postulated adrenal–androgen-stimulating hormone. The inset shows the independence of the two events in various clinical syndromes; one can occur without the other (*Source*: from Grumbach, 1980, with permission).

children show a pattern of gonadotropin secretion that is qualitatively similar to normal children, but quantitatively exaggerated, reflecting the absence of gonadal sex steroid inhibition.

A supersensitive feedback mechanism cannot, however, explain suppression of gonadotropin secretion in agonadal children during midchildhood. To do this one must involve a CNS inhibitory mechanism, independent of gonadal influences, that restrains GnRH secretion. It is postulated that precocious puberty resulting from hypothalamic lesions is a consequence of the impairment or destruction of this neural inhibitory mechanism.

Puberty, then, may be regarded as a maturational process in which the influence of these two mechanisms gradually wanes as shown in Figure 8.25. The FSH responsiveness in prepubertal girls is difficult to explain.

STEROID RECEPTORS

In Chapter 1, I presented the quandry posed by recent (1984) experimental evidence (p. 22) on estradiol receptors which indicated that they are located primarily in the nuclei of target tissues. Gorski has turned to an aqueous two-phase partioning system, which allows determinations in seconds following perturbations, to re-examine changes caused by ligand binding. He has also used cytochalasin-induced enucleation as an alternative approach to analysis of cytoplasmic and nuclear fractions. Although the results are still scanty, they are consistent with immunocytochemical results and extend the results to glucocorticoid receptors. The receptors for T_3 and 1,25-dihydroxycholecalciferol already conform to this model.

In the meantime, I present an overview of steroid action based on the old model, because much of that data probably is still relevant. This discussion expands upon that given in Chapter 1 so that differences among the various classes of receptors become evident. Later on, we may realize that some of these experimental results are artifacts.

My discussion will center around a general model (Fig. 8.26) that will need to be modified to suit each hormone.

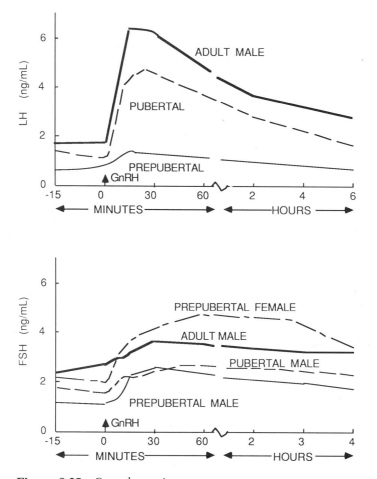

Figure 8.25 Gonadotropin secretory response to exogenous GnRH administration increases with age. There is a striking response to LH levels in pubertal and adult males and females, whereas the FSH response is less, except in prepubertal females (*Source*: from Grumbach, 1980, with permission).

Activation–Inactivation

Activation has not been proved for any steroid receptor, but there is considerable circumstantial evidence that the glucocorticoid receptor may exist in an inactive form requiring activation by phosphorylation as a precondition for binding.

Many factors may contribute to the loss of active aporeceptor. The most universally recognized factor is temperature. Although the instability of aporeceptors varies, all are sensitive to elevated temperatures (25°C). Some typical half-life values for loss of hormone-binding ability are 2 hr for L-cell and 4 hr for rat thymocyte glucocorticoid receptor, 3 hr for chick oviduct progesterone receptor, and 0.09 hr (at 30.8°C) for mouse kidney androgen receptor. The most labile appears to be the mouse mammary glucocorticoid receptor which inactivates rapidly at 4°C. Other inactivators of glucocorticoid receptors are salt, dilution, ammonium sulfate precipitation, alkaline phosphatase treatment, and sulfhydryl-blocking agents. Aporeceptors must vary in their structure because phosphatases have no effect on estrogen and progesterone receptors; sulfhydryl-blocking agents affect progesterone and 1,25-dihydroxycholecalciferol receptors.

Most of the inhibitors of inactivation are obvious. Keeping receptors at 4°C dramatically decreases the rate of inactivation, sometimes completely (the mouse mammary glucocorticoid receptor is an exception), suggesting either an enzymatic alteration or a conformational change in the receptor. Holoreceptors are much more stable, indicating protection of the ligand-binding site by bound hormone. The chick oviduct progesterone receptor is an exception to this rule. With glucocorticoid receptors, ATP will reactivate heat-inactivated receptors. And finally, low concentrations of molybdate (10 mM) stabilize a wide variety of aporeceptors including those of aldosterone, androgen, estrogen, dihydroxycholecalciferol, progesterone, and glucocorticoids; the mammary glucocorticoid receptor is an exception as is the progesterone holoreceptor. Molybdate may act, not only through phosphatase inhibition, but also by a direct action on the receptor itself.

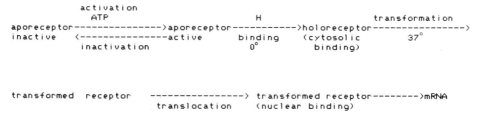

Figure 8.26   General model of the mechanism of steroid hormone action: H, hormone.

Transformation

There is a large body of evidence on transformation. The universal observation is the need for structural change before the attainment of nuclear and DNA-binding ability. For many receptors, transformation is associated with major changes, but for a few, the changes are more subtle. The evidence is summarized in Figure 8.27 and discussed in the following.

The cytosolic aporeceptor for estrogens exists in an 8S form that can be reversibly converted to a 4S form by increased ionic strength. Both forms bind [^{3}H]estradiol, neither is capable of translocation until transformation at 37°C to a 5S form occurs, and transformation will not occur in the absence of ligand. Transformation, which is only partially reversible, can also be produced by gel filtration, ultracentrifugation, or dialysis. The 5S form is indistinguishable from endogenous nuclear receptor and is capable of stimulating RNA synthesis in vitro.

The glucocorticoid receptor differs in that response to the same factors produces no change in sedimentation values: both transformed and untransformed receptors are 7S to 8S at low, and 3S to 4S at high, ionic strength. The only change detected so far is the isoelectric point which decreases by 1.0 pH unit upon transformation.

The progesterone receptor of chick oviduct can be transformed by warming, salt, dilution, or ammonium sulfate precipitation; only the first requires the presence of hormone. These treatments transform the native 7S–8S receptor form to 4S on low-salt gradients.

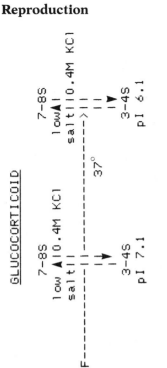

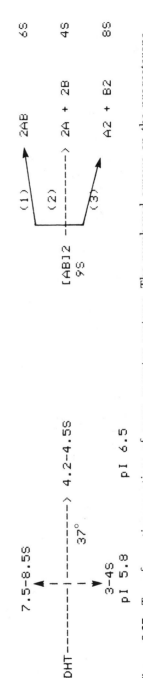

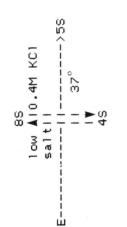

Figure 8.27 Transformation reactions of some receptor systems. The numbered arrows on the progesterone schema denote (1) spontaneous breakdown in tris buffer, (2) salt-dependent dissociation in tris buffer, and (3) salt-dependent dissociation in phosphate–molybdate buffer (*Source*: modified from Grody et al., 1982, with permission).

The dihydrotestosterone receptor of rat prostate is less well studied. There is a change in sedimentation value as well as change in pI, but there are too few reports to demonstrate a consensus.

Chick intestinal 1,25-dihydroxycholecalciferol receptor sediments at 3 to 3.5S. There is no change in sedimentation coefficient upon warming.

Rat kidney aldosterone receptor sediments at 8.5S in low-salt and at 4.5S in high-salt media. The receptors extracted from nuclei, however, are 3S. It is not known whether the 4.5S species is a transformation precursor or whether the 4.5S form is translocated and subsequently degraded to the 3S form.

These similarities and differences have promoted a large amount of speculation concerning the possible mechanism(s) of transformation. Grody et al. (1982) have concluded " . . . that there is no single mechanistic explanation for all these findings, and it is probably futile to insist on one." Some of the possible mechanisms are presented next.

Association/Dissociation of Subunits

Whenever there is a large change in sedimentation behavior, it is only natural to consider this hypothesis. Thus, the 4S-to-5S transformation of estrogen receptor is a second-order reaction. The estimated molecular weights are 80 kDa and 130 kDa, respectively, implying a molecular mass of the added unit of about 50 kDa. The 50-kDa protein may be equivalent to "estrogen receptor activation factor" identified by Thampan and Clark (1981), a 3S protein that binds to uterine nuclei, DNA cellulose, and native calf thymus DNA, but not to estradiol nor uterine 4S receptors. Transformation is reversible in 0.4 M KCl and 3 M urea with a half-life of the first-order reaction of 5 hr at 4°C.

The chick oviduct progesterone receptor is an example of transformation by dissociation (see Fig. 8.28). The native receptor is an AB protein dimer in which the two subunits possess kinetically identical hormone-binding sites but elute at different salt concentrations from several absorbents. They also differ in their binding affinity for nuclear constitutents, protein A binding with high affinity to a variety of DNAs but not to chromatin, whereas B binds strongly to chromatin from target cells and only weakly to DNA.

Even though the Stokes radius and calculated molecular mass were consistent with an AB dimer (A, 79 kDa; B, 108 kDa), for many years reconstitution experiments were unsuccessful, thereby casting doubt on the validity of the hypothesis. This occurred because apparently the standard treatments known to yield the 4S species (e.g., heat, 0.3 M salt, dialysis) are irreversible. Recently, however, the discovery that pyridoxal-5'-phosphate causes a reversible dissociation has allowed reconstitution of native dimer by several criteria. Pyridoxal phosphate not only dissociates the subunits, but it also blocks their binding to DNA, suggesting that primary lysyl amino groups may play a crucial role in dimerization as well as the binding of A protein to DNA.

There remains a major problem in that the native dimer is translocated into the nucleus, an apparent contradiction to current ideas about transformation. Higher relative molecular mass forms of the progesterone receptor (ca. 9S) can be demonstrated, but it is not known which form is the "native" form of the receptor.

Other candidates for transformation by subunit dissociation are the prostatic androgen receptor and the rat kidney aldosterone receptor.

Conformational Change

Whenever no apparent change in relative molecular mass can be demonstrated upon transformation, the simplest explanation is a conformational change, exposing additional positively charged residues, increasing its affinity for DNA (and other polyanions) and decreasing its isoelectric point. The characteristics of the rat hepatic glucocorticoid receptor ideally fit this description.

Addition or Removal of a Cytosolic Factor

Transformation by dilution or dialysis is most readily explained by this hypothesis. Even though no one has isolated such a factor, the evidence is strongly suggestive. Such a factor has been reported for the androgen, estrogen, and glucocorticoid receptors. For the progesterone receptor, reconstituted receptor aggregates are unusually resistant to retransformation unless crude cytosol is added.

Translocation

Translocation of the receptor–hormone complex from the cytosol to the nucleus, a process central to current models of hormone action, is a hypothesis supported only by circumstantial evidence. The underlying assumption that aporeceptors are found only in the cytoplasm has recently been questioned.

Nuclear Binding

The precise nature of the acceptor sites inside the nucleus remains unresolved. Usually there are several thousand high-affinity sites in each nucleus, as well as a much larger number of low-affinity sites. Whether all these high-affinity sites are biologically specific, or whether this is another case of redundancy, is not known. Some acceptor sites are DNAase-sensitive (glucocorticoids), others are not (progesterone). Chromosomal nonhistone proteins may also be part of the acceptor sites. Progesterone-binding specificity is conserved in reconstituted chromatin only if the target cell nonhistone proteins are used, the source of DNA and histone being less critical.

A clue to what the receptor might do comes from work on the avian oviductal progesterone receptor. Purified A-subunit exhibits several properties characteristic of a DNA helix-destabilizing protein, such as preferential binding to single-stranded or nicked DNA and conferring increased susceptibility of double-stranded DNA to nuclease S1, a single–strand-specific enzyme. The A-subunit protein also has DNA sequence specificity for cloned fragments of the chicken ovalbumin gene that it is believed to regulate.

Another unkown aspect of nuclear function is whether the receptor–acceptor acts catalytically or stoichiometrically. In other words, how long must a receptor remain in contact with a gene to stimulate it? Must the hormone remain bound for activity to be expressed?

And again, what is the fate of "used" receptors? Are they recycled or degraded? If the latter occurs, what is the signal for synthesis of new receptor? The basic problem is the lack of pure labeled receptor. Up to this point, the hormone has been labeled; as it dissociates from the receptor for any reason whatsoever, the label redistributes and becomes meaningless. The use of monoclonal antibodies to estrophilin and the recent cloning of human estrogen receptor cDNA may help in several ways.

CLINICAL

Amenorrhea

The most common complaint among women concerning reproduction is that of amenorrhea (absence of menses) or the closely related oligomenorrhea (*oligo-*, Greek meaning few or small) or dysmenorrhea (*dys-*, Greek meaning defective). Primary amenorrhea refers to the absence of menarche by the age of 18 years; secondary amenhorrhea refers to the absence of menstruation for 6 months or more in women who had previously menstruated.

The syndromes of amenorrhea may be subdivided (Table 8.8).

1. Anatomical defects of the uterus or vagina blocking menstrual flow
2. Failure of ovarian function, decreased estrogen production, and hence, inadequate endometrial development
3. Dysfunction of the hypothalamoadenohypohyseal system (either primary or secondary), leading to gonadal hypofunction

Category 1 is associated with primary amenorrhea; the other two may lead to either type.

Table 8.8 is more comprehensive than the following discussion because only those conditions attributable to defects in the basic biology discussed in this chapter are included here. Additionally, very rare disorders may be either omitted or mentioned only in passing.

Amenorrhea Resulting from Anatomical Defects

Whereas the cephalic end of the mullerian duct produces the fallopian tubes, the caudal end forms the uterus and upper two-thirds of the vagina. The syndrome of congenital failure of mullerian duct development is defined by an absent, bipartite, or rudimentary uterus, by absence of a vagina, and by normal ovaries. The

Table 8.8   Classification of Amenorrhea

1. Anatomical defects
   XX karyotype
      imperforate hymen
      absence of uterus
   XY karyotype
      disorders of embryonic development
         absence of uterus; presence of testes
            complete androgen insensitivity
            other forms of male pseudohermaphroditism (see Table 8.9)
2. Ovarian failure
   primary ovarian failure
      abnormal chromosome composition: 45,X karyotype
      gonadal dysgenesis
         46,XY karyotype
         46,XX karyotype
   secondary ovarian failure (see also 3)
      premature menopause with/without other autoimmune diseases
      secondary to oophoritis or pelvic inflammatory disease
3. Hypothalamoadenohypohyseal dysfunction
      hypothalamic amenorrhea
      pituitary/peripituitary lesions
         isolated gonadotropin deficiency
         hyperprolactinemia
      secondary to
         congenital adrenal hyperplasia
         Cushing's syndrome
         thyroid disease
         hirsutism–amenorrhea syndromes including polycystic ovarian
         syndrome

frequency of this disorder, about 1: 5000 female births, makes it second only to gonadal dysgenesis in importance.

Amenorrhea Resulting from Male Pseudohermaphroditism

The syndromes of male pseudohermaphroditism are all characterized by a male 46XY karyotype, a female phenotype, primary amenorrhea, the absence of a uterus, and the presence of testes. The testes, however, either fail to secrete testosterone or the peripheral end organs are insensitive to androgens; in either event, the defect may be partial or complete. Consequently, development of the wolffian system is inhibited or the external genitalia do not differentiate along male lines. The uterus is absent because the testes do secrete a mullerian-inhibiting hormone.

The impact of the defect is roughly proportional to the completeness of the defect (Table 8.9). Thus, phenotypes may extend from overtly feminine to ambiguous genitalia. Even when the initial phenotype is feminine, virilization may occur later, usually at puberty.

Androgen Insensitivity Syndrome

The androgen insensitivity syndrome (AIS), or feminizing syndrome, is divided into complete and incomplete variants. It is easier to describe the complete form (CAI) and then compare the incomplete form with it.

The syndrome of CAI (see Table 8.9) is characterized by a normal female phenotype with good breast development, a blind or absent vagina, no uterus, and the presence of testes in an individual with an XY karyotype. The syndrome is transmitted as an X-linked recessive disorder or a sex-limited autosomal-dominant disorder. Some patients lack androgen receptors, whereas others have a postreceptor defect. Members of the same family are, however, concordant in that they are all either receptor-positive or receptor-negative. Testosterone and dihydrotestosterone levels lie in the normal to high range for adult males and, as expected, there is no response to exogenous testosterone or dihydrotestosterone. Estradiol (benzoate), however, has a readily demonstrable effect. These facts are in accord with the observed breast development.

The LH levels are inappropriately high in these patients, indicating that androgen insensitivity extends to the hypothalamoadenohypophyseal system. The FSH levels, on the other hand, are only modestly elevated; presumably gonadal inhibin is selectively regulating FSH secretion. Gonadal tumors may develop in this syndrome, the prevalence being about 3.6% at 25 years and 33% at 50 years of age.

The syndrome of incomplete androgen insensitivity differs at the time of puberty in that pubertal changes include some degree

Table 8.9 Syndromes of Male Pseudohermaphroditism

Syndrome	Etiology	Phenotype	F sex char[a]	Virilization
Androgen action				
androgen insensitivity syndrome	No tissue receptors	Female	Present	Absent
	Action of androgen-receptor complex blocked	Female	Variable	Absent
familial incomplete male pseudo-hermaphroditism, type I	Decreased tissue receptor	Variable	Gynecomastia	Absent
	Action of androgen-receptor complex partially blocked	Usually, partial masculinization		
Androgen biosynthesis				
early defects				
testicular agenesis	Early complete failure	Female	Absent	Absent
testicular dysgenesis	Partial maturation	Variable	Absent	Variable
Leydig cell agenesis	Differentiation failure	Female	Absent	Absent
cholesterol 20, 22-desmolase	Combined adrenal and testicular defects	Variable	Absent	Absent
3β-ol DHGase[b]	Combined adrenal and testicular defects	Variable	Absent	Absent
17-hydroxylase	—	Female	Absent	Absent
late defects				
17β-ol DHGase[b]	Testicular defect	Female	Variable	Present
familial incomplete male pseudo-hermaphroditism, type II (5α-reductase lack)	Peripheral failure to convert T to DHT	Female	Absent	Marked virilization at puberty

[a]Secondary female sex characteristics.
[b]DHGase, dehydrogenase.

of virilization: hypertrichosis, clitoral hypertrophy, and scrotalization and pigmentation of the labia. These changes can only be avoided by early gonadectomy.

Familial, Incomplete Male Pseudohermaphroditism, Type I

This type of familial, incomplete male pseudohermaphroditism is a less-severe form of androgen insensitivity in individuals with a 46,XY karyotype. Phenotypic expression varies widely from mild defects in virilization to a normal female phenotype. Clinical features include ambigious external genitalia with various degrees of virilization, no uterus, and plasma testosterone levels that lie in the normal to high range for adult males. Some patients may be raised as males with surgical correction of their hypospadias (urethral orifice located somewhere between the tip of the penis and the perineum) and postpubertal gynecomastia, whereas others may be raised as females with gonadectomy and surgical correction of labioscrotal fusion.

Familial, Incomplete Male Pseudohermaphroditism, Type II

The type II form of this syndrome is characterized by male internal genitalia, whereas the external genitalia are feminine or ambiguous. The karyotype is XY, and virilization occurs at puberty.

The etiology lies in the lack of 5α-reductase activity. Thus, fetal testosterone promotes wolffian duct differentiation, but the external genitalia develop along feminine lines because of the block in synthesis of dihydrotestosterone. The most famous instance of this discovery occurred in a village in the Dominican Republic in which there was considerable intermarriage. Twenty-four examples of this syndrome were found in 13 families. At birth, affected males, who were usually reared as girls, had clitorallike phalluses, labialike scrota, and urogenital sinuses with a blind vaginal pouch. Testes were located in the inguinal canal or in the labia. At puberty, marked, but not complete, virilization occurred. The voice deepened, muscle mass increased, the phallus enlarged, the scrotum elongated and became hyperpigmented, the testes descended, and ejaculation could be induced by masturbation. On the other hand, the prostate remained small, beard growth was scanty, the hairline did not recede, and there was no acne. Psychosexual orientation was male. The defect occurs in both sexes, but it is expressed only in males.

What is responsible for the virilization that occurs at puberty? The answer is not known, but there may be a change in tissue sensitivity with time; external genitalia, although dihydro-testosterone-dependent in utero, may become testosterone-responsive at puberty.

Amenorrhea Resulting From Ovarian Failure

The syndrome of gonadal dysgenesis comprises a group of disorders in which the normal ovary is replaced by a white, fibrous streak. The most common form is monosomy X (45,X) in which one sex chromosome is lost. Other forms have a normal 46,XX, but there is a loss of either a short arm or a long arm of one X. Alternatively, there may be rearrangement. And finally, there may be mosaicism of 45,X with 46,XX or 46,XY or 47,XYY.

Monosomy X produces a complex syndrome involving the skin, skeletal, cardiovascular, and renal systems. Afflicted subjects are usually short (<152 cm in height), lack spatial perception, and frequently have an associated diabetes mellitus or thyroiditis.

Amenorrhea Caused By Pituitary or Hypothalamic Failure

Amenorrhea caused by hypogonadism may be primary or be secondary to a hypothalamic or a pituitary defect. The latter exists in several forms (see Chap. 2). Here we will discuss an isolated gonadotropin deficiency that encompasses hyposecretion of only FSH and LH and is often associated with anosmia. All of the available evidence points to the hypothalamus as being the origin of the syndrome; the pituitary gonadotropes are responsive to GnRH. The hypothalamic abnormalities include total absence of GnRH secretion as well as defects in the amplitude or in the frequency of GnRH secretion.

The syndrome has a familial aggregation with a complex mode of inheritence. Considering an equal involvement of the sexes, transmission without skipping generations, and expression in about 50% of the offspring, it may be transmitted as an autosomal-dominant trait with incomplete expressivity.

One recent treatment protocol emphasizes an important biochemical and physiological point. Whereas administration of GnRH two or three times daily produced no response, intermittent infusion every 2 hr by means of a small, portable pump did achieve ovulation. Thus, the reproduction of the natural rhythm was successful, and such a treatment clearly indicates that, at least here, the defect was located at a hypothalamic or higher level. (Conventional treatment uses FSH and hCG, bypassing the pituitary completely.)

Amenorrhea associated with hypofunction of the hypothalamus may occur for any of several reasons. Stress is probably the most common cause, and it may take any form from systemic disease to psychological and emotional stress. Often amenorrhea itself provokes profound anxiety, which further aggravates the problem. Even the stress of dieting may be sufficient to induce amenorrhea, and extreme weight loss, as in anorexia nervosa, may produce an amenorrhea with a reversion to immature patterns of response to GnRH.

Polycystic Ovarian Syndrome

The final cause of amenorrhea to be discussed has an uncertain etiology and a different history. Women with polycystic ovarian syndrome (PCOS) have a complex of signs consisting of amenorrhea, hirsutism, and obesity. Although they often have a history of oligomenorrhea, some have previously conceived. In PCOS, the ovaries are frequently enlarged (two to four times normal size). There is dysmaturation of the follicular complex with prominent theca cell hyperplasia with an occasional corpus luteum. This may be caused by an elevated LH/FSH ratio. The basis of the abnormal ratio may lie in an elevated follicular inhibin level and a low estradiol level which inhibits FSH more than LH secretion. Elevated plasma GnRH levels then promote the release of more LH than FSH.

The high LH concentration promotes androgen biosynthesis by the thecal cells, and indeed, the ovarian veins show a large concentration gradient of androstenedione. This is also, in part, due to the low FSH concentration and the consequent lack of induction of aromatase synthesis in the granulosa cells. Additionally, about 50% of POCS patients have elevated adrenal androgens. In spite of this increased ovarian and adrenal androgen production, urinary 17-oxosteroids are increased in less than 20% of PCOS patients; the majority, however, have elevated unbound androgens in the blood because of a depressed level of sex hormone-binding globulin.

In spite of the failure of ovarian estrogen synthesis, peripheral estrogen levels are elevated, especially that of estrone, which is produced peripherally from androstenedione. The obesity characteristic of this syndrome undoubtedly promotes this. Consequently, PCOS patients have a constant, low plasma level of estrogen.

The basic abnormality in PCOs is, therefore, the acyclicity of estrogen production and the predominance of estrone, a weak estrogen, providing acyclic feedback and inappropriate secretion of LH and FSH. All tissues respond appropriately to exogenous stimuli, i.e., ovarian and adrenal steroids suppress with a GnRH agonist or dexamethasone (see Chap. 9), respectively, and the LH preovulatory surge responds to exogenous estradiol.

Testicular Disorders

Primary Testicular Disorders

Primary testicular disorders are often associated with chromosomal abnormalities, usually with elevation of plasma FSH and LH concentrations, either singly or together (hypergonadotropic states). Seminiferous tubular dysgenesis is common (0.2%). A phenotypic male having two or more X chromosomes and at least one Y chromosome defines the syndrome. Although the 47,XXY karyotype is most common, there are many variants including 48,XXYY, 49XXXY, and 46XY/47,XXY mosaicism. In the 47,XXY karyotype, the duplicated X chromosome is derived from the maternal X chromosome.

The endocrine status in seminiferous tubular dysgenesis is notably variable. Plasma testosterone levels may range from normal to low, whereas LH and FSH levels are above normal. The testosterone response to hCG is blunted.

A profile of these patients shows that they are taller than average and infertile. Many have retarded facial, axillary, and pubic hair growth and decreased libido; about two-thirds have gynecosmastia. They are intellectually below average and often have behavioral disorders. It is not clear whether the latter has a genetic origin or is derived from feelings of inadequacy and inferiority.

Dysgenetic male pseudohermaphroditism comprises a spectrum of disorders (Table 8.10) associated with testicular dysgenesis that are explicable on the basis of the temporal relationship of the gonadal insult to the stage of testicular development. Thus, if gonadal failure occurs before organization of the genital tract, feminine internal and external genitalia form. If testicular failure occurs after the 16th week of gestation, the baby will appear to be a normal male, but at puberty he will fail to mature sexually. Other subgroups fall between these extremes (see Table 8.9).

Proper sexual development may also be compromised or diverted by a partial or, occasionally, even a complete loss of an enzyme involved in the biosynthesis of steroid hormones. Fortuntely, most of these defects are rare; only a deficiency of 21-hydroxyase is relatively common (see discussion of congenital adrenal hyperplasia in Chap. 9, p. 374). This genetic deficiency in cortisol synthesis leads to increased androgen biosynthesis which produces virilization of females and sexual precocity in males. On the other hand, a deficiency (or lack) of 17-hydroxylase or an enzyme needed at an earlier step in biosynthesis (see Fig. 8.9) will impede synthesis of any sex hormone. All affected individuals will be phenotypically female regardless of karyotype; puberty will not occur.

Hypogonadotropic Hypogonadism

The syndrome of hypogonadotropic hypogonadism was discussed earlier (p. 298) and is fully applicable to males.

Precocious Puberty

Pathologically, puberty may occur anytime after birth. Although the prevalence is low, it is a tragedy to those afflicted. The precise etiology is not known; however, the disease may be subdivided into gonadotropin-dependent and gonadotropin-independent groups. The former is amenable to treatment with a superagonist of GnRH, D-Try-6,Pro-9-ethylamide GnRH, at a dosage of 8 μg/kg daily. This amount, after an acute stimulation of gonadotropin secretion, suppresses pituitary release to nearly undetectable

Table 8.10 Dysgenetic Male Pseudohermaphroditism

Syndrome	Postulated defect	Clinical picture
XY gonadal dysgenesis	Failure of gonadal differentiation; absence of secretion of MIH and T; lack of HY antigen	Female phenotype with female internal genitalia; streak gonads; primary amenorrhea
Rudimentary testes ambiguous genitalia	Testes secretes MIH, but not enough T to induce male differentiation	Absence of mullerian structures; small phallus and fused labioscrotal folds
Hernia uteri inguinalis	Testes fails to secrete MIH, but does secrete T	Male external genitalia; inguinal hernia common
Mixed gonadal dysgenesis	Streak gonad on one side, testis on other; uterus and one tube may be present	Usually female external genitalia; phallus and partial labioscrotal fusion sometimes
Congenital anorchia	Loss of testicular function *after* differentiation	Male external genitalia; vas ends blindly; no mullerian elements; gynecomastia

Abbreviations used: DHT, dihydrotestosterone; MIH, mullerian-inhibiting hormone; T, Testosterone.

levels. Consequently, gonadal sex steroid levels fall into the prepubertal range, halting or even causing a regression of secondary sexual development and complete cessation of menses in girls. Growth velocity also diminishes, the skeletal maturation being retarded to a greater degree than linear growth.

Cancer

Epidemiological evidence of the involvement of steroids in cancer of their target tissues dates from the last century and experimental evidence from the 1940s. Because of the high incidence of breast cancer in women and of prostatic cancer in men, innumerable person-years of work and probably hundreds of millions of dollars have been expended trying to detect an imbalance in steroid metabolism that would account for the diseases. Recently (1985) Bradlow, Fishman and coworkers have found evidence in the mouse that may constitute a breakthrough.

Estrogens are metabolized differently from the neutral steroid hormones in that estrogens are modified mainly by further hydroxylation rather than by reduction. The major pathways of the oxidative metabolism of estradiol are hydroxylation at C-2 and C-16 and oxidation at C-17 to estrone. These activities are only minimally affected by age and do not differ significantly between pre- and postmenopausal normal women. In women with breast cancer, however, 16α-hydroxylation was specifically increased 50%, i.e., without any significant increase in 2-hydroxylation or in oxidation of estradiol to estrone.

Such results always raise the chicken-and-the-egg debate. Is increased 16α-hydroxylation the cause or the consequence of breast cancer? Although such questions are nearly impossible to answer in humans for ethical and other reasons, these investigators found an interesting correlation in mice. Certain strains of mice possess a mammary tumor virus that predisposes them to breast cancer. Bradlow and coworkers showed that the virus markedly enhanced the 16α-hydroxylation of estradiol but had no effect on 2-hydroxylation of estradiol or on the 16α-hydroxylation of androgen and progestin. Thus, they have established a relationship between genetics, hormonal factors, and mammary tumor virus, the three key factors in murine mammary tumorigenesis.

Prostatic cancer is the second leading cause of cancer deaths in man with 75,000 new cases being reported annually. Recently (1986), it was reported that combination treatment of patients, who had stage D2 (bone metastases) prostatic cancer and had had no previous treatment, with GnRH superagonist and the antiandrogen flutamide produced a 95% positive, objective response. The mortality at 2 years was 11% compared with 50% after standard hormonal therapy. Obviously, further testing is demanded.

SUMMARY

Hormonal regulation of reproduction is complex and still incompletely understood. Major control is exerted by the hypothalamoadenohypophyseal–gonadal system. This starts with gonadoliberin, a decapeptide having both the NH_2- and COOH-terminals blocked. Gonadoliberin is synthesized as a multigene product; the 92–amino acid prehormone contains a putative prolactin-inhibiting factor, as well as the customary signal peptide. GnRH binds to receptors on the pituitary gonadotropes and is eventually internalized. There is strong evidence that before internalization it generates a second-messenger system involving calcium–calmodulin rather than cAMP. Indirect evidence implicates diacylglycerol, inositol triphosphate, and protein kinase C.

Administration of GnRH and its analogues produces a biphasic effect. Small amounts given episodically induce a rise in GnRH receptors and promote the release and synthesis of gonadotropins. Extended administration produces down-regulation of GnRH receptors, desensitization of the pituitary to GnRH, depletion of the releasable LH pool, and reduced secretion of LH. Direct interactions of GnRH analogues with Leydig cells or ganulose cells impair their steroidogenic responsiveness to LH and to hCG. Gonadoliberin has a wide distribution in testis, corpus luteum, CNS, and gut, as well as in the hypothalamus.

There are two gonadotropins, luteotropin and folliculotropin. Both are subunit glycoproteins having α-subunits, nearly identical with those of TSH and hCG, and specific β-subunits. Both act through an adenylate cyclase mechanism.

Even though the names of the gonadotropins are derived from their functions in females, they function in both sexes; FSH might more appropriately be called gametotropin. In the ovary in the absence of progesterone, it stimulates the growth of granulosa cells in selected follicles as well the synthesis of the steroid aromatase enzyme, of inhibin, and of PRL receptors. In the testes, FSH acts on the Sertoli cells in the presence of testosterone to promote spermatogenesis and the synthesis of inhibin and of PRL receptors. Luteotropin regulates steroidogenesis. In theca interna cells of the growing follicles, it stimulates androgen production, which is aromatized to estradiol in the granulosa cells; in the corpus luteum, it stimulates progesterone production; and in the testicular Leydig cells, it promotes the production of androgen, mainly testosterone. In addition, the midcycle surge in LH plasma concentration is a prerequisite for ovulation. LH also increases PRL and β-adrenergic receptor formation, down-regulates its own receptor, and increases the secretion of plasminogen activator, prostaglandins, and relaxin.

The steroidogenic tissues include the gonads, corpus luteum, adrenal cortex, and during pregnancy, the fetoplacental unit, as well as the liver and kidney (in 1,25-dihydroxycholecalciferol synthesis). Steroid synthesis follows a basic pattern, with the enzymic complement of each tissue determining the secretory products. Steroid hydroxylases, of which there are at least eight (excluding bile acid synthesis), are all mixed-function oxidases, requiring cytochrome P_{450}, NADPH, and molecular oxygen. The three lyases have the same requirements. There are at least three oxidoreductases, which reversibly oxidize–reduce oxygen, an isomerase, and an esterase. The use of these five key reactions in a selected sequence produces half-a-dozen steroid hormones from a common precursor, cholesterol.

The rate-limiting step is usually side-chain cleavage of cholesterol, a mitochondrial reaction, which is regulated by ACTH in the zona fasciculata or zona reticularis of the adrenal cortex, by angiotensin II and III in the zona glomerulosa of the adrenal cortex, and by LH in the gonads and corpus luteum. Corticotropin and LH apparently act through adenylate cyclase, cAMP, and a cAMP-dependent protein kinase which may phosphorylate a labile protein. This phosphoprotein may in an undetermined manner facilitate side-chain cleavage.

Because steroid hormones are not stored, cholesterol must be supplied to the mitochondria at a rate in excess of side-chain cleavage. As I pointed out in Chapter 1, most cholesterol is transported into steroidogenic tissues on LDL and stored in lipid droplets in the form of cholesterol esters, principally the arachidonate ester in humans. Activation of cholesterol esterase requires the synergistic action of ACTH–LH and γ_3-MSH.

Testosterone, the principal testicular androgen, is a prehormone for certain target tissues in which a reductase produces 5α-dihydrotestosterone, a more potent androgen than testosterone.

The process of recruitment of primordial follicles is initiated by FSH and limited by folliculostatin, but the process of selection of the one (or more) destined to produce an ovum (ova) is not known. Asymmetrical ovarian function is an inherent characteristic of monotocous species.

Events in the menstrual cycle of women are timed by the ovary, which has a preset follicular phase of about 14 days with considerable variation (one to several weeks) and a preset luteal phase of 14 days, normally, with little variation. Estradiol synthesized in the growing follicles modulates the sensitivity of the adenohypophyseal gonadotropes to GnRH, which is normally released from the hypothalamus in unvarying pulses occurring every 2 hr day and night. Estradiol, exceeding its critical concentration of 150 pg/ml for more than 36 hr, produces an LH surge (day 0) and ovulation between days 1 and 2 as evidenced by a rise in basal body temperature. A marked increase in circulating progesterone during the luteal phase suggests that ovulation occurred. Menses follow the decrease in plasma progesterone and estradiol, and the cycle restarts.

Gametogenesis in men is continuous rather than cyclic, taking 72 days. Luteotropin stimulates testosterone production in the Leydig cells, which diffuses into the Sertoli cells, as well as escaping into the circulation. Follicle-stimulating hormone and testosterone act together in the Sertoli cells to promote spermatogenesis.

A biological function of the pineal gland and its product, melatonin, is well established in seasonal breeders in which short photoperiods increase melatonin synthesis and suppress gonadal function. Melatonin is produced by modification of tryptophan, the final step, the methylation of N-acetylserotonin, being photosensitive. Although the same reactions occur in nonseasonal breeding animals, the physiologic role of melatonin is not clear.

Prolactin release from the pituitary is inhibited tonicly by dopamine and possibly other factors and is stimulated by a prolactin-releasing factor. While TRH and VIP possess this activity, their physiological relevance is not established. The function of prolactin depends upon the species; in primates, it is required for lactation. There are probably other functions, for hyperprolactininemia in either sex produces infertility.

A number of placental hormones are probably critical to fetal development. Human chorionic gonadotropin, which is produced in large amounts during the first trimester, is similar to LH in structure and is functionally identical. The production of human chorionic somatomammotropin increases directly with the placental mass, and the plasma concentration of hCS is used clinically as a measure of placental function. In humans, its rate of secretion (1 g/day at term) is the greatest of any protein hormone, accounting for 10% of all placental protein production at term.

Steroid hormone production by the fetoplacental unit is also remarkable, especially that of progesterone and estrogens. Before the eighth week of gestation, hCG produced by the trophoblasts stimulates the corpus luteum to produce progesterone and estradiol. Thereafter, progesterone biosynthesis from LDL cholesterol in the maternal plasma is autonmous, limited only by the number of LDL receptors on the surface of the trophoblasts. Progesterone has an anesthetic effect on the uterine myometrium and suppresses lactation. Similarly, the capacity of placental trophoblasts to convert androgens to estrogens is so great that the placental aromatase cannot be saturated. Dehydroepiandrosterone sulfate from both maternal and fetal adrenals is the principal androgen. The fetal liver and, to a lesser

extent, the fetal adrenal glands hydroxylate DHEA sulfate extensively. In the placenta, the sulfate conjugates are hydrolyzed, and
both 16α-hydroxyDHEA and DHEA are aromatized to estriol and
estradiol, respectively.

Sexual development during ontogeny is driven by the sex
chromosomal pair XX in females and XY in males. Male development is initiated earlier than the female counterpart, and female
development is innate. In other words, if the H–Y antigen does
not initiate gonadal differentiation into testes at 5 to 6 weeks of
gestational age, a week later they will develop as ovaries.

The testicular Sertoli cells produce antimullerian hormone, a
dimeric glycoprotein that causes the mullerian duct system to
disappear, leaving the wolffian ducts to grow into the epididymis,
vas deferens, seminal vesicles, and ejaculatory duct. If this does
not occur, then a little later, the wolffian duct regresses (rem-
nants remain), and the mullerian duct develops into the fallopian
tubes, uterus, and upper portion of the vagina.

The external genitalia of both sexes arise from common
antecedents. In the XY fetus, hCG promotes androgen biosynthesis in the testicular Leydig cells which, in turn, causes the
genital folds to fuse and elongate to form a penis and urethra and
the genital swellings to fuse to form the scrotum. These changes
require the conversion of testosterone to 5α-dihydrotestosterone
in these tissues. In the absence of an androgenic signal, these
tissues later form the clitoris, labia majora, and labia minora.

Although the aforementioned steps are apparently initiated
by the Y chromosome, participation of several autosomes is required for successful completion. The process is complex. If it
proceeds normally, the phenotypic sex of the neonate will match
its chromosomal sex. If any errors occur, the two do not match
(pseudohermaphroditism of various degrees of severity).

The hormones that participate in parturition are numerous:
relaxin, oxytocin, prostaglandins, cortisol, estradiol, and progesterone. Their roles differ sharply with the species, and some of
them may not be involved whatsoever in a given species. In
humans, these relationships are still not clear.

The mammary gland is a complex organ requiring many hormones for its preparation and function. Again, there are marked
species' variations. In vivo, estrogens promote the development

of the duct system and, perhaps, in conjunction with progesterone, the lobuloalveolar system as well. During pregnancy, further development occurs under the influence of prolonged elevated levels of estrogens, progestins, and prolactin. Adipose tissue is replaced by epithelial components, and milk synthesis is inhibited by progesterone. In organ culture, insulin and glucocorticoids are indispensable for maintaining viability, growth, and differentiation, and STH is required for maximum response; thyroid hormones play a permissive role.

After birth, progesterone disappears, and prolactin and T_3 prevail. Lactose synthetase is a dimeric enzyme consisting of galactosyltransferase and α-lactalbumin, the regulatory subunit. Its synthesis is stimulated by a combination of prolactin and T_3 and suppressed by progesterone. Oxytocin, a milk letdown factor, acts on the smooth muscle of the milk ducts to cause expression of milk during suckling.

Puberty is the time of transition from the quiescence of childhood to the productive capability of adulthood. It occurs in two discrete steps called adrenarche and gonadarche, the former preceding the latter by about 2 years. Adrenarche is associated with the differentiation and growth of the zona reticularis of the adrenal cortex, with an increased secretion of DHEA and its sulfate by the adrenal, and with the growth of axillary or pubic hair. Gonadarche is initiated by a sleep-associated increase in the episodic secretion of LH, first at night and then spreading to the day, until an adult pattern of 12 discrete bursts over a 24-hr period with no diurnal variation is attained. Puberty then may be regarded as a maturational process in which the zona reticularis develops its full potential and a supersensitive negative-feedback control and a CNS inhibition of the hypothalamoadeno-hypophyseal–gonadal system are lost.

Experimental evidence starting in 1984 has indicated that the dogma concerning steroid receptors may be partially incorrect, that is, like T_3 receptors, cytosolic receptors for estradiol and glucocorticoids may be secondary. Nevertheless, until the overall picture clarifies, the older model cannot be discarded. It is discussed in terms of each steroid hormone under the headings of activation–inactivation, transformation, translocation, and nuclear binding.

SUPPLEMENTAL BIBLIOGRAPHY

The Gonadoliberin–Gonadotropin–Gonadal Hormone System

Adelman, JP, AJ Mason, JS Hayflick, and PH Seeburg. Isolation of the gene and hypothalamic cDNA for the common precursor of gonadotropin-releasing hormone and prolactin release-inhibiting factor in human and rat. *Proc Natl Acad Sci USA 83*: 179–183, 1986.

Aron, C. Mechanisms of control of the reproductive function of olfactory stimuli in female mammals. *Physiol Rev 59*:229–284, 1979.

Bardin, WC, N Musto, G Gunsalus, N Kotite, S-L Cheng, F Larrea, and R Becker. Extracellular androgen binding proteins. *Annu Rev Physiol 43*:189–198, 1981.

Barraclough, CA, PM Wise, and Mk Selmanoff. A role for hypothalamic catecholamines in the regulation of gonadotropin secretion. *Recent Prog Horm Res 40*:487–520, 1984.

Bellvé, AR and LA Feig. Cell proliferation in the mammalian testis: Biology of the seminiferous growth factor (SGF). *Recent Prog Horm Res 40*:531–561, 1984.

Cardinali, DP. Melatonin, a mammalian pineal hormone. *Endocr Rev 2*:327–346, 1981.

Catt, KJ. Regulation of peptide hormone receptors and gonadal steroidogenesis. *Recent Prog Horm Res 36*:557–622, 1980.

Channing, CP, FW Schaerf, LD Anderson, and A Tsafriri. Ovarian follicular and luteal physiology. *Int Rev Physiol 22*:117–201, 1980.

Clayton, RN and KJ Catt. Gonadotropin-releasing hormone receptors: Characterization, physiological regulation and relationship to reproductive function. *Endocr Rev 2*:186–209, 1981.

Conn, PM. The molecular basis of gonadotropin-releasing hormone action. *Endocr Rev 7*:3–10, 1986.

diZerega, GS and GD Hodgen. Folliculogenesis in the primate ovarian cycle. *Endocr Rev 2*:27–49, 1981.

Ferin, M, D Van Vugt, and S Wardlaw. The hypothalamic control of the menstrual cycle and the role of endogenous opioid peptides. *Recent Prog Horm Res 40*:441–480, 1984.

Fink, G. Feedback actions of target hormones on the hypothalamus and pituitary with special reference to gonadal steroids. *Annu Rev Physiol 41*:571–586, 1979.

Franchimont, P. Inhibin: From concept to reality, *Vitam Horm 37*: 244–302, 1979.

Freidinger, RM, DF Veber, and DS Perlow. Bioactive conformation of luteinizing hormone-releasing hormone: Evidence from a conformationally constrained analog. *Science 210*:656–658, 1980.

Hsueh, AJW, EY Adashi, PBC Jones, and TH Welsh, Jr. Hormonal regulation of the differentiation of cultured ovarian granulosa cells. *Endocr Rev 5*:76–127, 1984.

Hulting, A-L, JA Lindgren, T Hokfelt, P Eneroth, S Werner, C Patrono, and B Samuelsson. Leukotriene C4 as a mediator of luteinizing hormone release from rat anterior pituitary cells. *Proc Natl Acad Sci USA 82*:3834–3838, 1985.

Jacobi, GH and UK Wenderoth. Gonadotropin-releasing hormone analogues for prostatic cancer: Untoward side effects of high-dose regimens acquire a therapeutic dimension. *Eur Urol 8*:129–134, 1982.

Knobil, E. The neuroendocrine control of the menstrual cycle. *Recent Prog Horm Res 36*:53–88, 1980.

Leung,PCK and DT Armstrong. Interactions of steroids and gonadotropins in the control of steroidogenesis in the ovarian follicle. *Annu Rev Physiol 42*:71–82, 1980.

Lieberman, S, NJ Greenfield, and A Wolfson. A heuristic proposal for understanding steroidogenic processes. *Endocr Rev 5*:128–148, 1984.

Li, CH, RG Hammonds, Jr, K Ramasharma, and D Chung. Human seminal inhibins: Isolation, characterization, and structure. *Proc Natl Acad Sci USA 82*:4041–4044, 1985.

Lincoln, DW, HM Fraser, GA Lincoln, GB Martin, and AS McNeilly. Hypothalamic pulse generators. *Recent Prog Harm Res 41*:369–410, 1985.

Ling, N, S-Y Ying, N Ueno, F Esch, L Denoroy, and R Guillemin. Isolation and partial characterization of a M_r 32,000 protein with inhibin activity from porcine follicular fluid. *Proc Natl Acad Sci USA 82*:7217–7221, 1985.

McGuffin, VL and RN Zare. Femtomole analysis of prostaglandin pharmaceuticals. *Proc Natl Acad Sci USA 82*:8315–8319, 1985.

Means, AR, JR Dedman, JS Tash, DJ Tindall, M vanSickle, and MJ Welsh. Regulation of the testis Sertoli cell by follicle-stimulating hormone. *Annu Rev Physiol 42*:59–70, 1980.

Parvinen, M. Regulation of the seminiferous epithelium. *Endocr Rev 3*: 404–417, 1982.

Pierce, JG and TF Parsons. Glycoprotein hormones: Structure and function. *Annu Rev Biochem 50*:465–495, 1981.

Plant, TM. Gonadal regulation of hypothalamic gonadotropin-releasing hormone release in primates. *Endocr Rev 7*:75–88, 1986.

Preslock JP. Steroidogenesis in the mammalian testis, *Endocr Rev 1*: 132–139, 1980.

Reiter, RS. The pineal and its hormones in the control of reproduction in mammals. *Endocr Rev 1*:109–131, 1980.

Rothchild, I. Regulation of the mammalian corpus luteum. *Recent Prog Horm Res 37*:183–283, 1981.

Rouzer, CA and B Samuelson. On the nature of the 5-lipoxygenase reaction in human leukocytes: Enzyme purification and requirement for multiple stimulatory factors. *Proc Natl Acad Sci USA* 82:6040–6044, 1985.

Sanborn, BM, JJ Heindel, and GA Robison. The role of cyclic nucleotides in reproductive processes. *Annu Rev Physiol* 42:37–58, 1980.

Shinohara, O, M Knecht, and KJ Catt. Inhibition of gonadotropin-induced granulosa cell differentiation by activation of protein kinase C. *Proc Natl Acad Sci USA* 82:8518–8522, 1985.

Simpson, ER, GE Ackerman, ME Smith, and CR Mendelson. Estrogen formation in stromal cells of adipose tissue of women: Induction by glucocorticoids. *Ann NY Acad Sci* 78:5690–5694, 1981.

Yen, SSC. Neuroendocrine regulation of the menstrual cycle, In *Neuroendocrinology* (DT Krieger and JC Hughes, eds). Sinauer Associates, Sunderland, Mass, 1980, pp. 259–272.

Conception and Pregnancy

Dorner, G. Sexual differentiation of the brain. *Vitam Horm 38*: 325–381, 1980.

Epel, D. The program of fertilization. *Sci Am 237*:128–138, 1977.

Hussa, RO. Biosynthesis of human chorionic gonadotropin. *Endocr Rev 1*:268–293, 1980.

Jaffe, RB, M Seron-Ferre, K Crickard, D Koritnik, BF Mitchell, and ITH Huhtaniemi. Regulation and function of the primate fetal adrenal and gonad. *Recent Prog Horm Res* 37:41–96, 1981.

Jones, GS. Update of in vitro fertilization. *Endocr Rev 5*:62–75, 1984.

Josso, N, J-Y Picard, and D Tran. The anti-Mullerian hormone. *Recent Prog Horm Res 33*:117–162, 1977.

Kelly, PA, J Djiane, M Katoh, LH Ferland, L-M Houdebine, B Teyssot, and I Dusanter-Fourt. The interaction of prolactin with its receptors in target tissues and its mechanism of action. *Recent Prog Horm Res 40*:379–435, 1984.

Lippes, J. Applied physiology of the uterine tube. *Obstet Gynecol 4*: 119–166, 1975.

Martini, L. The 5α-reduction of testosterone in neuroendocrine structures. Biochemical and physiological implications, *Endocr Rev 3*:1–25, 1982.

Rosen, JM, RJ Matusik, DA Richards, P Gupta, and JR Rodgers. Multihormonal regulation of casein gene expression at the transcriptional and posttranscriptional levels in the mammary gland. *Recent Prog Horm Res 36*:157–187, 1980.

Seron-Ferre, M and RB Jaffe. The fetal adrenal gland. *Annu Rev Physiol 43*:141–162, 1981.

Shiu, RPC and HG Friesen. Mechanism of action of prolactin in the control of mammary gland function. *Annu Rev Physiol 42*:83–96, 1980.

Tai, HH. Biosynthesis and metabolism of pulmonary prostaglandins, thromboxanes and prostacyclin. *Clin Resp Physiol 17*:626–646, 1981.

Turek, FW, J Swann, and DJ Earnest. Role of the circadian system in reproductive phenomena. *Recent Prog Horm Res 40*:143–177, 1984.

Thorburn, GD and JRG Challis. Endocrine control of parturition. *Physiol Rev 59*:863–918, 1979.

Vigier, B, J-Y Picard, and N Josso. A monoclonal antibody against bovine anti-Mullerian hormone. *Endocrinology 110*:131–137, 1982.

Wilson, JD, JE Griffin, FW George, and M Leshin. The role of gonadal steroids in sexual differentiation. *Recent Prog Horm Res 37*:1–33, 1981.

Puberty

Cutler, GB, Jr, FG Cassoria, JL Ross, OH Pescovitz, KM Barnes, F Comite, PP Feuillan, L Laue, CM Foster, D Kenigsberg, M Caruso-Nicoletti, HG Garcia, M Uriarte, KD Hench, MC Skerda, LM Long, and DL Loriaux. Pubertal growth: Physiology and pathophysiology. *Recent Prog Horm Res 42*:443–465. 1986.

Grumbach, MM. The neuroendocrinology of puberty. In *Neuroendocrinology* (DT Krieger and JC Hughes, eds). Sinauer Associates, Sunderland, Mass, 1980, pp. 249–258.

Ojeda, SR, WW Andrews, JP Advis, and SS White. Recent advances in the endocrinology of puberty. *Endocr Rev 1*:228–257, 1980.

Parker, LN and WD Odell. Control of adrenal androgen secretion. *Endocr Rev 1*:392–410, 1980.

Steroid Receptors

Clark, JH, B Markaverich, S Upchurch, H Ericksson, JW Hardin, and EJ Peck, Jr. Heterogeneity of estrogen binding sites: Relationship to estrogen receptors and estrogen action. *Recent Prog Horm Res 36*:89–125, 1980.

Gorski, J, WV Welshons, D Sakai, J Hansen, J Walent, J Kassis, J Shull, G Stack, and C Campen. Evolution of a model of estrogen action. *Recent Prog Horm Res 42*:297–322, 1986.

Grody, WW, WT Schrader, and BW O'Malley. Activation, transformation and subunit structure of steroid hormone receptors. *Endocr Rev 3*:141–163, 1982.

Katzenellenbogen BS. Dynamics of steroid hormone receptor action. *Annu Rev Physiol 42*:17–36, 1980

Liao, S and D Witte. Autoimmune anti-androgen-receptor antibodies in human serum. *Proc Natl Acad Sci USA 82*:8345–8348, 1985.

McEwen, BS. Binding and metabolism of sex steroids by the hypothalamic–pituitary unit: Physiological implications. *Annu Rev Physiol 42*:87–110, 1980.

Schrader, WT, ME Birnbaumer, MR Hughes, NL Weigel, WW Grody, and BW O'Malley. Studies on the structure and function of the chicken progesterone recepor. *Recent Prog Horm Res 37*:583–629, 1981.

von der Ahe, D, S Janich, C Scheidereit, R Renkawitz, G Schutz, and M Beato. Glucocorticoid and progesterone receptors bind to the same sites in two hormonally regulated promoters. *Nature 313*:706–709, 1985.

Walter, P, S Green, G Greene, A Krust, J-M Bornert, J-M Jeltsch, A Staub, E Jensen, G Scrace, M Waterfield, and P Chambon. Cloning of the human estrogen receptor cDNA. *Proc Natl Acad Sci USA 82*:7889–7893, 1985.

Clinical

Boepple, PA, MJ Mansfield, ME Wierman, CR Rudlin, HH Bode, JF Crigler, Jr, JD Crawford, and WF Crowley, Jr. Use of a potent, long acting agonist of gonadotropin-releasing hormone in the treatment of precocious puberty. *Endocr Rev 7*:24–33, 1986.

Bradlow, HL, RJ Herschcopf, CP Martucci, and J Fishman. Estradiol 16α-hydroxylation in the mouse correlates with mammary tumor incidence and presence of murine mammary tumor virus: A possible model for the hormonal etiology of breast cancer in humans. *Proc Natl Acad Sci USA 82*:6295–6299, 1985.

Handelsman, DJ. Hypothalamic–pituitary gonadal dysfunction in renal failure, dialysis and renal transplantation. *Endocr Rev 6*:151–182, 1985.

Horwitz, KB, LL Wei, SM Sedlacek, and CN D'Arville. Progestin action and progesterone receptor structure in human breast cancer: A review. *Recent Prog Horm Res 41*:249–308, 1985.

Labrie, F, A Dupont, A Belanger, R St-Arnaud, M Giguere, Y Lacourciere, J Emond, and G Monfette. Treatment of prostate cancer with gonadotropin-releasing hormone agonists. *Endocr Rev 7*:67–74, 1986.

Manni, A, R Santen, H Harvey, A Lipton, and D Max. Treatment of breast cancer with gonadotropin-releasing hormone. *Endocr Rev 7*:89–94, 1986.

Mittwoch, U. Whistling maids and crowing hens—hermaphroditism in folklore and biology. *Perspect Biol Med 24*:595–606, 1981.

Santoro, N, M Filicori, and WF Crowley, Jr. Hypogonadotropic disorders in men and women: Diagnosis and therapy with pulsatile gonadotropin-releasing hormone. *Endocr Rev 7*:11–23, 1986.

Snyder, PJ. Gonadotroph cell adenomas of the pituitary, *Endocr Rev 6*: 552–653, 1985.

9

Fuel Metabolism

Insulin   316
    Chemistry   316
    Regulation of insulin secretion   318
    Regulation of metabolism   326
    The insulin receptor   331
Glucagon   334
    Chemistry   334
    Regulation of secretion   334
    Effects   334
Glucocorticoids   338
    Corticoliberin   339
    Corticotropin   340
    Steroidogenesis   342
    Regulation of the hypothalamoadenohypophyseal–
        adrenocortical axis   346
    Biological effects of glucocorticoids   349
Epinephrine   351
    Chemistry   351
    Regulation   352
    Effects   353
    Adrenergic receptors   354
Integration   357
Clinical Aspects   364
    Diabetes mellitus   364
    Malfunctions of the adrenal cortex   370
    Malfunctions of the adrenal medulla   380
Summary   382
Supplemental Bibliography   387

Normally, fatty acids (from triglycerides) are the principal fuel of the body. During starvation and in certain disease states, however, amino acids (from body proteins) also become an important source of energy. The hormones regulating energy metabolism are principally glucagon and insulin, but epinephrine, glucocorticoids, somatotropin (STH), and others play important roles. The interplay among these hormones is quite complex, with dependence upon such variables as time, stress, nutritional status, age, and others. Although there is a vast quantity of literature pertaining to this area, the surface of knowledge, especially that relating to hormonal interrelationships, is barely scratched.

INSULIN

Chemistry

Insulin, first isolated in 1921, is an "old" hormone with a modern history. The "native" hormone isolated by Banting and Best contains two dissimilar polypeptide chains having a 21-residue A-chain and a 30-residue B-chain joined by two disulfide linkages, A7–B7 and A20–B19. There is also an intrachain disulfide (A6–A11). The fact that these bonds will not reform in good yield upon (air) oxidation of reduced insulin was the first clue that insulin is a processed polypeptide. Several decades passed, however, before the precursor, proinsulin, was isolated.

Insulin structure is highly preserved throughout many phyla of vertebrates. In many mammalian species, except the coypu and guinea pig, the sequence is nearly identical, there being only one to six differences from human insulin (see Appendix D and Fig. 9.1). Human insulin (5807 Da) has an acidic isoelectric point (5.35) and a specific activity of 24 IU/mg. Because of its acidity, insulin readily forms salts with basic proteins and with zinc that remarkably change its properties.

The cystallographic structure of Zn insulin shows an α-helix at A2-8, an irregular right-handed helix at A13-18 lying antiparallel to that at A2-8 and another α-helix at B9-19. B1-7 and B24-30 have an extended conformation. Insulin forms dimers through an antiparallel pleated sheet structure involving residues B24-26 and nonpolar contacts at B12, 16, 24, 25, and 26. The hexamer forms by coordination of two zinc atoms with the B10 histidines and by dimer–dimer interaction through B1, 4, 6, 14, 17, and 20 and A13 and 14. Monomer–receptor interaction is thought to occur at A1, 5, 19, and 21 and B25.

NUMBER OF DIFFERENCES

	1	2	3	4	5	6	7	8	9	10	11	12	13	14	15	16	17	18
1 COYPU		17	20	19	20	20	21	22	22	22	22	23	23	23	24	24	25	27
2 GUINEA PIG	33		18	17	18	18	17	18	18	20	21	25	21	20	21	21	20	25
3 MOUSE	38	35		2	3	4	6	7	6	10	10	14	19	16	17	17	14	20
4 SPINY MOUSE	37	33	4		1	2	4	5	4	8	8	12	18	15	16	16	12	20
5 RABBIT	38	35	6	2		1	3	4	3	7	7	11	17	16	15	15	11	19
6 HUMAN	38	35	8	4	2		2	4	3	7	6	12	17	16	15	15	11	19
7 ELEPHANT	40	33	12	8	6	4		2	4	7	6	12	17	16	15	15	11	19
8 SHEEP	42	35	14	10	8	8	4		2	6	7	12	17	16	15	15	11	19
9 SPERM WHALE	42	35	12	8	6	6	8	4		5	7	11	17	16	15	15	11	19
10 CHICKEN/ TURKEY	42	39	20	16	14	14	14	12	10		3	8	15	14	13	13	8	18
11 DUCK	42	41	20	16	14	12	12	14	14	6		8	15	14	13	13	8	19
12 RATTLESNAKE	44	49	27	24	22	24	24	24	22	16	16		19	19	18	18	15	22
13 TOADFISH	45	42	38	36	34	34	34	34	34	30	30	38		4	6	6	13	20
14 COD	44	39	31	29	31	31	31	31	31	27	27	27	8		4	4	11	19
15 ANGLER FISH	46	41	33	31	29	29	29	29	29	25	25	35	12	8		2	10	18
16 TUNA	46	41	33	31	29	29	29	29	29	25	25	35	12	8	4		9	17
17 BONITO	49	40	28	24	22	22	22	22	22	16	16	30	26	22	20	18		17
18 ATLANTIC HAGFISH	52	49	39	39	37	37	37	37	37	35	37	43	40	37	35	33	34	

PERCENT DIFFERENCE

Figure 9.1 A summary of differences in the sequence of insulin. Note the small number of differences for mammalian species except for the coypu and guinea pig. (The sequences are shown in Appendix D) (*Source*: from the *Atlas of Protein Sequence and Structure*, 1976, p 129).

In solution, insulin forms a concentration-dependent mixture of monomer and polymers, obeying physical chemical laws. At physiologic concentrations in plasma, it is believed to be a

mixture of monomer and dimer On the plasma membrane receptor, however, a condition more closely resembling the solid state
may prevail. It is interesting that the contact points for dimer formation differ from those for insulin–receptor interaction; this
has led to a proposal for receptor aggregation.

Steiner's discovery of proinsulin by radiolabeling an in-
sulinoma preparation was the first prohormone to be detected. It
is a single polypeptide having the structure, $H_2N.B$-chain-Arg-Arg-
C-peptide-Lys-Arg-A-chain-OH. The connecting (C-) peptide contains about 30 amino acid residues. The proinsulin sequence,
although containing the necessary information for the correct
pairing of cysteinyl residues, has little biological activity. Proteolytic processing in the storage granules of the pancreatic
β-cells produces insulin plus C-peptide. Although the
crystallographic structure of proinsulin is not yet known, the fact
that proinsulin cocrystallizes with insulin suggests that the
C-peptide may be located on an exterior face of the crystal. The
sequence of the C-peptide is less well preserved through evolution than that of native insulin (compare Appendix D and E and
Figs. 9.1 and 9.2).

As one would expect (see Chap. 1), translation of the proinsulin gene in a wheat germ ribosomal system or the sequencing
of the cDNA prepared from the mRNA of rat islets of Langerhans
reveals the presence of a 23-amino acid signal peptide attached to
the NH,-terminus of proinsulin. Thus, preproinsulin is a single
polypeptide containing about 109 amino acid residues.

Regulation of Insulin Secretion

The pancreas is mainly an exocrine organ regulated by
gastrointestinal hormones (see Chap. 3). Scattered through it,
however, are small islands of endocrine tissue called islets of
Langerhans. In fact, there are two types of islet tissue. In one
type, the centrally located insulin-secreting (β) cells are surrounded by numerous glucagon-secreting (α) cells and scattered
somatostatin-containing (δ) cells (Fig. 9.3). The other type has the
same central core, but it is surrounded by abundant pancreatic
polypeptide-containing (PP) cells and fewer δ-cells. This
phenomenon may be related to differing embryonic origins of the
pancreas. The glucagon-rich cells are restricted to that portion of

		1	2	3	4	NUMBER OF DIFFERENCES 5	6	7	8	9
1	RAT 2		4	30	13	13	16	18	19	31
2	RAT 1	5		31	14	14	17	18	20	32
3	GUINEA PIG	37	38		29	28	29	33	33	45
4	HUMAN	15	16	35		7	9	12	17	29
5	DOG	18	19	38	9		8	9	13	23
6	HORSE	20	21	35	11	11		10	16	30
7	PIG	21	21	40	14	12	12		15	31
8	BOVINE	22	23	41	20	18	20	17		28
9	DUCK	38	39	55	35	31	37	38	34	

PERCENT DIFFERENCE

Figure 9.2 A summary of differences in the sequence of proinsulin. The larger number of differences here (compared with Fig. 9.1) reflect the lower degree of homology of the C-peptide. (The sequences are shown in Appendix E) (*Source*: from the *Atlas of Protein Sequence and Structure*, 1976, p 127).

the pancreas derived from the dorsal primordium, whereas the PP-rich cells come from the ventral primordium. The vascularization of the two portion of the pancreas also differs.

Somatostatin, which inhibits the secretion of both insulin and glucagon, is considered a paracrine substance. Its physiological function in the islets is still not understood.

There are three phases to insulin secretion; basal, phase I (acute phase), and phase II (prolonged phase). A basal state is difficult to define rigorously. Certainly it means "unstimulated," but often there may be a low concentration of glucose, other substrates, parasympathetic and sympathetic neural tone, and

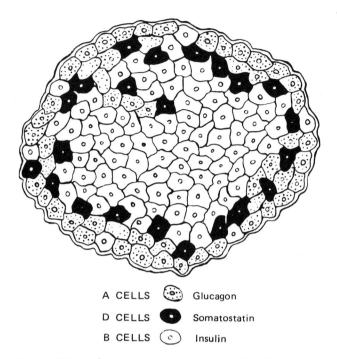

A CELLS   Glucagon

D CELLS   Somatostatin

B CELLS   Insulin

Figure 9.3 Schematic representation of an islet of Langerhans showing distribution of glucagon-, somatostatin-, and insulin-producing cells. Islet cell types having no firmly established function are omitted (*Source*: from Orci, L and RH Unger, *Lancet* 2:1243, 1975).

hormones present. Yet, in vitro, there is still a basal release in defined medium with no nutrients present (Fig. 9.4). Addition of glucose above a critical concentration (>5.5 mM) produces an increase in plasma insulin concentrations within 3 min, followed by a return toward baseline within 6 to 10 min. It is assumed that the acute phase reflects the release of preformed insulin. The second phase of insulin release responds more slowly, is directly related to the degree and duration of hyperglycermia, and persists until the hyperglycemia is terminated. This phase is believed to be partially dependent upon the synthesis of insulin because inhibitors of protein synthesis blunt the response.

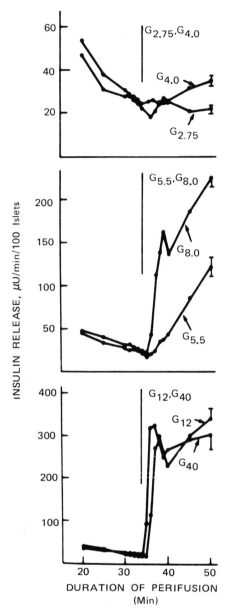

Figure 9.4 Glucose-induced release of insulin from isolated, perifused rat islets. Groups of 50 islets were perifused for 30 min with no added substrate and then for 20 min at the indicated glucose concentrations. Note that the threshold for insulin release occurs at 4 mM and the maximum response at 12 mM glucose. At 8 mM and higher glucose concentrations, a biphasic response is seen (*Source*: from Sawalich, 1979).

Some studies of the mechanism of insulin secretion fail to recognize these phases. One phase may be absent while the other remains intact. For example, type II diabetic patients, who are noninsulin-dependent and have measurable basal levels, do not have phase I insulin responses to glucose stimulation, but they do have second-phase responses. On the other hand, they do have phase I responses to nonglucose insulin secretagogues, such as arginine, glucagon, tolbutamide, and isoproterenol. Failure to recognize these differences may lead to either false conclusions or to inconclusive results.

There are many substances controlling insulin secretion (Table 9.1). The primary control is exerted by D-glucose, probably the α-anomer (D-glucose is normally present as a mixture of 36% α- and 64% β-anomer); it causes an increase in both phases of insulin secretion above a threshold concentration of 5.5 mM (see Fig. 9.4). The K_m for glucose stimulation is about 8.0 mM.

Other substances as well neural stimulation provoke insulin secretion (Table 9.1), but their action is always secondary to that of glucose, i.e., there is no response unless there is glucose present. Moreover, the insulin response to a constant amount of stimulant, such as isoproterenol or arginine, is dependent upon the plasma glucose concentration, increasing rather sharply at lower glucose concentrations and reaching a plateau at about 25 mM glucose.

Normal pancreatic islets appear capable of adapting to environmental changes in such a way as to minimize the effect of the change, at least in the short term. For example, infusion of nondiabetic men with glucose for 20 hr leads to a consistent increase in the sensitivity of the β-cells. Specifically, insulin concentrations as well as insulin responses to intravenous arginine, measured at three glucose levels and matched to preinfusion control levels, undergo greater potentiation by glucose than do controls. Incidentally, there is a concomitant decrease in glucagon and glucagon responses to arginine. Thus, both the α-cells and β-cells demonstrate adaptation to hyperglycemia in a way such that the degree of hyperglycemia is minimized.

The β-cell is also capable of adapting to the insulin resistance that accompanies obesity or excessive concentrations of glucocorticoids. However, this ability is gradually lost with aging, which may provide a partial explanation of the increased

Table 9.1   Substances Controlling Insulin Release from Pancreatic β-Cells

Stimulatory		Inhibitory
D-Gluose[a]		
threshold	4 mM	
½ maximal release	7–8 mM	
maximal release	12 mM	
Ten amino acid mixture[b]	100%	
arginine	86	
lysine	64	
leucine	34	
phenylalanine	32	
valine	12	
methionine	11	
Glycerol	(indirect)	
Ketone bodies	(in dogs, not in man)	
Hormones		
cholecystokinin		Epinephrine
gastrin		Glucocorticoids
GIP		Norepinephrine
glucagon		Prostaglandin E
secretin		Somatostatin
somatotropin		
VIP		
Neural factors		
β-adrenergic		α-Adrenergic
parasympathetic (vagal)		

[a]See Figure 9.4.
[b]Infusion of 30 g of an individual or mixture of amino acids.

prevalence of glucose intolerance and noninsulin-dependent diabetes mellitus (NIDDM) among those over 60 years of age.

A group of essential amino acids (see Table 9.1) composes the principal secondary insulin secretogogues. Of these, arginine and lysine are the most potent. They affect both the first and second phase of insulin secretion but by a different mechanism than glucose does. The evidence for this is the differential response to inhibitors cited earlier, and the glucose-induced phase I of insulin secretion is absent in NIDDM patients, but arginine-induced phase I is not.

A rather large group of hormones may affect insulin secretion (see Table 9.1). Several of them are gastrointestinal hormones, and one may argue that the function of these hormones, released during digestion, is the preparation of the body, through the release of insulin, for the incoming flood of nutrients. However logical this argument may seem, evidence for the physiological importance of these hormones as insulin secretogogues is very uneven. Gastric inhibitory peptide (GIP) is firmly established. Oral glucose is a more effective stimulator of insulin secretion than is intravenously injected glucose because the former stimulates GIP release which, in humans, provokes the release of insulin (see Chap. 3).

Turmoil is the one word best characterizing prostaglandin research. It is difficult to attain even a consensus on any point because of a combination of factors. Investigators use different species or different tissues from the same species, different assays, and different experimental conditions; then, they try to make *generalized* conclusions. The following statements should be read with the reservation that they are probably sound, but not universally accepted:

1. The pancreatic islet synthesizes arachidonic acid metabolites.
2. PGE_2 . . . inhibit[s] glucose-induced [phase I] insulin secretion and worsen[s] glucose homeostasis.
3. Virtually all inhibitors of the cyclooxygenase pathway, with the sole exception of indomethacin, . . . augment glucose-induced [phase I] insulin secretion and improve glucose homeostasis.
4. Defective glucose-induced first-phase insulin secretion in type II diabetic patients can be partially restored by inhibitors of the cyclooxygenase pathway.
5. Virtually all lipoxygenase inhibitors inhibit secretion caused by glucose and most other secretagogues. [Robertson, 1986]

There is also neural control of insulin secretion (see Table 9.1). Adrenergic control by epinephrine or norepinephrine is inhibitory. These two are considered to act as α-adrenergic stimulants because phentolamine, but not propranolol, prevents epinephrine from inhibiting glucose-induced release of insulin. Epinephrine is ineffective, however, in inhibiting the arginine-induced release of insulin.

The relative contribution of vagal stimulation, which is stimulatory, is not known. Furthermore, although islet (β?) cells have muscarinic receptors binding N-methylscopolamine with a K_d of 2–3 nM, there are no good antagonists. Most experiments have used 1–2 mM carbamylcholine, a 1 million-fold molar excess of inhibitor! Do such large concentrations have some nonspecific effects?

The mechanism of control of insulin secretion is not understood. There are two models: (1) according to the substrate site or metabolism hypothesis, a trigger substance(s) that stimulates insulin secretion is formed in the β-cell during the metabolism of fuel molecules; or (2) in the receptor or regulator site hypothesis, initiation of insulin secretion by fuel molecules is the result of direct interaction of intact fuel molecules with receptors on the β-cell plasma membrane. There is considerable evidence supporting a substrate-site hypothesis.

1. At nonstimulatory concentrations of glucose, fractional usage in the glycolytic pathway of rodent islets is greater than 90%, and it increases at higher glucose levels that stimulate insulin secretion.
2. Inhibitors of glycolysis, such as mannoheptulose, 2-deoxyglucose, and iodoacetate, block insulin secretion in response to increased glucose levels.
3. Inhibitors of glycolysis fail to alter insulin secretion in response to 2-oxoisocaproate, which is metabolized intramitochondrially.

Such results are interpreted as mitochondrial generation of a "trigger," although there is no consensus on what that trigger might be.

On the other hand, the secretory resonse of β-cells may be affected by the intact molecular structure of fuel molecules. For example, certain amino acids in the presence of glucose (arginine, leucine) stimulate insulin secretion. $(-)2-$Aminobicyclo[2,2,1]heptane−2−carboxylic acid, a nonmetabolizable analogue of leucine, also stimulates insulin secretion. It is asserted, however, that this substance increases the metabolism of endogenous amino acids by activation of glutamate dehydrogenase.

Recently, two fractions of islet cell glucokinase with K_m for glucose of 5.7 and 4.5 mM have been described. The characteristics of this enzyme are consistent with the concept that it serves as a glucose sensor of islet β-cells.

In summary, any mechanism proposed for the secretion of insulin must incorporate a host of factors: glucose, nonglucose secretagogues, hormones, neural stimulation and inhibition, cAMP, and Ca^{2+}. The last will probably also draw in inositol triphosphate, diacylglycerol, and protein kinase C. Obviously, the mechanism must be complicated—perhaps, a cascade allowing different factors to activate or inhibit at different levels. There may also be more than one pool of insulin, reflecting the fact that only a small number of β-cells abut a δ-cell.

Regulation of Metabolism

Transport

Insulin is the anabolic hormone, promoting the storage of energy in the form of glycogen, triglycerides, and protein. It promotes glucose transport into fat and muscle cells down a concentration gradient (passive transport). The following properties differentiate carrier-mediated transport (facilitated diffusion) from simple diffusion:

1. Saturation kinetics
2. Stereospecificity
3. Competition between pairs of sugars for transport
4. Counterflow

Uptake of glucose by rat heart muscle, for example, is saturable, having a V_{max} of 380 μmol/g/hr with a K_m of 6.6 mM. The V_{max}, but not the K_m, is increased by insulin. The favored conformation for transport is a pyranose ring having the largest number of hydroxyl groups in the equatorial position. For D-glucose, this means the chair conformation; α-D-glucose is preferred over β-D-glucose.

The order of affinity for a series of sugars is D-glucose > D-galactose >D-xylose > L-arabinose > D-arabinose > L-xylose, L-galactose, and L-glucose. D-3-O-Methylglucose and 2-deoxyglucose also have a high affinity for the carrier. Most, if not all, of these share a common transport system.

Countertransport clearly differentiates passive transport from simple diffusion. For example, 3-O-methylglucose, a nonmetabolized glucose analogue, rapidly enters heart cells and approaches equilibrium distribution (Figure 9.5). The addition of glucose at this point causes a decline in the tissue concentration of 3-O-methylglucose, indicating that it has been transported out of the cell against a concentration gradient. This can be explained as follows: Initially 3-O-methylglucose combines with the carrier and rapidly enters the cells. After a few minutes when intra- and extracellular concentrations are equal, efflux equals influx, and net transport ceases. When glucose is added at a concentration well above its K_m, influx of 3-O-methylglucose is competitively inhibited. Because glucose is rapidly phosphorylated, it does not accumulate within the cell and cannot interfere with the efflux of 3-O-methylglucose. Because efflux of 3-O-methyglucose exceeds influx, its intracellular concentration falls until the flux rates are again equal. Countercurrent transport occurs when two substances share a common carrier, when a concentration gradient of one substrate can be maintained across the membrane, and when efflux and influx pathways do not interfere with each other.

Insulin-sensitive hexose transport systems are responsive to a wide variety of agents, such as oxidants, polyamines, hypertonicity, sulfhydryl reagents, lectins, antireceptor antibodies, antimembrane antibodies, proteases, phospholipases, and neuraminidase. Because it is almost inconceivable that all of these agents share a common feature, their usefulness in providing insight into insulin action is correspondingly slight.

In contrast, amino acid transport is active and involves several transport systems. That for neutral amino acids is coupled with the gradient of sodium concentration across the membrane. Insulin increases the accumulation of some amino acids, but the physiological significance of this effect is doubtful.

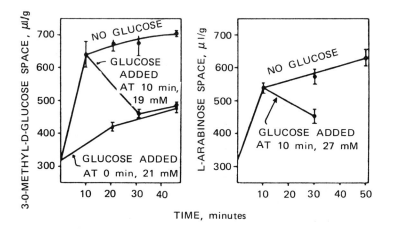

TIME, minutes

Figure 9.5 Countertransport of 3-O-methyl-D-glucose and L-arabinose in isolated, perfused rat hearts on addition of D-glucose to the perfusate Hearts were perfused with oxygenated buffer containing 3-O-methyl-[¹⁴C] D-glucose (0.75 mM) (a) or L-arabinose (13 mM) (b). In some groups in (a), additional glucose was added as indicated. (b)One group perfused with L-arabinose for 10 min was perfused for an additional 20 min with buffer containing 13 mM l-arabinose and 27 mM D-glucose. Distribution of 3-O-methylglucose and L-arabinose is expressed as the sugar "space," i.e., the volume of tissue water required to dissolve the sugar found in the heart at the concentration of sugar in the perfusate. The vertical line through each point indicates 2 SEM; N = 6 (*Source*: from Morgan et al., 1972).

Regulation of Enzymatic Activity

A second way in which insulin can control energy fluxes is control of the enzymatic activity of key regulatory enzymes in the glycolytic and fatty acid synthesis pathways. Our discussion will be centered on three major tissues, liver, muscle, and adipose tissue (Table 9.2), but one should not infer from this that insulin has no effect on other tissues. The activities of the enzymes affected (Table 9.3) are modified either by phosphorylation or dephosphorylation. The mechanism is not known, but it is generally accepted that adenylate cyclase is not involved (see p. 328).

The net effect of these coordinated changes is an increased flux of glucose through the glycolytic pathway, producing

Table 9.2 A Summary of Some Anabolic[a] Effects of Insulin

Liver	Adipose tissue	Muscle
Glycogen synthesis	Glucose transport	Glucose transport
Fatty acid synthesis	Glycerol synthesis	Amino acid transport
Triglyceride synthesis	Fatty acid synthesis	Glycogen synthesis
	Triglyceride synthesis	Protein synthesis

[a]All factors are increased.

Table 9.3 Enzymatic Activities Affected by Insulin

Enzyme	Increase/decrease	Comment
Fructose-1,6-bisphosphatase	↓	Glycolysis
Glycogen synthase	↑	Gylcogen deposition
Pyruvate kinase	↑	Glycolysis
Pyruvate dehydrogenase	↑	AcetylCoA formation
AcetylCoA carboxylase	↑	Fatty acid synthesis
Citrate lyase	↑	Fatty acid synthesis

glycogen and acetyl-CoA. Any excess of the latter over the body's needs for energy is diverted into fatty acid synthesis through the two key enzymes, citrate lyase and acetyl-CoA carboxylase.

Protein synthesis is also increased by insulin, but here it is difficult to single out one or two key enzymes. Certain ribosomal fractions involved in protein synthesis are, however, phosphorylated as a result of insulin action. This, coupled with increased transport of amino acids, may be sufficient to account for the increase in protein synthesis. This leads logically to the next topic.

Regulation of Enzyme Biosynthesis

Insulin can increase the concentration (Table 9.4) of certain key enzymes and thereby their total activity. Occasionally, it can both increase the activity of existing enzyme and synthesize new enzyme (pyruvate kinase).

Table 9.4 Enzymes Reacting to Insulin by Increased Synthesis

Enzyme	Comment
Hexokinase II	Especially in adipose tissue
Glucokinase	Especially in hepatic tissue
Glycogen synthase	
Pyruvate kinase	
Phosphoenolpyruvate carboxykinase	
Lipoprotein kinase	

The three ways in which insulin can effectuate its action have three different time scales. Insulin increases glucose transport (V_{max}) by causing a translocation of glucose transporters from an intracellular pool to the plasma membrane within seconds of insulin binding. This effect may be linked to an even more rapid effect on ion flux and membrane potential, for altering membrane potential by other means produces a similar change in glucose transport. Recruitment of glucose transporters is not instantaneously synonymous with transport of glucose itself; there is a 30-sec lag period (Fig. 9.6) followed by a rapid increase, reaching a maximum in 5 min.

Regulation of enzymatic activity implies the involvement of a second messenger. All manner of compounds have been implicated—peptides, glycopeptides, phospholipids, and even prostaglandinlike compounds—but none have been proved. Even so, it is already apparent that the response time may be somewhat longer (a minute or so) because it is generally assumed that a biochemical reaction must generate the second messenger. Synthesis of enzymes, on the other hand, must certainly take hours to days.

Similarly, the three different responses to insulin have three different mechanisms. Although the path to the glucose transporter appears to be straightforward, that to the second messenger for modification of enzymatic activity appears to be threading its way through a maze, and that requiring gene expression of selected enzymes is indiscernible.

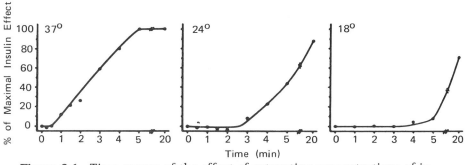

Figure 9.6 Time course of the effect of saturating concentrations of insulin on the rate of uptake of 3-O-methylglucose by adipocytes. Both the lag and stimulation phases are temperature-dependent. *Source*: R Horuk and JM Olefsky. *Diabetes/Met Rev 1*:83, 1985; reprinted by permission of the copyright owner, John Wiley & Sons, Inc.

The Insulin Receptor

Knowledge of the insulin receptor is relatively advanced. Three approaches to the elucidation of its structure were used. Cuatrecasas and Jacobs isolated the receptor in a highly purified form using affinity chromatography as a major purification step. Because of the low concentration of this receptor in tissue, a 250,000-fold purification was required, and it was difficult to accumulate sufficient purified receptor for analysis. Yip and coworkers affinity-labeled the receptor using 4-azidobenzoyl-[125I]iodoinsulin as a ligand. Czech and his colleagues avoided the chemical modification of insulin by use of the cross-linking reagent, bis-N-hydroxysuccinimidyl suberate, on the [125I]iodoinsulin-receptor complex. These last two approaches used the specificity of the binding reaction and the sensitivity of radiolabeling to avoid the unfavorable logistics of isolation.

These and other groups agree on the essential characteristics of the insulin receptor (Fig. 9.7). In four species and three tissues, the receptor has the form B-A-A-B, which is held together by disulfide bonds between the subunits. Upon mild reduction, each AB-dimer still binds insulin. High-affinity binding is lost upon further reduction to the basic subunits.

Recently (1985), the isolation of the cDNA encoding the complete sequence of the proreceptor has confirmed and extended

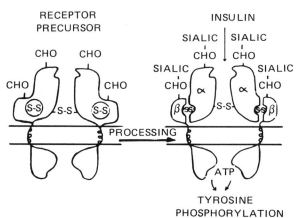

Figure 9.7 General features of the insulin receptor complex deduced from structural studies on the isolated or affinity-labeled complex and from the nucleotide sequence of its cDNA. The proreceptor is a single-chain, incompletely glycosylated polypeptide. Cellular processing leads to a heterotetrameric, disulfide-linked receptor complex. The α subunit binds insulin with high affinity, whereas the β subunit is a transmembrane polypeptide having tyrosine kinase activity. *Source*: MP Czech, KT Yu, RE Lewis. Diabetes Met Rev *1*:34, 1985; reprinted by permission of the copyright owner, John Wiley & Sons, Inc.

these conclusions. The proreceptor is synthesized as a single polypeptide that contains one predicted transmembrane sequence of about 23 amino acids located approximately 400 amino acid residues from the carboxyl terminus. The precursor, which is cotranslationally glycosylated, to a limited extent, and does not bind insulin with high affinity, is processed in several steps. These include the formation of both intramolecular and inter-molecular disulfide bonds, cleavage to form two subunits with polypeptide masses of 83 and 70 kDa, further glycosylation, and finally capping with sialic acid to form the mature receptor subunits of 130 and 90 kDa. A portion of the B-subunit is cytoplasmic, and a portion is exofacial, whereas the entire A-subunit, which contains an insulin-binding site, is exofacial (see Fig. 9.7).

That the gene for the insulin receptor should have considerable homology with those for other growth factors, such as epidermal growth factor (EGF) and insulinlike growth factor (IGF-II), is not surprising, but the homology with various oncogenes was unexpected. After the fact, one can point out that oncogenes promote abnormal growth, and therefore, growth is the thread that runs through the entire family.

As I mentioned before, insulin promotes phosphorylation and dephosphorylation of specific enzymes. Of special interest is a tyrosine kinase that is a part of the cytoplasmic portion of the B-subunit of the insulin receptor. This, again, is a property that is shared with other receptor systems as well as with several oncogenic viruses. Although the tyrosine(s) (of the insulin receptor) that are phosphorylated are not yet rigorously identified, they are part of the cytoplasmic B-subunit (autophosphorylation), and the phosphorylated insulin-receptor complex is more effective in promoting insulin's actions than the nonphosphorylated complex. Some serine and threonines also appear to be phosphorylated, and they appear to inhibit tyrosine kinase.

To date, there is no evidence that the intact insulin receptor is the physiologically active form. Although it is hard to determine this fact, it is easy to test whether or not modification of the receptor changes its binding and kinase properties. Removal of sialic acid from the purified receptor enhances both properties, and trypsin treatment activates kinase activity. The monomeric AB form of the receptor, formed by mild reduction, exhibits much higher kinase activity. Such results are suggestive and intriguing.

Like the low-density lipoprotein (LDL) receptor (see Chap. 2), the insulin-receptor complex is internalized. Unlike the LDL receptor, however, internalization is not an integral step in hormone action. (The status of growth-promoting effects of insulin in this regard are not clear.) The evidence for this conclusion comes from several directions. Responses in hexose transport and enzyme activation are more rapid than the rate of internalization. The rapid actions of insulin are seen even though internalization is chemically blocked. And in vitro, insulin's actions can be demonstrated, even when the insulin is chemically bonded to large aggregates in such a way that pinocytosis is precluded. According to current thinking, the purpose of internalization is the degradation of insulin and a loss of receptors from the sur-face of the cell (down-regulation). The receptor itself recycles back to the plasma membrane several times in its relatively brief life.

GLUCAGON

Chemistry

Glucagon, being a 29-amino acid polypeptide with no cysteine residues, has a simpler structure than insulin (Fig. 9.8). Never-theless, fewer comparisons between species have been made, and the sequence of proglucagon (18 kDa) is largely unknown. Pro-glucagon is unusual in having not only a large NH_2-terminal por-tion but, also, a COOH-terminal octapeptide addition to glucagon (see Fig. 9.8).

Glicentin, a polypeptide isolated from porcine gut, has 100 amino acid residues and glucagonlike immunoreactivity. The par-tial sequences identified so far are identical with those of pan-creatic glucagon.

Regulation of Secretion

Like insulin, the primary regulator of glucagon secretion is glucose, but unlike insulin, glucose's action is inhibitory with a K_i of about 5 mM. Maximum suppression of glucagon release occurs at 9 to 10 mM glucose concentrations.

Glucogenic amino acids directly stimulate glucagon secretion in isolated islets. Because glucagon promotes lipolysis and ketogenesis, it is logical that ketogenic amino acids do not stimulate secretion. On the other hand, high free fatty acid con-centrations depress α-cell secretion, suggesting that they may engage in direct negative-feedback control.

Neural control of the release of the two hormones is also linked. Epinephrine (and norepinephrine) inhibits glucose-induced insulin release and augments glucagon secretion.

Effects

The overall action of glucagon opposes that of insulin. Whereas in-sulin lowers blood glucose by increasing its transport into muscle

```
     1                 5               10              15
....his.ser.gln.gly.thr.phe.thr.ser.asp.tyr.ser.lys.tyr.leu.asp.ser.

           20            25        29
arg.arg.ala.gln.asp.phe.val.gln.trp.leu.met.asn.thr.lys.arg.asn.asn.

lys.asn.ile.ala
```

Figure 9.8 The structure of pancreatic proglucagon. The prohormone consists of a large NH$_2$-terminal polypeptide, the 29-amino acid polypeptide of glucagon and a COOH-terminal octapeptide commencing with a Lys-Arg dipeptide. Note that glucagon contains no cysteine, has seven hydroxyamino acid residues and a basic dipeptide (Arg-17–Arg-18) that apparently is more stable to proteolysis than is the Lys-30–Arg-31 dipeptide.

and fat tissue, glucagon raises blood glucose by increasing hepatic glycogenolysis and gluconeogenesis. Because hepatic glycogen stores are small and muscle (protein) mass is enormous, the latter mechanism predominates; the former is important, however, for a "quick fix." Whereas insulin promotes lipogenesis, glucagon stimulates lipolysis and ketone body formation, thereby offering the tissues an alternative form of energy and minimizing gluconeogenesis which, in turn, spares the muscle needed to obtain the next meal. These opposing actions of insulin and glucagon have led to the concept that the insulin/glucagon ratio is more important than the absolute concentrations of the two hormones.

The molecular mechanisms of glucagon action are known, to various degrees. All, however, presumably involve adenylate cyclase and cAMP. The steps leading to activation of glycogen phosphorylase are now classic textbook material and will not be repeated here. Glucagon also activates hormone-sensitive triglyceride lipase by phosphorylation, the liberated fatty acids (bound to albumin) and glycerol being transported to the liver. There the rate-limiting step in β-oxidation of the fatty acids is transport across the inner mitochrondrial membrane. Again glucagon increases the activity of carnitine palmitoyltransferase I through a decrease in the activity of acetyl-CoA carboxylase and a consequent decrease in the concentration of malonyl-CoA, a potent inhibitor of transferase I. The major portion of the acetyl-CoA generated is made into acetoacetate through hydroxymethyl-glutaryl-CoA; reduction yields D-3-hydroxybutyrate. These two substances plus acetone constitute the ketone bodies: water-soluble, easily oxidizable substances available as an alternate energy source to peripheral tissues. They are normal fuels of metabolism at all times and become quantitatively important in the fasting (or diabetic) state (Table 9.9). Indeed, heart muscle and the renal cortex preferentially metabolize acetoacetate rather than glucose, and even the brain adapts to their utilization during starvation.

Gluconeogenesis requires glucagon (or accompanying conditions) to do two things: turn off glycolysis while turning on gluconeogenesis to prevent futile cycling. Glycolysis is controlled at the three rate-limiting steps: (1) conversion of glucose to glucose-6-phosphate; (2) conversion of fructose-6-phosphate to

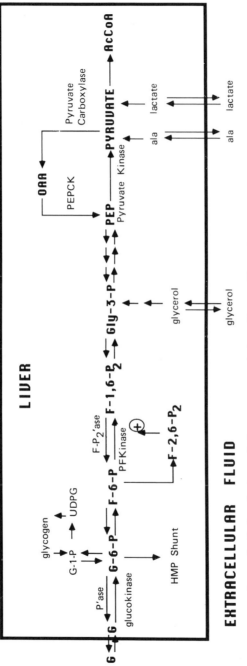

Figure 9.9 Control of glycolysis and gluconeogenesis in a liver cell.

fructose-1,6-bisphosphate, and (3) conversion of phospho-enolpyruvate to pyruvate (Fig. 9.9). Because the major site of gluconeogenesis is the liver (the renal cortex produces about one-tenth as much glucose), this discussion is confined to that organ.

The liver contains both a hexokinase and glucokinase; hex-okinase has a much smaller K_m and V_{max}, whereas glucokinase is induced by insulin. In the well-fed state, glucokinase is responsi-ble for the preponderant part of phosphorylation of glucose; dur-ing starvation, it virtually disappears, and hexokinase maintains a low level of phosphorylation. The reverse action is promoted by glucose-6-phosphatase. The activity of this enzyme increases in starvation. The role that glucagon plays, if any, is not known.

6-Phosphofructo-1-kinase controls the major rate-limiting step in glycolysis—the conversion of fructose-6-phosphate to fructose-1,6-bisphosphate. Although most texts state that this en-zyme is allosterically stimulated by ADP and AMP (and inhibited by ATP and citrate), more recent evidence indicates that fructose-2,6-bisphosphate is a more powerful activator. This syn-thesis is catalyzed by a 6-phosphofructo-2-kinase and reversed by a corresponding phosphatase. Glucagon administration rapidly decreases the level of fructose-2,6-bisphosphate, thereby effec-tively shutting off glycolysis.

Pyruvate kinase catalyzes the third irreversible reaction in glycolysis A two-step reaction is required to reverse it. Pyruvate carboxylase forms oxaloacetate from pyruvate; phosphoenol-pyruvate carboxykinase then completes the reversal. The level of these two enzymes is increased in starvation; the role of glucagon, if any, is not known.

The source of pyruvate is muscle lactate returning to the liver (Cori cycle) or transamination of alanine. The synthesis of alanine transaminase may be induced by cortisol. Glycerol returning to the liver from adipose tissue, which does not possess a glycerol kinase, is phosphorylated and enters the gluconeogenic pathway at the level of 3-phosphoglyceraldehyde.

GLUCOCORTICOIDS

The glucocorticosteroids are those steroids made by the adrenal cortex that influence (among other things) carbohydrate metabolism. The two natural products are corticosterone and cortisol (hydrocortisone). The ratio of the two depends upon the species involved; for example, rats make only the former, whereas humans make both in a ratio of about 1:5 corticosterone/cortisol, respectively; (see Table 8.2).

Corticoliberin

Corticotropin-releasing hormone (CRH), a polypeptide having 41 amino acid residues (Fig. 9.10), has been sequenced from sheep, pig, rat, and human, the last being determined from the sequence of its cDNA. The NH$_2$-terminus is not needed as CRH4–41 has complete activity, whereas the COOH-terminus is very sensitive to alteration. The CRH1–41 segment with a free terminal alanine carboxyl group or CRH1–39-NH$_2$ possesses less than 0.1% potency. The maximum response to CRH is equal to that of 8-bromo-cAMP; norepinephrine or Arg(8)-vasopressin exhibit only 30 to 50% and 10 to 20% of the intrinsic activity of CRH, respectively (but see later discussion). Both natural and synthetic CRH cause a dose-dependent release of corticotropin (ACTH) and β-lipotropin (LPH) that is inhibited by glucocorticoid.

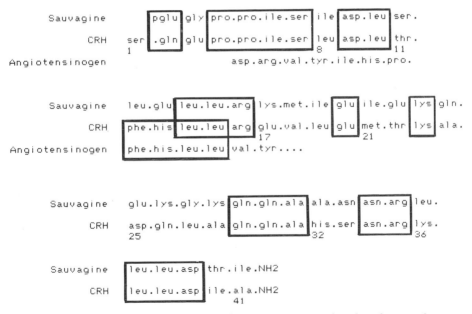

Figure 9.10 Primary sequence of ovine CRH and related peptides (*Source*: from Vale et al., 1981).

The three hormones, CRH, vasopressin (VP), and neurophysin (VP), are contained within the same neurosecretory vesicles in the median eminence; hence, coordinate secretion is obligatory. Both CRH and VP are found in portal blood, and VP potentiates the effect of CRH on ACTH secretion from anterior pituitary cells in vitro. These data support the hypothesis that CRH and VP act synergistically in vitro to promote secretion of ACTH. Secretion is calcium-dependent.

Corticotropin-releasing hormone contains regions homologous with other peptides (see Fig. 9.10). It shares the tetrapeptide, Phe-His-Leu-Leu, with angiotensinogen, the precursor of angiotensin II and III. More intriguing is the extensive homology with sauvagine, a peptide from frog skin! There is almost 50% homology, and an additional 12 amino acids could represent single-base changes. Remember that other mammalian hormones or hormonal candidates, such as thyrotropin-releasing hormone (TRH) and bombesin, also occur in frog skin.

Corticotropin

Adrenocorticotropin (ACTH), a 39-amino acid polypeptide, is one of the hormones controlling the synthesis of steroids in the zona fasciculata and reticularis of the adrenal cortex. The first 25 amino acid residues, the portion that carries the biological message, are invariant among mammals (Fig. 9.11). Even the dogfish has only three conservative changes. The message is read by plasma membrane receptors that, in turn, control the synthesis of glucocorticoids and androgens (see p. 340).

The detection and isolation of proinsulin led to a search for large precursor molecules of other hormones. The one for ACTH was initially missed because it was larger than expected. In fact, it was the first of the multigene hormones in which the gene product contains several hormones linked in series through basic dipeptides. In ACTH, it is found in a 3l-kDa (265-amino acid) polypeptide containing α-, β-, and γ-melanocyte-stimulating hormone (MSH), corticotropinlike intermediate lobe polypeptide (CLIP), β- and γ lipotropin (LPH), β-endorphin (endorphin = *endo*genous m*orphine*) and met-enkephalin, as well as ACTH itself (Fig. 9.12). There is no official name for the conglomerate, but the name proopiomelanocortin (POMC), which sums its principal

```
            1              5                        10
Human       ser.tyr.ser.met.glu.his.phe.arg.trp.gly.lys.pro.val.gly.
Porcine
Ovine/bovine
Dogfish                                                         met


            15            20                       25
Human       lys.lys.arg.arg.pro.val.lys.val.tyr.pro.asn.gly.ala.glu.
Porcine
Ovine/bovine
Dogfish     arg                   ile                    ser.phe


            30            35                       39
Human       asp.glu.ser.ala.glu.ala.phe.pro.leu.glu.phe.
Porcine                  leu
Ovine/bovine                 gln
Dogfish                  val     asn.met.gly.pro       leu
```

Figure 9.11 Primary structure of ACTH from several species.

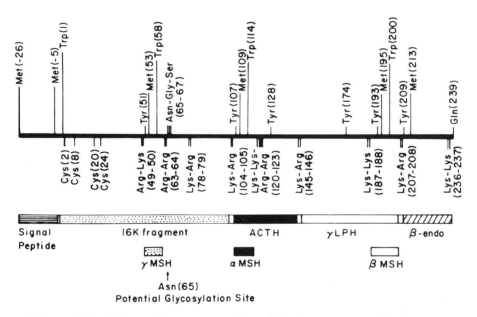

Figure 9.12 Schematic representation of bovine proopiomelanocortin. The numbering starts with ACTH, positive to the right and negative to the left. Met-(−131) is assumed to be the translational initiation site. The location of known component peptides is shown by shaded bars (*Source*: from Nakanishi et al., 1979).

341

parts, is widely accepted. The end products vary with the cells in which processing occurs. In the corticotropes of the adenohypophyseal gland, ACTH and β-LPH are released from POMC in equimolar quantities.

The α-MSH and β-MSH, portions of ACTH and LPH, respectively, are synthesized in the intermediate lobe of the pituitary, a tissue that humans do not have. These hormones provoke the aggregation of melanin granules in integumental melanocytes, thereby enabling certain species to change their protective coloration rapidly. The γ-MSH form was discovered when the cDNA of POMC was sequenced. It was subsequently isolated from several species; the sequence of the human 76-amino acid glycopeptide contains two disulfide bridges (Cys 2 to 8 and Cys 20 to 24) and two glycosylation sites (Asn-65 and possibly Thr-45) flanking the γ-MSH sequence (Tyr-51 to Gly-62)(Fig. 9.13). Furthermore, the length of the glycopeptide apparently varies with the species, being shortest (74 residues) for the rat and longest (80 residues) for the pig.

Unexpectedly, the NH$_2$-terminal glycopeptide of POMC has significant homology with calcitonins from seven species, varying from 16 to 28%. Interestingly, the human glycopeptide has the lowest homology with human calcitonin and the highest homology with porcine calcitonin. Both the human and porcine glycopeptides are also equipotent with ACTH in stimulating the release of aldosterone from human adrenal tumor cells.

Steroidogenesis

I previously (Chap. 2) discussed the fact that most steroid production is derived from LDL cholesterol deposited in steroidogenic cells as lipid droplets containing cholesterol esters, mainly the arachidonate ester in humans. Obiovusly, hydrolysis of ester and transport of the hydrophobic cholesterol molecule into the mitochondria is a prerequisite to side-chain cleavage. Although ACTH, through a cAMP mechanism, does stimulate cholesterol esterase, the degree of stimulation is not consonant with the V_{max} of steroidogenesis. Pedersen and Brownie tested the ability of a series of fragments of POMC to synergize with submaximal concentrations of ACTH in activating cholesterol esterase. Only the NH$_2$-terminal 16-kDa fragment was active (minimally), but a

```
                  ┌─────────────────────────────┐         10
(h)   H2N.TRP.CYS.LEU.GLU.SER.SER.GLN.CYS.GLN.ASP.LEU.THR.THR.GLU.SER.
(b)
(p)                                                              SER
(rat)
```

```
                       20 ┌───────────────────┐               30
(h)        ASN.LEU.LEU.GLU.CYS.ILE.ARG.ALA.CYS.LYS.PRO.ASP.LEU.SER.ALA.
(b)                     ALA
(p)                     ALA
(rat)                   ALA                         ARG.LEU
```

```
                                                               Y
                                40                             │
(h)        GLU.THR.PRO.MET.PHE.PRO.GLY.ASN.GLY.ASP.GLU.---.GLN.PRO.LEU.THR.
(b)                     VAL                          ---
(p)                     VAL                       GLX.ALA
(rat)                   VAL                          ---
```

```
                        │<─────────────── ɣ-MSH ───────────────
                        50 │                                60
(h)        GLU.ASN.PRO.ARG.LYS.TYR.VAL.MET.GLY.HIS.PHE.ARG.TRP.ASP.ARG.
(b)
(p)
(rat)
α-MSH              CH3.CO.SER      SER     GLU              TYR.GLY.LYS.
β-MSH(b)           ASP.SER.GLY.PRO LYS     GLU              TYR.GLY.SER.
```

```
           ------>│              Y
                  │              │              70
(h)        PHE.GLY.ARG.ARG.---.ASN.SER.SER.SER.SER.GLY.SER.SER.GLY.ALA.GLY.
(b)                         ASN.GLY                   VAL.GLY         ALA
(p)                         ASN GLY       GLY.GLY     GLY.GLY
(rat)              PRO       ASX ----------           SER.ALA.GLY     SER.ALA
α-MSH      PRO.VAL.OH
β-MSH      PRO.PRO.LYS.ASP.OH
```

```
(h)        GLN.OH
(b)
(p)
(rat)
```

Figure 9.13 Sequence of several pro-γ-MSHs and a comparison with α-and βMSH. The rat sequence is not known before residue 19 of the human peptide; in the porcine peptide, replace all Glu and Gln with Glx and Asp and Asn with Asx. Note the 100% homology within the γ-MSH region of pro-γ-MSH and the very high homology at the NH₂-terminal end of this peptide.

trypsin digest of this fragment was quite active. Eventually this activity was traced to the γ_3-MSH liberated (γ_3-MSH consists of γ-MSH plus some additional COOH-terminal amino acids, the human and rat polypeptides containing 25 and 27 amino acids, respectively). The physiological significance of this observation must still be established.

The rate-limiting reaction promoted by ACTH is always side-chain cleavage (see Chap. 8). Beyond this point, the products of the inner zones of the adrenal cortex differ from those of the zona glomerulosa (see Chap. 6) because they contain a slightly different complement of enzymes: namely, the inner zones lack an 18-hydroxylase and possess a 17-hydroxylase (Fig. 9.14). Most of the pregnenolone formed from cholesterol is converted to 17-hydroxypregnenolone which is, in turn, converted to the two principal products of the adrenal cortex (on a quantitative basis): dehydroepiandrosterone (DHEA) and cortisol. The former is formed by a second side-chain cleavage, the latter by dehydrogenation at C-3 and consecutive hydroxylations at C-21 and C-11. Corticosterone is also formed by the latter sequence but omitting the 17-hydroxylation.

Note, that of the reactions described, all are irreversible and that there are alternative pathways at many points. Thus, if there is a deficiency or lack of a particular hydroxylase (see p. 362), the substrate for that enzyme accumulates, and an alternative pathway is utilized to produce quantities of products usually present in minor amounts.

Metabolism of all 4-en-3-one–type hormones proceed reductively. Four protons are added in ring A to produce saturated alcohols; 20-oxo groups are also reduced. These two reactions are unordered. On the other hand, 11β- and 17β-hydroxyl groups are readily oxidized. The 11β-ol to 11-oxo reaction is readily reversible so that parental administration of cortisone is equivalent to administration of cortisol (Fig. 9.15). If cortisone is given intrasynovially, however, it is ineffective because absorption from the joint cavity is slow.

Cortisol, as well as progesterone, is tranported in the blood bound to a specific, high-affinity, low-capacity β-globulin called transcortin (52 kDa). The association constant is about 2×10^7 M^{-1} at 37°C and 3×10^8 M^{-1} at 4°C, with little difference between the affinity of the two ligands, which displace each other

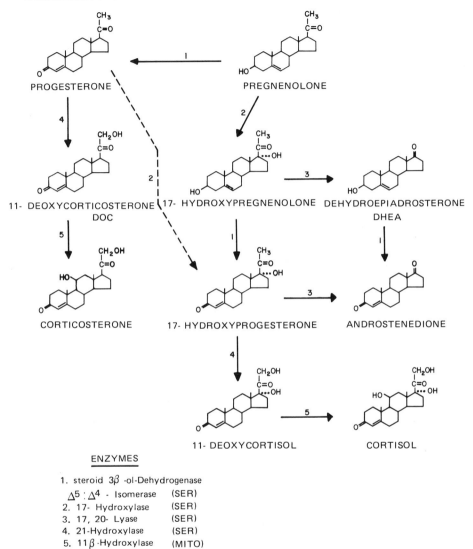

ENZYMES

1. steroid 3β -ol-Dehydrogenase
   Δ5 : Δ4 - Isomerase   (SER)
2. 17- Hydroxylase   (SER)
3. 17, 20- Lyase   (SER)
4. 21-Hydroxylase   (SER)
5. 11β -Hydroxylase   (MITO)

Figure 9.14 Steroidogenesis in the zona fasciculata and reticularis. Most DHEA synthesis is believed to occur in the zona reticularis which does not complete its development until the age of adrenarche (see Chap. 8). All hydroxylases are mixed-function oxidases. They, as well as the lyase, require NADPH, O_2, and cytochrome P_{450}, as well as steroid substrate. The hydroxylations are ordered reactions that follow the sequence 17, 21, 11.

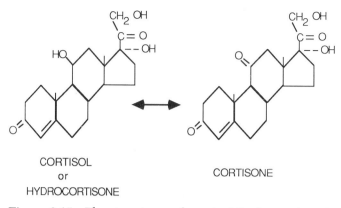

CORTISOL
or
HYDROCORTISONE

CORTISONE

Figure 9.15 The structures of cortisol (hydrocortisone) and cortisone.

from a single binding site. This high binding means that about 90% of cortisol is bound and 10% is unbound at 37°C. There is no satisfactory explanation of how a hydrophobic and a hydrophilic ligand can each bind to a common site with nearly the same affinity. There is also no published evidence for two separate interacting sites. Estrogens increase the plasma concentration of transcortin.

Regulation of the Hypothalamoadenohypophyseal–adrenocortical Axis

The simple concept of negative-feedback first mentioned (see Fig. 1.1). must now be enlarged to explain all the observations made. This system responds to stress in all of its forms: physical and surgical trauma; noxious chemical and biological agents; extreme hypoglycemia, exercise, or cold; highly emotional states, such as crucial examinations or solo performances; and many others. Some of the stresses applied experimentally are swimming in water at 4°C, ether anesthesia, laparotomy, immobilization or injection of histamine, endotoxin, or insulin. Corticosteroids, usually corticosterone, cortisol, or dexamethasone, a synthetic, potent analogue, exert a negative-feedback in a complex way, both temporally and mechanistically. Endogenous corticosteroids may have their primary actions in vivo at the level of the brain and of the hypothalamus, whereas synthetic glucocortocoids that do not bind to transcortin may act primarily on corticotropes and regions of the brain that lie outside the blood–brain barrier.

There appear to be three major time frames of corticosteroid feedback action: fast (0–30 min), intermediate (1–8 hr), and slow (8 hr to days). The fast feedback of stimulated ACTH response occurs if a stimulus is applied soon after injection of steroid and is dependent upon the *rate* of rise of plasma glucocorticoids. This rate is minimally 13 μg/L/min (38 nM/min) in male rats (higher in females) and 27 μg/L/min (75 nM/min) in hypoadrenocortical humans. This feedback action affects both stimulated CRH and ACTH secretion. Although the mechanism is not known, its rapidity suggests an effect on hormone release rather than hormone synthesis, i.e., a membrane effect. Both 11-deoxycorticosterone and 11-deoxycortisol antagonize the fast-feedback effect of corticosterone.

Delayed feedback of corticosteroids on stimulated ACTH response occurs if a stimulus is applied at least 1 hr, but better, 2 to 4 hr after the start of glucocorticoid infusion. This response is sensitive to the integrated steroid concentration (plasma steroid concentration $\times$ time). 11-Deoxycorticosterone and 11-deoxycortisol are agonists of this action, indicating a different pathway for delayed feedback. Intermediate or delayed corticosteroid feedback inhibits ACTH release but not its synthesis, and both release and synthesis of CRH.

Prolonged exposure (>1 day) to corticosteroids inhibits both the release and synthesis of ACTH, probably through a reduction in the level of mRNA for POMC. The translational efficiency of mRNA for POMC or the processing of POMC to ACTH is not affected by glucocorticoid treatment. The half-time for disappearance of POMC and its mRNA is 16 hr with a maximum (80%) effect occurring with 48 hr of steroid treatment of AtT20 cells (a murine pituitary cell line).

Figure 9.16 summarizes these observations. Note that in vivo there is a "silent" period extending from 30 min to 60 to 90 min in which no inhibition occurs; this silent period does not exist at the level of the corticotropes. In summary, under conditions of stimulation, ACTH secretion is inhibited in a dose-dependent manner by glucocorticoids in all three time domains, albeit through different mechanisms.

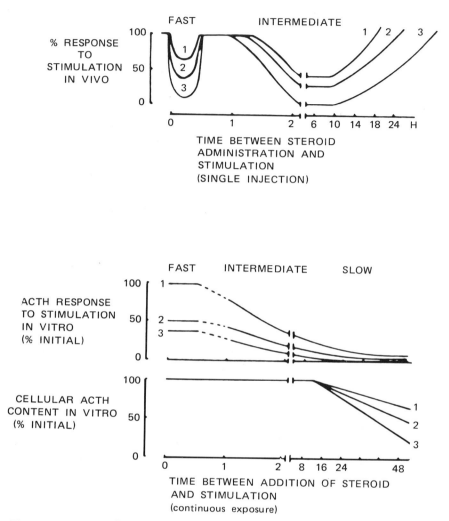

Figure 9.16 Time frames of corticosteroid inhibition of ACTH secretion in vivo. Increasing amounts of steroid injected (3 > 2 > 1) increases the rate of plasma corticosteroid concentration and produces increasing degrees of inhibition to a stimulus during the period of fast-feedback. Increasing the dose also increases the level of circulating steroid achieved and the duration of that level; these produce increasing degrees and duration of inhibition during the period of intermediate-feedback. Little or no inhibition occurs if the stimulus is applied during the "silent" period between the times of fast- and intermediate-fastback (*Source*: from Keller-Wood and Dallman, 1984).

Most endocrine organs exhibit a basal secretion of hormone, i.e., a secretion independent of any stimulatory hormone. With ACTH, basal secretion follows a different set of rules than stimulated secretion. In both humans and rats, glucocorticoids inhibit basal ACTH secretion during the silent period, as well as at other times. Because spontaneous release in vitro is not inhibited (by reasonable concentrations of glucocorticoids), inhibition of the CRH neuron or of its afferent pathways may be mediating the inhibition of basal ACTH release in vivo.

Synthesis and secretion of glucocorticoids in an unstressed state is both episodic and diurnal. The peak secretion of cortisol occurs in the early morning hours just before or after awakening, i.e., it is sleep-entrained. As the day progresses, the frequency and amplitude of secretory bursts diminish until by evening the adrenal is dormant and plasma cortisol concentrations approach the limit of detection—unless stressful events intervene. Changing one's sleep pattern by moving swiftly across several time zones or going on to a night shift produces a listlessness, sometimes called "jet lag," which lasts for a few days to a week until the body becomes accustomed to a new sleep pattern.

What is the physiological significance of such complexity? Fast, rate-sensitive feedback may control the rate and magnitude of ACTH and corticosteroid responses to stimuli before delayed feedback has a chance to become operative, thus preventing exaggerated responses. Moreover, multiple stimuli in the fast-feedback domain are not necessarily additive. For example, rats are unresponsive to a second application of ether vapor applied within 15 min of the first one or to a second immobilization applied within 5 min of the first one. This effect is not demonstrable in the delayed-feedback time domain, perhaps because of the sensitization of the adrenocortical system by a prior stress.

Biological Effects of Glucocorticoids

Cortisol, in nonstress situations, has no demonstrable function. In fact, an addisonian (a person with no, or minimal functioning adrenal cortex) has no problems with daily life until stressed. In stressful situations, however, it is essential for life. The major effects are summarized in Table 9.5. In addition, cortisol plays a permissive role in adipose tissue, allowing other hormones (epinephrine, glucagon) to mobilize fatty acids.

Table 9.5 Pharmacological Actions of Glucocortcoids

Increased	Decreased
Nitrogen (urea) excretion	Protein synthesis
Gluconeogenesis	Glucose transport into muscle/fat
Neutrophils	Eosinophils
RBCs	Basophils
Mineralocorticoid activity (mild)	Inflammatory reaction
Phenylethanolamine-N-methyl transferase	Hypersensitivity reaction
Transaminases	Histamine synthesis
Tryptophan-2,3-dioxygenase	Release of CRH and ACTH

The diversity of effects presented in Table 9.5 challenges scientists to devise a unifying theory. So far, no one has been equal to the challenge. The most recent (1984) hypothesis by Munck and coworkers postulates that the major action of glucocorticoids in response to stress is the suppression of the mediators of the body's defense mechanisms to avoid their over-shooting and creating damage. They are careful to distinguish between basal, permissive levels of glucocorticoids, on the one hand, and abnormal changes on the other, and their discussion pointedly excludes them. The unifying basis of all glucocorticoid action is the presence of uniform, high-affinity glucocorticoid receptors in essentially every nucleated cell in the body. Munck's hypothesis is attractive because it unifies the physiology of the adrenocortical system on a rational basis and provides the framework within which new experiments can be planned and interpreted.

EPINEPHRINE

Chemistry

The catecholamines include the neurotransmitters, norepinephrine, epinephrine, and dopamine. Dopamine tonicly inhibits prolactin secretion, while epinephrine is the principal hormone released from the arenal medulla, as long as the adrenal cortex makes cortisol. Norepinephrine and dopamine are widely distributed in the CNS.

Synthesis of epinephrine in the adrenal medulla beginning with tyrosine requires two hydroxylations, a decarboxylation and a transmethylation. The rate-limiting step is the first (Fig. 9.17 and 9.18). The level of tyrosine hydroxylase is controlled mainly by neuronal impulses releasing acetylcholine. The last step is also controlled, this time by glucocorticoid through capillary transport from the surrounding cortex. It induces the transcription of DNA and synthesis of phenylethanolamine-N-methyl transferase (PNMT) which transfers a methyl group from S-adenosylmethionine (SAM). Obviously, synthesis will stop at the norepinephrine state unless a critical and rather high concentration of glucocorticoid prevails.

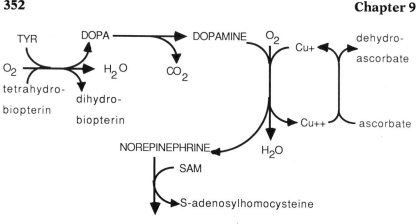

Figure 9.17 Biosynthesis of the catecholamines, dopamine (as an intermediate), norepinephrine, and epinephrine from tyrosine. Note that synthesis requires two different mixed-function oxidases, neither of which utilizes cytochrome P_{450}. Tyrosine hydroxylase and L-amino acid decarboxylase are cytoplasmic enzymes.

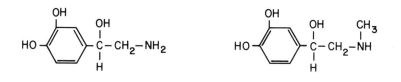

Figure 9.18 Structures of adrenomedullary catecholamines. The naturally occurring D-forms are 15 to 20 times more potent than the L-isomers.

Regulation

The medulla, which arises embryologically in the neural crest, remains a functional part of the nervous system and may be considered as a specialized sympathetic ganglion innervated by the customary long preganglionic neurons. There is a cholinergic synapse with chromaffin cells in the medulla.

    The catecholamines are contained mostly in chromaffin granules, a subcellular organelle within the chromaffin cells. The catecholamine concentration in the granules (0.55 M) can be as much as 30,000 times higher than that in the cytoplasm. A number of proteins have been identified in the granule membrane. Some of these are dopamine β-hydroxylase (EC 1.14.17.1), H^+-ATPase (EC 3.6.1.3), NADH:(acceptor)oxidoreductase (EC 1.6.99.3), phosphatidylinositol kinase (EC 2.7.1.67), cytochrome B_{561}, and α-actinin. Addition of ATP to a suspension of chromaffin granules results in the generation of a membrane potential of 80 to 100 mV, positive inside, which provides the driving force for amine influx through a reserpine-sensitive carrier coupled to proton efflux. The carrier protein for monoamine transport has not been characterized.

Discharge of catecholamines into the circulation is a response elicited by a wide variety of stimuli. Impulses from the CNS converge into a final common pathway arising in the hypothalamus and in the midbrain. The pathways in the CNS appear to involve catecholamines as well as other transmitters. For example, catecholamines in the arcuate nucleus are selectively decreased in animals subjected to the stresses of immobilization, formalin injection, or exposure to cold. Other stimuli include hypoglycemia, or histamine, or bradykinin injection..

Effects

The metabolic responses concern carbohydrate and lipid metabolism. At physiologic concentrations, epinephrine produces glycogenolysis and the accumulation of lactic acid in muscle. The latter is used by the heart as an energy source and by the liver in gluconeogenesis. At considerably higher (pathologic) concentrations, epinephrine will also produce hepatic glycogenolysis. The mechanism through cAMP is now a classic textbook example of a cascade amplification. Norepinephrine has about one-fifth the activity of epinephrine.

A major target of both epinephrine and norepinephrine is adipose tissue. In the presence of cortisol, they activate hormone-sensitive triglyceride lipase through a cAMP mechanism. The fatty acids so liberated serve as an alternative energy source in a stressful situation.

Epinephrine and norepinephrine differ in their effects on blood vessels and on the heart. Epinephrine constricts cutaneous and renal arterioles but dilates skeletal muscle vessels. Norepinephrine is a more potent general vasoconstrictor, although less potent cutaneously. On the other hand, the increased rate and force of cardiac contraction is attributable solely to epinephrine.

Adrenergic Receptors

The actions of these two catecholamines are mediated by α-receptors and β-receptors; these responses may be similar or different (Table 9.6). The major β-adrenergic responses are contraction of most smooth muscle, relaxation of intestinal smooth muscle, inhibition of insulin secretion, stimulation of salivary K^+ and water excretion, aggregation of platelets, and stimulation of hepatic glycogenolysis in some species.

Actually, the subject is more complicated than I have represented it to be because each category can be further subdivided on the basis of the pharmacological actions of inhibitors, and now on the basis of neurobiochemistry. For example, epinephrine, isoproterenol, and norepinephrine all stimulate myocardium. The first two also stimulate bronchial muscle, but epinephrine does not. Obviously the two tissues have different kinds of β-receptors, the myocardial receptor now being called β_1 and the bronchial β_2. Both β-receptors bind to Ns, the stimulatory guanine nucleotide-binding protein of the adenylate cyclase complex (see Chap. 1), in hormone-sensitive tissues.

Similarly, α-receptors may be subdivided. α_2-Receptors bind to Ni, the inhibitory guanine nucleotide-binding protein of the adenylate cyclase complex (see Chap. 1), in hormone-sensitive tissues. α_1-Receptors stimulate the Ca^{2+}–protein kinase C pathway.

In comparison with the β-adrenergic system, work on the α_1-adrenergic mechanisms is just beginning because only recently have specific labeled α_1-antagonists ([³H]dihydroergocryptine and [³H]WB-4104) and an α_1-agonist ([³H]clonidine) become available. Therefore, the following statements are tentative conclusions based on a small number of observations. As work on more tissues and more species is reported, some conclusions may be modified or perhaps abandoned.

α-Receptors appear to be located on plasma membranes of target cells. It is speculated that binding of an α_1-agonist activates a plasma membrane enzyme, releasing a primary intracellular signal (a second messenger that is not a cyclic nucleotide) that

Table 9.6 Characteristics of α- and β-Adrenergic Receptors

Characteristics	α-Receptors	β-Receptors
Sensitivity to agonists	Epi > nor > phenyl > iso	Iso > epi > nor > phenyl
Typical antagonists	Phentolamine	Propranolol
	Phenoxybenzamine	Dichlorisoproterenol
	Ergot alkaloids	Alprenolol
Typical responses		
most smooth muscles	Contraction	Relaxation
intestinal smooth muscle	Relaxation	Relaxation
salivary glands	K^+ and H_2O excretion	Amylase excretion
cardiac muscle	Increased contractility	Increased contractility and heart rate
platelets	Aggregation	Inhibition of aggregation
pancreas	Inhibition of insulin secretion	Stimulation of insulin secretion
adipose tissue	Inhibition of lipolysis	Lipolysis
liver	Glycogenolysis	Glycogenolysis
skeletal muscle		Glycogenolysis

Abbreviations used: epi, epinephrine; nor, norepinephrine; phenyl, phenylephrine; iso, isoproterenol.
Source: modified from Exton, 1981.

promotes the release of calcium from the endoplasmic reticulum. Phosphatidylinositol breakdown is an early response preceding a change in cytosolic calcium concentration. Although it is not known for certain whether this is a prerequisite to calcium release or simply a concomitant, unrelated event, our discussion in Chapter 1 would lead us to expect the critical enzyme to be phospholipase C, the second messenger to be inositol triphosphate, and the relationship to be significant.

Recently, reports on the structure of adrenergic receptors have begun to appear (Table 9.7). As expected, work on the β-adrenergic receptors is more advanced. The β-receptor may be subdivided into β_1- receptors and β_2-receptors based on differential affinity to selected antagonists. All physicochemical characterizations, such as pI, Stokes radii, and radiation inactivation analysis, also indicate a difference, with the β_1-receptor being smaller and more acidic than the β_2-receptor. The latter has recently been cloned and sequenced. The gene contains no introns and produces a 418-amino acid polypeptide that contains no signal·sequence. The peptide resembles the visual protein opsin and is homologous with it. Both have seven hydrophobic regions 20 to 25 amino acids long, that may be transmembrane segments, both are involved in signal transduction, and both are phosphorylated.

Table 9.7 Molecular Characteristics of β-Adrenergic Receptors

Characteristic	β_1 Receptor	β_2 Receptor
Endogenous ligand	Epinephrine, norepinephrine	Epinephrine
pI (isoelectric point)	5.5 (Turkey RBCs)	4.2 (Canine lung)
Stokes radius	4.2 (Canine heart) 4.3 (Turkey RBCs)	5.8 (Dog lung, liver)
Hydrodynamic mol. mass	65 kDa (Turkey RBCs & canine heart)	90 kDa (Dog lung, liver)
SDS-PAGE mol. mass	65–70 kDa (Turkey RBCs) Smaller subunits or fragments	55–58 kDa (Dog, calf lung) 114 kDa Intact receptor
Radiation inactivation	90 kDa (Turkey RBCs)	109 kDa (Canine lung)

Source: modified from Venter and Fraser, 1983.

A comparison of the α_1-adrenergic receptor and α_2-adrenergic receptor shows that they have the same size and share immunogenic determinants, indicating that they may have evolved as a result of gene duplication.

INTEGRATION

Human glucose counterregulation is commonly believed to pit glucagon, catecholamines, somatotropin, and cortisol against insulin. [Pure STH should *not* be counterregulatory as the somatomedins produced by its action possess *insulinlike* properties (see Tables 4.3 and 4.4)]. But are they equally effective? Gerich and colleagues answered this question for *acute* (90 min) responses to insulin-induced hypoglycemia in normal and adrenalectomized subjects. They used an infusion of somatostatin to suppress both glucagon and STH release or they infused somatostatin plus either glucagon or STH. Similarly, they infused phentolamine plus propranolol (complete α- and β-blockade) with, or without, somatostatin. These experiments showed that restoration of normoglycemia after insulin-induced hypoglycemia primarily is due to a compensatory increase in glucose production; that intact glucagon secretion, but not STH or cortisol secretion, is necessary for normal glucose counter-regulation; and that adrenergic mechanisms are not normally involved but become important whenever glucagon secretion is impaired. In *chronic* hypoglycemia, such as starvation, there can be no doubt of the importance of cortisol in inducing transaminases to supply the precursors for gluconeogenesis.

Another implication of the aforementioned experiments as well as of many other experiments is the importance of coordinate control of metabolism. You have already learned about futile cycling in one-step reactions, such as the importance of not having 6-phosphofructokinase and fructose-1,6-bisphosphate phosphatase both active at the same time. The same reasoning applies to whole sequences, such as glycolysis and gluconeogenesis, or lipogenesis and lipolysis and ketone body formation. Although the importance of coordinate control here is axiomatic, the details of the mechanisms remain obscure. The mechanism of mobilizing fuel in, say, a fight-or-flight situation must be rapid and must, I assume, use covalent modification of enzymatic activity. On the other hand, chronic stimuli may use either this method of response or enzyme induction.

Because of the interplay of hormonal systems in intact animals, it is difficult to sort out these two responses to extended stimuli. The recent introduction of cell culture techniques employing *defined* media (no serum) permit a more direct approach. For example, Spence and Pitot using primary cultures of adult male rat hepatocytes showed indirectly that either T_3 (10 μM) or insulin (1 μM) produced a two- to threefold increase in several lipogenic enzymes, namely, glucose-6-phosphate dehydrogenase, malic enzyme, ATP-citrate lyase, acetyl-CoA carboxylase, fatty acid synthetase, and stearoyl-CoA desaturase. [Oddly, fructose or glycerol (5 mM) without hormone did the same thing.] Note that such experiments tell us what is possible, not what happens under physiologic conditions. It is another tool that will be used more frequently in the future to define the limits of reality.

A summary of changes in key enzymes *as we understand them today* appears in Table 9.8.

In the well-fed state (Fig. 9.19), the insulin/glucagon ratio is high because the high serum glucose concentration suppresses glucagon and stimulates insulin secretion. As a result, anabolic reactions predominate. The synthesis and the activation of key enzymes in glycolysis and lipogenesis (see Table 9.8) promote the conversion of glucose to triglycerides, the major fuel depot of the body. Glycogen stores in muscle and liver are also repleted. Amino acids are incorporated into protein. The early "fasting" state (Fig. 9.20) represents that period between regular meals when digestion has ended (normally 2–3 hr after eating) and the portal vein is no longer presenting the liver with large quantities of nutrients. Consequently the insulin/glucagon ratio drops. Glucose is mobilized from glycogen stores. The absence of glucose-6-phosphatase in muscle tissue prevents the escape of glucose from that tissue. Rather, it is glycolized to pyruvate and converted largely to lactate and alanine for transport to the liver and gluconeogenesis.

The supply of glycogen is limited, however, compared with that of triglycerides (760 vs. 135,000 cal in a normal 70-kg subject; in obese subjects, the latter may be as large as 700,000 cal).

Table 9.8   Key Enzymes in Metabolism

| Enzyme | Covalent modification | | | |
| | Well-fed state | | Starvation | |
	Form	Active	Form	Active
Glycolysis				
glucokinase	—	—	—	—
6-P-fructo-1-kinase	−P	Yes	+P	No
6-P-fructo-2-kinase	−P?	Yes?	+P?	No?
pyruvate kinase	−P	Yes	+P	No
Lipogenesis				
G-6-P dehydrogenase	—	—	—	—
6-P-gluconate DHGase	—	—	—	—
Malate enzyme	—	—	—	—
pyruvate DHGase	−P	Yes	+P	No
ATP-citrate lyase	—	—	—	—
acetylCoA carboxylase	−P	Yes	+P	No
fatty acid synthase	—	—	—	—
stearoylCoA desaturase	—	—	—	—
lipoprotein lipase	—	—	—	—
HMGCoA reductase	−P	Yes	+P	No
Gluconeogenesis				
aminotransferase	—	—	—	—
pyruvate carboxylase	—	—	—	—
PEPCK	—	—	—	—
fructose-1,6-bis-phosphatase	—	—	—	—
G-6-Pase	—	—	—	—
Miscellaneous				
glycogen phosphorylase	−P	No	+P	Yes
glycogen synthase	−P	Yes	+P	No
triglyceride lipase	−P	No	+P	Yes
carnitine palmitoyltransferase I	—	—	—	—

Abbreviations used: DHGase, dehydrogenase; −P, dephosphorylated from; +P, phosphorylated form.

Therefore, as glycogen stores are depleted, the body turns to fat stores for its energy needs and to protein stores for its obligatory glucose needs (Fig. 9.21). The insulin/glucagon ratio decreases still further. The activation of hormone-sensitive triglyceride lipase promotes the release of large amounts of fatty acids into the blood (tenfold increase, Table 9.9). Carnitine palmitoyl transferase I becomes active in the presence of decreased levels

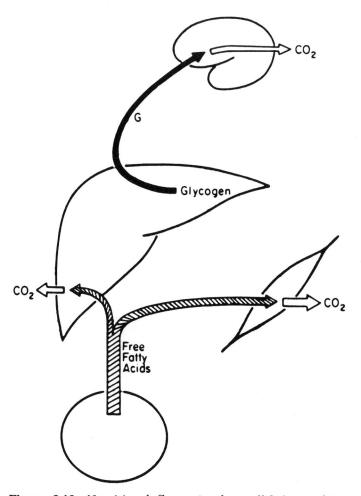

Figure 9.19 Nutritional fluxes in the well-fed state. Between meals, glucose for brain is provided by hepatic glycogenolysis, and free fatty acids released from adipose tissue become the predominant fuel for muscle. High glucagon and low insulin levels promote hepatic glycogenolysis, diminished glucose entry into muscle and an increased level of free fatty acids (*Source*: from Cahill. *Clin Endocrinol Metab* 5:402, 1976 with permission).

of malonyl-CoA [acetyl-CoA carboxylase is phosphorylated and rendered inactive (see Table 9.8)], thus enabling the mitochondria to process fatty acyl-CoA into acetyl-CoA. A portion of the latter is used for the generation of ATP, but most of it is diverted into the

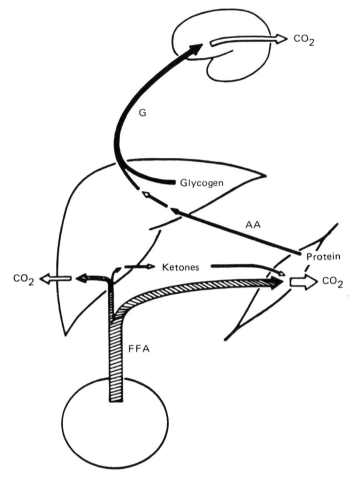

Figure 9.20 Nutritional fluxes in the early-fasting state. With a fast of over 12 hr, as liver glycogen becomes depleted, gluconeogenesis from amino acids originating in muscle provides glucose for brain. Ketoacid production by liver becomes more prominent (*Source*: from Cahill. *Clin Endocrinol Metab* 5:403, 1976 with permission).

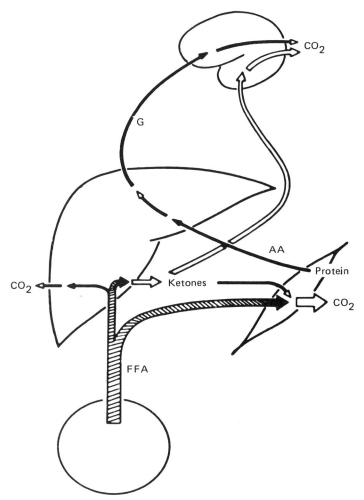

Figure 9.21 Nutritional fluxes in the fasting state. In prolonged fasting, glucose utilization by the brain decreases, thereby requiring less protein catabolism. Bodily energy requirements are reduced so that ketoacid utilization by muscle is diminished. Brain glucose is provided by gluconeogenesis from glycerol derived from lipolysis of adipose triglyceride and from amino acids derived from muscle (*Source*: from Cahill *Clin Endocrinol Metab* 5:406, 1976 with permission).

Table 9.9 Substrate and Hormone Levels in Four Nutritional States

Hormone or substrate (units)	Well-fed	12-h fast	3-d fast	2-w fast
Insulin (μU/mL)	40	15	8	6
Glucagon (pg/mL)	80	100	100	120
Insulin/glucagon ratio	0.5	0.15	0.05	0.05
Glucose (mM)	6.1	4.8	3.8	3.6
Fatty acids (mM)	0.14	0.6	1.0	1.4
Acetoacetate (mM)	0.04	0.05	0.4	1.3
β-Hydroxybutyrate (mM)	0.03	0.10	1.4	6.0
Lactate (mM)	2.5	0.7	0.7	0.6
Pyruvate (mM)	0.25	0.06	0.04	0.03
Alanine (mM)	0.8	0.3	0.3	0.1
ATP equivalents (mM)	313	290	380	537

only pathway available, namely, ketogenesis. The concentrations of water-soluble acetoacetate and β-hydroxybutyrate may increase 30- to 50-fold during prolonged starvation (see Table 9.9), providing muscle and cardiac tissue with much of their energy.

In the meantime, hypoglycemia has increased cortisol secretion. In addition to its permissive action on lipolysis, its antianabolic action in muscle provides a source of amino acids. Many of them are metabolized to pyruvate and transaminated to alanine for transport to the liver (alanine cycle). Starvation induces the synthesis of key enzymes of gluconeogenesis, namely: pyruvate carboxylase, phospho*enol*pyruvate carboxykinase, and glucose-6-phosphatase. The alanine entering the liver is transaminated to pyruvate, the nitrogen is excreted as urea, and the pyruvate is converted to glucose for utilization by those organs unable to use fatty acids or ketone bodies, namely: blood cells, brain, testes, and a few other tissues. Fortunately, after 2 to 3 days of starvation, ketonemia has increased sufficiently so that the brain can utilize some ketoacid, thus conserving glucose and, indirectly, muscle protein.

Now go back and reread Chapter 1. You can now begin to appreciate the wondrous complexities designed into our bodies so that we can cope with the most hostile environment and the most threatening insults that life thrusts upon us from time to time.

CLINICAL ASPECTS

Diabetes Mellitus

The Greek name implies a catastrophic, catabolic disease. But modern medicine tells us that this disease, known from antiquity, is more complex than that. Even when its metabolic aspects are, more or less, well controlled, the disease progresses in certain selected tissues, none of which can be considered target tissues of insulin. They are the eyes, kidneys, cardiovascular system, neural system, and the skin and feet. Pathologic changes in one or more of these organs or tissues shorten the lives of diabetics.

Diabetes mellitus (DM) is a complex disease, and there have been several attempts to classify subgroups. Early attempts focused on urinary and blood glucose values and results of an oral glucose tolerance test (OGTT) (see below) Later on, age at *onset* of the disease became the prime variable, and currently, the degree of insulin dependence is the controlling factor (Table 9.10).

Tests

Measurement of fasting (overnight) plasma or blood glucose by the glucose oxidase method is specific for hexose, whereas measurement of reducing sugars includes additional monosaccharides. A value greater than 140 mg/dl on two occasions is one diagnostic criterion for DM. (Plasma values are about 15% higher than blood values.)

An oral glucose tolerance test (OGTT) is a more sensitive indicator of DM. Measurements of plasma glucose taken hourly or half-hourly after ingestion of a glucose load (50–100 g), especially if accompanied by plasma insulin measurements (by RIA), are very revealing (Fig. 9.22). For example, note that the obese and average-weight individuals handle a glucose load identically, but that the obese person must secrete much more insulin to do so (an example of insulin resistance). Values of plasma glucose in excess of 200 mg/dl at 2 hr and one other time between zero and 2 hr is another diagnostic criterion of DM.

Classic clinical symptoms of DM are polyuria, polydipsia, ketonuria, and rapid weight loss.

Table 9.10 Classification of Diabetes Mellitus

Class	Former terminology	Clinical characteristics
Type I insulin-dependent type (IDDM)	Juvenile onset DM; ketosis-prone DM; low-output β cell failure	Dependent upon injected insulin to prevent ketosis and preserve life; youthful onset, but may occur at any age; insulinopenia
Type II noninsulindependent type (NIDDM) subdivisions nonobese NIDDM obese NIDDM	Maturity-onset DM; ketosis-resistant, stable DM: high-output β cell failure	Not ketosis prone, but it may develop with infection or stress; onset usually after 40, but may occur at any age; 60–90% are obese; serum insulin may be low, normal, or high
Associated syndromes pancreatic disease Cushing's syndrome acromegaly pheochromocytoma glucagonoma drug-induced insulin receptor abnormalities certain genetic syndromes	Secondary diabetes	Requires two diagnoses: DM and presence of associated syndrome

Abbreviations used: DM, diabetes mellitus.

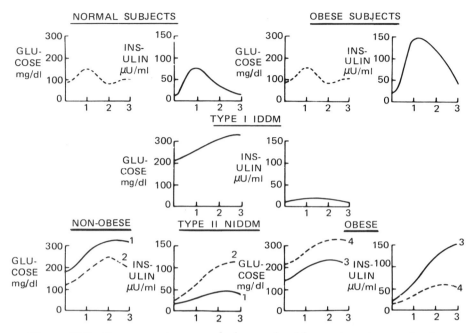

Figure 9.22   Responses to an oral glucose load by various types of subjects. Note that the obese group react with hyperinsulinism to attain a normal plasma glucose response. The type I IDDM group has no response, and the type II NIDDM group has a delayed response that is heterogeneous, i.e., some subjects are subnormal while others exhibit hyperinsulinism.

Type I, Insulin-Dependent Diabetes Mellitus

Type I, insulin-dependent diabetes mellitus (IDDM), also known as juvenile-onset diabetes, has a rather explosive onset, usually with no previously detected abnormality of glucose metabolism. Patients are initially seen with florid hyperglycemia, weight loss, polyuria, nocturia, frequently with ketosis, dehydration, and sometimes even coma.

   The etiology has a stong genetic component. There is about a 50% concordance of IDDM between monozygotic twins. More recently, certain histocompatibility antigens are found with greater frequency among those with IDDM. Antigen HLA-D3 or HLA-D4 occur in 95% of Caucasian type I patients versus 40% of the control population. Genetic analysis indicates that the gene is recessive with a penetrance of 50%. Thus, we can conclude that, although genetics is an important factor in the etiology of IDDM, there must be additional components.

The HLA data suggest an autoimmune mechanism, and there are reports to confirm it. For example, there is an association between IDDM and several disorders of putative autoimmune causality, namely, Addison's disease, thyroid disease, and pernicious anemia. The prevalence of islet cell antibodies in the circulation of patients with IDDM is quite variable, the largest number reported being 80%. Antibodies decrease in concentration with time, and some of the variability in reported values may be attributed to the time of sampling relative to the onset of the disease. Antibodies are present in the circulation for a number of years before the disease can be detected clinically.

For many years, investigators have tried to link viral infection with the onset of IDDM. Although the evidence in animals is strong, that in humans is not. Rubella and coxsackie viruses have been studied the most. About 29% of children born with congenital rubella have DM later.

Whatever the cause, the net result is a loss of mass of islet tissue, which is about 1 million in the normal human pancreas, with a marked diminution in β-cells. Indeed about 50% of IDDM patients whose pancreas was evaluated by autopsy had no recognizable β-cells. Insulin and C-peptide levels are low to undetectable in the serum of those first seen with IDDM disease. The T lymphocytes are believed to be the major determinant of β-cell destruction. The loss of glucose-induced phase I insulin secretion accompanies β-cell destruction and precedes hyperglycemia.

There is no accepted treatment. Cyclosporine, which selectively blocks the activation of T lymphocytes, has shown some promise in initial trials. Other clinicians are testing alternate-day therapy with prednisone, a synthetic glucocorticoid with immunosuppressant activity.

Type II Noninsulin-Dependent Diabetes Mellitus

Noninsulin-dependent diabetes mellitus (NIDDM) is such an insidious disease that millions of people are said to be unaware that they have it. Frequently, it is detected upon routine examination or upon complaint concerning one of the complications of DM. Most notable is the correlation of the disease with obesity: 60 to 90% of patients with NIDDM are obese. (Obesity is often defined as being more than 15 or 20% overweight, using actuarial mortality tables as the definition of normality. There is some debate about the validity of this definition, but none, however, concerning the seriousness of obesity.) Ketosis does not usually occur unless infection or other stress is present. Because NIDDM usually occurs after the age of 40 it is sometimes called adult-onset, or maturity-onset DM.

Obesity and genetics are strongly implicated in the etiology of NIDDM. There is 100% concordance between diabetic identical twins when the index case is diagnosed after the age of 50 years. There is also a correlation with HLA typing. The presence of obesity with its attendant hyperinsulinism (see Fig. 9.22) and insulin resistance undoubtedly contributes to an exhaustion of the β-cells in type II diabetics. Naturally, there are concomitant histological changes including some degeneration of β-cells or invasion of the islets by amyloid or by fibrous tissue.

Obesity is not the sole environmental factor compromising β-cell function. Pregnancy may produce gestational diabetes, which usually disappears after parturition. A similar result may follow a pathologic increase in the secretion of an "anti-insulin" hormone, such as glucagon, glucocorticoid, or somatotropin (see Table 9.10). Barring tumors, the role, if any, of these hormones in the etiology of type II DM remains controversial. There is hypersecretion of STH and glucagon in poorly controlled diabetics in the face of hyperglycemia. Although there is no question that this is inappropriate, it may be secondary because insulin therapy usually normalizes the relationship between plasma glucose and hormonal secretion.

A recent contribution to this controversy by Press and coworkers takes advantage of modern technology. Well-controlled, type I diabetics receiving insulin-pump therapy were given exogenous STH for 45 hr such that the plasma concentrations of STH doubled to 16 ng/ml, values equal to those of poorly controlled diabetics. Plasma glucose concentrations rose from a baseline of 86 mg/dl to 204 at 18 hr and 240 mg/dl at 42 hr. The hyperglycemia was mainly due to increased hepatic glucose production without a change in circulating levels of insulin and glucagon. Levels of circulating free fatty acids, ketone bodies, and branched-chain amino acids were also increased. Thus, the whole spectrum of abnormal fuel concentrations that earmark poor diabetic control were reproduced by modest elevation of STH concentrations, despite optimized insulin treatment.

An earlier classification scheme had four groups into which to place diabetics: potential, latent, chemical, and overt. Although this scheme is no longer used, it does serve to illustrate the progression of DM. A person with *potential diabetes* had a genetic predisposition (family history) to the disease and a normal ability to handle glucose. In *latent diabetes*, there is normal glucose tolerance under usual circumstances, but a stress, such as pregnancy, or another disease, such as Cushing's syndrome, may reveal an abnormal response. In *chemical diabetes*, the patients remain asymptomatic, but they now consistently have an abnormal glucose tolerance. In the final stage, there is frank fasting hyperglycemia. Ketosis is usually absent unless it is precipitated by a severe stress. Type I patients may also march through these steps, but at a greatly accelerated pace. Carbohydrate intolerance can be uncovered by prospective testing in the siblings of patients with IDDM.

In summary, IDDM patients have insulinopenia and an acute, life-threatening form of the disease. Those with NIDDM retain some β-cell function; their plasma insulin concentrations may range from low to high (see Fig. 9.22). This accounts for the lack of ketosis, for triglyceride synthesis is more responsive (sensitive) to insulin than is glucose transport.

Type II diabetics do not respond immediately to glucose, i.e., the "early" peak of insulin release is absent whenever the fasting blood glucose concentration is higher than 125 mg/dl. The delayed phase of insulin release is usually retained so that peak insulin concentrations are attained later than normally (see Fig. 9.22). Other insulin secretagogues often retain their effect, although it may be subnormal. For example, administration of a protein meal, infusion of arginine, or administration of the β-adrenergic agonist, isoproterenol, initiates a rise in plasma insulin in most type II patients, even when there is no response to a 5-g glucose load. These examples illustrate the retention of at least partial β-cell function in type II diabetics.

Metabolically, there is a marked similarity between diabetes mellitus and starvation (see Fig. 9.21), the major exception being the plasma glucose concentration. The muscle and adipose cells of diabetics are bathed in a glucose solution so that they are "starving" in the midst of plenty and turn to the metabolism of triglycerides and ketone bodies as an alternative source of energy. As long as some insulin is present, ketosis remains low to moderate and acidosis, dehydration, and coma do not ensue.

Malfunctions of the Adrenal Cortex

Laboratory Tests

Before discussion of adrenopathies, it is essential to understand the biochemical and physiological limitations of the tests employed to differentiate between abnormality and normality. The student must also appreciate the differences between the black-and-white, normalized (physiology's classic "70-kg man") people of a test and those of the real world. First of all, the fact that people are not inbred is obvious but often overlooked. Therefore, the range of "normality" is so large that it may overlap the pathologic range. Second, the normals quoted for many procedures usually represent a limited group (characteristically white medical or nursing students), and the values may not apply to pediatric, geriatric, black, Asiatic, or other populations. Third, normal values usually assume a lean body mass. Values for obese subjects, for example, often appear abnormal until normalized, commonly for surface area. Fourth, a clinician must never rely solely on laboratory data; to be acceptable, laboratory data must be congruent with "clinical impressions," a vague term covering the composite of medical history, physical examination, medications being taken, pregnancy, drug abuse. Judicious synthesis of laboratory data and clinical impressions is particularly important when the former are located on the borderline between normality and abnormality.

The laboratory tests that may be requested include urinary 17-hydroxycorticosteroids (17-OHCS; Porter-Silber chromogens), urinary 17-ketogenic steroids (17-KGS), urinary free cortisol, and plasma cortisol. No one test is clearly superior to the others, each having its own advantages and disadvantages; hence, they are all widely used. Collection of 24-hr urine specimens is notoriously unreliable; hence, results should be expressed in terms of creatinine excretion. Even so, many physicians prefer the assurance of a phlebotomy. Plasma assays, however, reflect an instantaneous value of cortisol (or ACTH), whereas urinary assays are integrative.

The first two urinary assays (17-OHCS and 17-KGS) are measurements of conjugated metabolites of cortisol. Cortisol is metabolized mostly in the liver by reduction. The 4-en-3-oxo group is reduced in two steps to a saturated 3α-alcohol, and the 20-ketone is reduced more slowly to an alcohol (Fig. 9.23). The

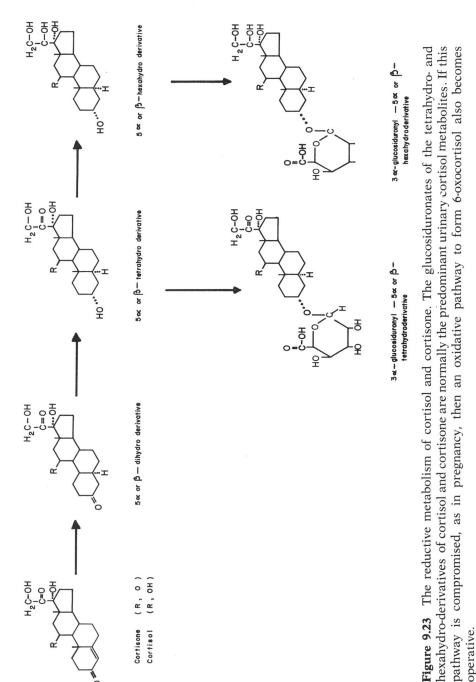

Figure 9.23 The reductive metabolism of cortisol and cortisone. The glucosiduronates of the tetrahydro- and hexahydro-derivatives of cortisol and cortisone are normally the predominant urinary cortisol metabolites. If this pathway is compromised, as in pregnancy, then an oxidative pathway to form 6-oxocortisol also becomes operative.

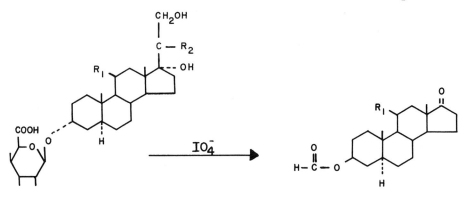

R_I , R_2 HO– or O=

Figure 9.24 Oxidation of vicinal glycols and ketols by periodate in the 17-KGS method. Note that one must compensate for glucosuria.

tetrahydro-derivatives (in ring A) are measured by the 17-OHS assay, whereas both groups of derivatives are measured by the 17-KGS assay.

The 17-KGS assay involves treatment of urine with sodium periodate, a gentle oxidizing agent that works only on vicinal glycols or ketols with scission of a C-C bond (Fig. 9.24). This reagent quickly removes the side-chain of the steroid producing a 17-ketosteroid (17-oxosteroid), the process described by the name of the assay, *and* it digests the glucuronic acid moiety, leaving only a formate ester at C-3. The ester is hydrolyzed by brief exposure to alkali. After extraction, the 17-ketosteroids (17-KS) are quantitated spectrophotometrically after reaction with *m*-dinitrobenzene and strong alkali to yield a magenta color (Zimmerman reaction). Endogenous 17-KS are either measured separately or destroyed by a reductive pretreatment with sodium borohydride.

The 17-OHCS assay enzymatically hydrolyzes the glucuronic acid moiety of the cortisol metabolites. Many drugs, including aspirin, are also excreted as glucosiduronates, and they compete for the β-glucuronidase. If large quantities are present, hydrolysis of steroid conjugates will be incomplete, and the assay will be erroneously low. After extraction, treatment of the organic residue with alcoholic sulfuric acid produces a yellow color which is "specific" for compounds containing the dihydroxyacetone group (Porter-Silber reaction), i.e., the side-chain of cortisol and its tetrahydro-derivatives.

The 17-KGS assay is preferable to the 17-OHCS assay. Because it is a purely chemical assay, it is more robust, more reliable, and faster. The values obtained (5–20 mg/day) are higher than the 17-OHCS values (1.9–6.5 mg/g creatinine per day) and more closely approximate the cortisol secretion rate (6–18 mg/m^2 per day) (the body surface area of an average adult is about 1.5 m^2).

Plasma cortisol assays, measured by radio immunoassay (RIA), give the total cortisol concentration in plasma at one time point. Because of episodic secretion and diurnal rhythm, one measurement has a limited value except in conjunction with certain tests that are to be discussed next.

Clinical Tests

Once a dysfunction of the hypothalamo–pituitary–adrenocortical (HPA) system is suspected, tests of the reserve capacity of the system and of the adrenal cortex should be applied. These include administration of metyrapone (Fig. 9.25), which tests the intactness of feedback control; a stress, such as an insulin tolerance test; and an ACTH test, which assesses adrenocortical reserve capacity. In patients with suspected hypercortisolism, a suppression test using dexamethasone (see Fig. 9.25) is also useful. Each test is now briefly described.

Metyrapone inhibits 11β-hydroxylase, the last enzyme acting in the synthesis of cortisol (see Fig. 9.14). The product secreted by the adrenal cortex is then 11-deoxycortisol, which is ineffective in feedback control of the hypothalamus and adenohypophysis. As a consequence, ACTH secretion is controlled exclusively by the positive-feedforward signals of the CNS. Because the RIA of plasma ACTH is troublesome and not widely available, adrenocortical response is usually measured instead. This takes the form of a plasma 11-deoxycortisol assay by RIA or a urinary 17-KGS or 17-OHCS assay. The most common variant involves oral administration of metyrapone (30 mg/kg) at 23:00 or 24:00 hr followed 8 hr later by a venepuncture. At this time, 11β-hydroxylase activity is fully depressed, and a single determination of plasma 11-deoxycortisol is reliable.

The ability of the HPA system to respond to stress is critical for survival. One of the tests used for assessing the response to

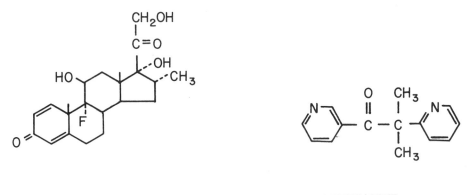

DEXAMETHASONE   METYRAPONE

Figure 9.25 Structures of dexamethasone and metyrapone.

stress is the insulin tolerance test. Regular insulin (0.15 U/kg) injected intravenously produces a rapid fall in plasma glucose, reaching a nadir 20 to 30 min postinjection. In response, plasma cortisol should rise, reaching a maximum 40 to 60 min later (60—90 min postinjection). The response is inversely correlated with the degree of hypoglycemia produced (slope, -0.43 μg/mg between glucose concentrations of 70 and 30 mg/dl); the response should be greater than -0.2 μg/mg. Because the response to insulin is individual, one must know the degree of hypoglycemia produced to interpret this test fully.

It is sometimes useful to measure one component of the HPA system. Infusion of synthetic 1-24-ACTH (0.25 mg/8 hr) will assess the reserve capacity of the adrenal cortex; the plasma cortisol concentration should double at some point (4–8 hr) during the infusion. A positive response combined with an inadequate resonse to metyrapone or to insulin, or to both, indicates a defect located at the pituitary–hypothalamic level. Failure to respond to the ACTH infusion does not necessarily indicate permanent adrenocortical insufficiency. Long-term, glucocorticoid therapy, as in treatment of inflammatory processes or in immunosuppressive steroid therapy, may have produced such profound atrophy of the adrenal cortex that response to a single infusion of

ACTH has become impossible. An ACTH stimulation test given on 3 successive days will differentiate the pathologic from the iatrogenic condition.

The dexamethasone (see Fig. 9.25) suppression test is used in cases of hypercortisolism to differentiate adrenal from pituitary Cushing's syndrome. Adrenal (and ectopic) tumors are much more resistant to feedback regulation; they will not suppress, even with 2 mg/day (0.5 mg qid) of dexamethasone.

Syndromes

Three types of problems will be discussed next: Cushing's syndrome as an example of hyperfunction; congenital adrenal hyperplasia (CAH), sometimes also called adrenogenital syndrome, as an example of dysfunction; and Addison's disease, as an example of hypofunction.

Hyperadrenocorticism is both more complicated and more common than hypofunction. Most (68%) patients with hyperfunction have pituitary Cushing's syndrome, sometimes called Cushing's disease. Although most have a pituitary tumor, many do not; the etiology of the latter is unknown. A small (17%) number have adrenal Cushing's syndrome caused by an adrenal tumor (adenoma or carcinoma), and a nearly equal number (15%) have ectopic Cushing's syndrome. For unknown reasons, ectopic tumors are concentrated in lung, pancreas, thymus, or medullary thyroid tissue.

The syndrome, described by Cushing in 1932, is characteristically variable. Clinical features include the following (with average frequency expressed as percent): obesity (88), plethoric face (75), hypertension (74), hirsutism (64), muscle weakness (61), menstrual disorders (60), acne (45), bruising (42), mental disorders (42), and backache (osteoporosis) (40). The natural course of the disease is also unpredictable, varying from a rapidly progressive, disabling disease culminating in death to spontaneous remission. The hormonal basis of the clinical features remain largely unknown. Only obesity and mental disorders occur with about equal frequency in patients given glucocorticoids. Excess production of testosterone in women contributes to three other features, namely hirsutism, menstrual disorders, and acne. In men with pituitary Cushing's syndrome, on the other hand, the suppression of LH and FSH secretion leads to impaired testosterone secretion and loss of libido, impotence, and oligospermia.

The diagnosis of Cushing's syndrome proceeds in two steps. The first step is a screening procedure; *sustained* hypersecretion of cortisol *must* be demonstrated to confirm a clinical impression of Cushing's syndrome, i.e., values of plasma cortisol in blood samples taken in the morning and evening should both be inappropriately high (assuming a stressless day) to sustain the diagnosis. Urinary 17-KGS or unbound cortisol values need not be inappropriately high, although they usually are. Thus, the loss of diurnal rhythm in cortisol secretion is the basis of the syndrome.

The second step must differentiate among the three sources of hypercortisolemia—namely, adrenal, pituitary, or ectopic tumor (Fig. 9.26). Cushing's syndrome of adrenal origin is clearly distinguished by low or undetectable levels of plasma ACTH; the autonomous adrenal tumor, secreting excessive amounts of cortisol, has suppressed pituitary secretion of ACTH. On the other hand, a high concentration of ACTH ($>$200 pg/ml, as shown) by RIA, clearly demonstrates an ectopic tumor. In spite of the high levels of ACTH, the patient may be only slightly cushingoid or occasionally asymptomatic. This occurs because the ectopic tumor may have inadequate levels of the enzyme that produces ACTH and β-lipoprotein (and other fragments) from proopiomelanocortin. The prohormone is biologically inactive (see Chap. 1), but the antibody recognizes the ACTH portion of the prohormone released by the tumor into the circulation.

In about one-third of cushingoid patients, ACTH concentrations fall in a range (100–200 pg/ml) that fails to distinguish pituitary from ectopic Cushing's syndrome. Some of the tests described previously as well as x-rays and computerized tomographic studies are used to resolve these cases.

The two names, congenital adrenal hyperplasia and adrenogenital syndrome, together describe the properties of a family of congenital diseases of varying severity. The observation is a partial to total inability to complete one of the three hydroxylations required to convert pregnenolone to cortisol (see Fig. 9.14). The basic defect remains unknown, i.e., whether it is deletion of (all or part of) relevant genetic material, a mutation that makes the gene product inactive, a reading-frame shift, a change

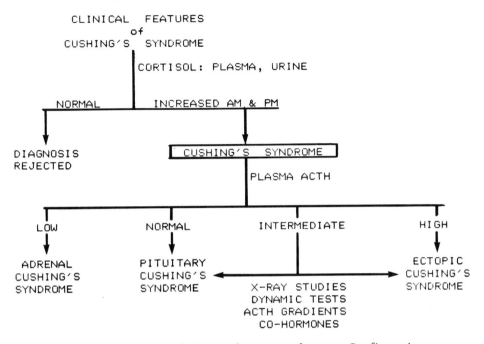

Figure 9.26 Diagnosis of the Cushing's syndromes. Confirmation requires the demonstration of *sustained*, excessive cortisol production. Differentiation is based on plasma ACTH, although distinction of pituitary from ectopic syndromes may require additional procedures (*Source*: from Gold, 1979).

in regulatory operons, or whether there are multiple foci, constitute unanswered questions. Here we will consider what is known about only the most common variant, 21-hydroxylase deficiency. The other two forms, 11β-hydroxylase and 17-hydroxylase deficiency, are rarer and consequently little investigated.

The consequences of a 21-hydroxylase deficiency depend upon its severity. A partial loss compromises cortisol synthesis (see Fig. 9.13) but not that of aldosterone (see Fig. 6.6). Thus, this syndrome may be divided into salt-losing (complete loss) and non–salt-losing forms. The former obviously produces an acute situation that, if not recognized, ends quickly in the death of the baby. The latter varies greatly in severity, depending upon the degree of loss. In both forms, the failure to produce adequate amounts of cortisol releases negative-feedback on the hypothalamoadenohypophyseal unit and causes an increase in ACTH secretion that, in turn, produces adrenocortical hyperplasia and stimulation of synthesis in the steps before the enzymatic block. As precursors accumulate, they are forced into pathways that are normally little used (Fig. 9.27). Side-chain cleavage of 17-hydroxyprogesterone produces the androgens, androstenedione and testosterone, which are responsible for virilizing effects. Hepatic metabolism of 17-hydroxyprogesterone escaping from the adrenal yields the metabolite, pregnanetriol glucosiduronate, normally a trivial urinary compound; it is, in fact, diagnostic of 21-hydroxylase deficiency.

The non–salt-losing form of CAH is a nonacute disease that varies greatly in its clinical expression. A severe deficiency produces virilization of both sexes in utero. It may interfere with normal sexual development to the extent that XX individuals are born with ambiguous genitalia (clitoral enlargement and labioscrotal fusion so extensive that they may be assigned a male gender). Less severe deficiency may cause virilization during childhood, producing premature puberty in boys and failure to develop secondary sex characteristics and to menstruate in girls. In both sexes, there may be an initially rapid growth followed by premature closure of the epiphyses with resultant short stature. In the mildest cases, the condition may never be detected in men and only in adult women complaining of hirsutism and acne.

Congenital adrenal hyperplasia is a rather common autosomal-recessive trait, being detected in about 1:5000 births. Although it is associated with the HLA antigens, there appears to be a random association between alleles of the HLA loci and the 21-hydroxylase deficiency occurring as the result of multiple, unrelated mutations that are relatively common. Homozygous individuals show the trait, whereas heterozygous persons show a greater increase in 17-hydroxyprogesterone secretion in response to the administration of ACTH than to a control population or homozygous unaffected siblings. The typing of cells obtained by amniocentesis enables obstetricians to counsel parents about the outcome of pregnancy.

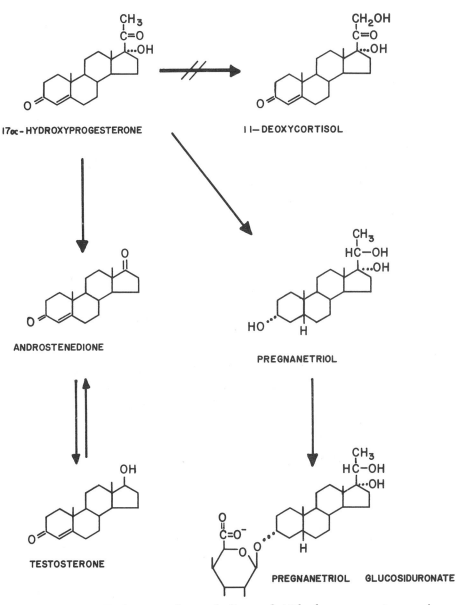

Figure 9.27 Pathways of metabolism of 17-hydroxyprogesterone in CAH. Note that the minor pathway of androgen biosynthesis has become important and that much of the 17-hydroxyprogesterone escapes from the adrenal and is metabolized by the liver to pregnanetriol glucosiduronate. Both pathways are further driven by high ACTH concentrations as a result of diminished negative-feedback by cortisol.

Hypoadrenocorticism may be primary (adrenal origin), secondary (pituitary origin), or tertiary (hypothalamic origin). The primary disease is a rare syndrome, called Addison's disease, that may be caused by an autoimmune response or, less frequently today (ca. 20%), by tuberculosis of the adrenal glands. Basal secretion of cortisol is usually low or low-normal (rather than undetectable); the prime attribute of hypoadrenocorticism is an inability to respond to stress. This is demonstrated by a lack of response of plasma or urinary cortisol to a stress, such as insulin-induced hypoglycemia or to administration of ACTH (plasma ACTH is already high because of the absence of feedback from cortisol).

In panhypopituitarism (the lack of all adenohypophyseal hormones) or in an isolated deficiency of ACTH, endogenous ACTH is absent or inappropriately low, and the adrenal gland is severely atrophied. It will respond, however, if ACTH is administered on 3 consecutive days, allowing the trophic action of ACTH to rebuild the adrenal cortex.

People with hypoadrenocorticism may lead uncomplicated lives unaware of their disease until they are stressed. Then a rapid series of events may culminate in death unless adequate replacement thereapy with cortisol or a synthetic steroid is initiated. The amount of steroid administered must be proportional to the stress. Thus, the addisonian patient on steroid replacement therapy must continually adjust the dose to compensate for the varying amount of stress present in their daily lives.

Malfunctions of the Adrenal Medulla

Laboratory Tests

Epinephrine and norepinephrine are metabolized (Fig. 9.28) extremely rapidly in the plasma. The half-life is about 1 to 2 min. Although vanillylmandelic acid (VMA), the principal urinary metabolite, is the one usually assayed, its presence cannot differentiate between a medullary and a peripheral pheochromocytoma. Assay of metanephrine and normetanephrine can do this, although admittedly the assay is more difficult.

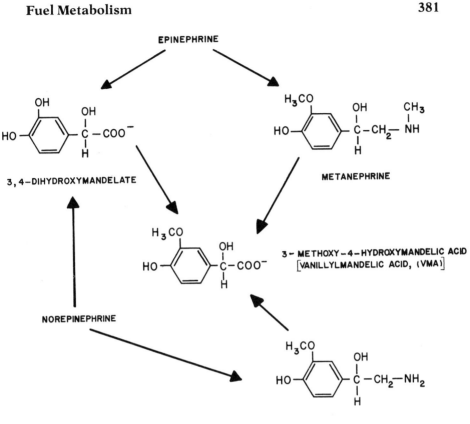

Figure 9.28 The metabolism of epinephrine and norepinephrine involves two, unordered reactions, one a methyl transfer from SAM and the other an oxidative deamination.

Clinical

Pheochromocytomas are rare lesions, with a prevalence of less than 0.1% among all hypertensive people; over 90% are benign. The syndrome may be familial, inherited as an autosomal-dominant trait as part of the syndrome of multiple endocrine neoplasia type II (see p. 218). It is completely curable. Although the tumors may occur any time from infancy to old age, the greatest frequency occurs during the fourth and fifth decade of life.

The symptoms are too numerous to detail here, but they include hypertension, often with very wide fluctuations, and spells of nervousness, apprehension, profuse sweating, headache, severe palpitations of the heart, and pain. Total plasma catecholamines exceed 2000 pg/ml, and urinary unconjugated catecholamines, metanephrine, and VMA exceed 115, 1300, and 7000 μg/24 hr, respectively. The most sensitive assay is the one for urinary metanephrine.

SUMMARY

The principal fuel of the body is fatty acids (from triglycerides), but during starvation and in certain disease states, amino acids (from body proteins) also become an important source of energy. In addition, the plasma concentration of glucose must be maintained reasonably constant because red and white blood cells are totally dependent upon glucose for their energy supply, and neural tissue is partially dependent upon it. The hormones involved are insulin, glucagon, epinephrine, and glucocorticoids.

The chemistry of insulin is well established. It was the second hormone to be isolated, the first polypeptide hormone to be sequenced, and the first to be analyzed by x-ray crystallography—all Nobel laureate work. The preprohormone is synthesized as a single polypeptide, the excision of the C-peptide from the midportion of the prohormone producing the double-chain mature form.

Regulation of insulin synthesis and secretion is complex. There are three phases: basal, phase I (a short phase involving the release of preformed insulin), and phase II (prolonged phase that, of necessity, must include protein synthesis). It is axiomatic that different mechanisms must be involved in these responses, but it is not obvious that certain stimuli may affect these phases differently. For example, type II diabetics, who are noninsulin-dependent and have measurable basal levels of insulin, do not have phase I insulin respnses to glucose stimulation, but they do have phase II responses. On the other hand, they do have phase I responses to nonglucose secretagogues, such as arginine, glucagon, tolbutamide, and isoproterenol.

Primary control of insulin secretion is exerted by D-glucose; it causes an increase in both phases above a threshold concentration of 5.5 mM. The K_m for glucose is about 8.0 mM. Although many other substances also regulate insulin secretion, every one is glucose-dependent. There are numerous hormones that possibly exert some control. Of the seven that are said to stimulate insulin secretion,however, only one, GIP, has established physiological relevance. Of the five inhibitory hormones, only the catecholamines have been established as physiologically important; PGE_2 is nearing that status. Cyclic cAMP and Ca^{2+} are also integral parts of the secretory mechanism.

Insulin is the anabolic hormone, promoting the storage of energy in the form of glycogen, triglycerides, and protein. It promotes glucose transport into fat and muscle cells by facilitated diffusion. It controls the enzymatic activity of key regulatory enzymes by phosphorylation–dephosphorylation, and of certain other enzymes by induction of their synthesis. The net effect of these coordinated changes is an increased flux of glucose through the glycolytic pathway, producing glycogen and acetyl-CoA. Any excess of the latter over the body's needs for energy is diverted into fatty acid synthesis through two key enzymes, citrate lyase and acetyl-CoA carboxylase. Protein synthesis is also increased, but here it is difficult to single out one or two key enzymes.

The insulin receptor is synthesized as a single polypeptide, which does not bind insulin, and is then processed in several steps. These include glycosylation, formation of intra- and intermolecular disulfide bonds, cleavage to form subunits, and capping with sialic acid to form the mature receptor subunits of 130 and 90 kDa. The final tetrameric receptor has the form B-A-A-B held together by disulfide bonds between the subunits. A portion of the B-subunit is cytoplasmic and a portion exofacial, whereas the entire A-subunit, which contains an insulin-binding site, is exofacial. The gene for the insulin receptor has considerable homology with those for EGF and IGF-I as well as with those for some oncogenes.

Another feature that the insulin receptor shares with several others is a tyrosine kinase that is part of the cytoplasmic portion of the B-subunit of the insulin receptor. The phosphorylated insulin-receptor complex is more effective in promoting insulin's actions than the nonphosphorylated complex.

Glucagon is a single-chain, 29-amino acid residue polypeptide with no cysteines. The sequence of proglucagon (18 kDa) is still unknown. Glucose inhibits glucagon secretion from the α-cells of the islets of Langerhans with a K_i of about 5 mM and maximal suppression of 9 to 10 mM. Glucogenic amino acids stimulate, and free fatty acids suppress, glucagon secretion in isolated islets.

The overall action of glucagon opposes that of insulin. Whereas insulin lowers blood glucose by increasing its transport into muscle and fat tissue, glucagon raises blood glucose by increasing hepatic glycogenolysis in the short-term and gluconeogenesis in the long-term. Whereas insulin promotes lipogenesis, glucagon stimulates lipolysis and ketone body formation, thereby offering the tissues an alternative form of energy and minimizing gluconeogenesis. The insulin/glucagon ratio may be more important than their absolute concentrations in the regulation of energy fluxes.

Glucagon acts through adenylate cyclase, cAMP, and cAMP-dependent protein kinase to activate glycogen phosphorylase and inactivate glycogen synthetase, to activate hormone-sensitive triglyceride lipase and to inactivate acetyl-CoA carboxylase. The last-mentioned enzyme is the key enzyme in fatty acid synthesis, and its inactivation decreases the concentration of malonyl-CoA and, thereby, increases the activity of carnitine palmitoyltransferase I, the regulatory enzyme in fatty acid oxidation. Glucagon shuts off glycolysis by decreasing the hepatic concentration of fructose-2,6-bisphosphate, the most powerful activator of 6-phosphofructo-1-kinase. Gluconeogenesis is stimulated by an increased flux of precursors: glycerol from lipolysis of triglycerides, alanine from muscle (which requires cortisol), and muscle lactate.

Cortisol and corticosterone are the principal glucocorticosteroids, the ratio of the two produced being species-specific. Their synthesis is controlled by ACTH, and the concentration of ACTH in the blood is regulated by the hypophysiotrophic hormone, corticoliberin, a polypeptide having 41 amino acid residues. An amidated COOH-terminal peptide is essential for its maximal activity. Corticotropin-releasing hormone, VP, and neurophysin-VP are contained within the same neurosecretory vesicles in the median eminence; hence, coordinate secretion is obligatory. The CRH and VP probably act synergistically to promote secretion of ACTH.

The hormone form of ACTH is a large glycopeptide called proopiomelanocortin that contains within its 265 amino acid residues several hormones: α-, β-, and γ-MSH, CLIP, β- and γ-LPH, β-endorphin, and met-enkephalin. The end products vary with the cells in which processing occurs. In the corticotropes of the adenohypophysis, ACTH and β-LPH are released from POMC in equimolar quantities.

Synthesis of glucocorticoids occurs in the zona fasciculata and reticularis and closely resembles steroidogenesis, as discussed in Chapters 6 and 8, with the following exceptions: There is no 18-hydroxylase, and there are 17- and 11β-hydroxylases. Hydroxylations follow the order 17, 21, and 11β to form cortisol and 21 and 11β to form corticosterone.

Cortisol as well as progesterone are transported in the blood bound to a specific, high-affinity, low-capacity β-globulin, called transcortin, and also to albumin. In the blood, about 90% of cortisol is protein-bound. That which is bound cannot enter cells.

The hypothalamoadenohypophyseal–adrenocortical system responds to stress in all forms: physical and surgical trauma; noxious chemical and biological agents; extreme hypoglycemia, exercise, or cold; and highly emotional states. Endogenous corticosteroids may have their primary actions at the level of the brain and of the hypothalamus while synthetic glucocorticoids may act primarily on corticotropes and regions of the brain that lie outside the blood–brain barrier.

There appear to be three major time frames of corticosteroid feedback action: fast (0–30 min), intermediate (1–8 hr), and slow (8 hr to days). The physiological significance of such complexity is not completely clear. Fast, rate-sensitive feedback may control the rate and magnitude of ACTH and corticosteroid responses to stimuli before delayed feedback has a chance to become operative, thus preventing exaggerated responses. Moreover, multiple stimuli in the fast-feedback domain are not necessarily additive.

Cortisol in nonstress situations has no demonstrable function. In stressful situations, however, it is essential for life. The diversity of effects—from metabolic actions to effects on blood cells and the immune system—is so wide that no one has yet proposed an acceptable unifying theory. This chapter, however, considers mainly the metabolic actions. These are an inhibition of protein synthesis, except for an induction of transaminases, leading to gluconeogenesis and increased urea excretion. There is also an inhibition of glucose transport into muscle and fat cells that, in certain pathologic or pharmacologically induced cases, can become so severe as to produce "steroid" diabetes.

The catecholamines, epinephrine and norepinephrine, are synthesized from tyrosine in the adrenal medulla. The rate-limiting step is the first one, the hydroxylation of tyrosine to dihydroxyphenylalanine. The level of tyrosine hydroxylase is mainly controlled by neuronal impulses releasing acetylcholine. The last step is controlled by the capillary transport of glucocorticoid from the surrounding cortex. It induces the synthesis of phenylethanolamine-N-methyl transferase which transfers a methyl group from S-adenosylmethionine to norepinephrine, forming epinephrine.

The medulla may be considered as a specialized sympathetic ganglion innervated by the customary long preganglionic neurons. There is a cholinergic synapse with chromaffin cells. Stresses of all types produce a discharge of catecholamines, principally epinephrine, from the medulla.

Carbohydrate and lipid metabolism are affected by catecholamines. At physiologic concentrations, epinephrine produces glycogenolysis and the accumulation of lactic acid in muscle. The latter is used by the heart as an energy source and by the liver in gluconeogenesis. At pathologic concentrations, epinephrine will also produce hepatic glycogenolysis. In both the muscle and liver, action occurs through a cAMP mechanism. In the presence of cortisol, both epinephrine and norepinephrine activate hormone-sensitive triglyceride lipase through a cAMP mechanism.

The two catecholamines have four adrenergic receptors: β_1-and β_2-receptors bind to Ns, the stimulatory guanine nucleotide-binding protein of the adenylate cyclase complex in hormone-sensitive tissues, whereas α_2-receptors bind to Ni, the inhibitory counterpart. α_1-Receptors stimulate the Ca^{2+}–protein kinase C pathway.

Work on the structure of the four receptors has progressed unevenly. The β_1-receptor is smaller and more acidic than the β_2-receptor. The gene for the latter contains no introns, and the 418-amino acid polypeptide produced contains no signal peptide. This peptide is homologous with the visual protein opsin in that both have seven hydrophobic regions 20 to 25 amino acids in length that may be transmembrane segments; both are involved in signal transduction, and both are phosphorylated. The α_1- and α_2-receptors have the same size and share immunogenic determinants.

In summary, insulin, the anabolic hormone, is counter-balanced by glucagon, cortisol, and epinephrine. The counter-regulatory hormones are not equivalent. In a complex, short experiment (90 min) performed on human subjects made hypoglycemic by insulin injection, intact glucagon secretion, but not STH or cortisol secretion, was necessary for normal glucose counterregulation; adrenergic mechanisms are not involved unless glucagon secretion is impaired. In chronic hypoglycemia, such as prolonged fasting or starvation, however, there can be no doubt of the importance of cortisol in inducing transaminases to supply the precursors of gluconeogenesis.

These principles were demonstrated in three examples showing energy fluxes in the well-fed, early-fasting, and starvation states.

SUPPLEMENTAL BIBLIOGRAPHY

Insulin

Amatruda, JM, JN Livingston, and DH Lockwood. Cellular mechanisms in selected states of insulin resistance: Human obesity, glucocorticoid excess and chronic renal failure. *Diabetes Metab Rev* *1*:293–317, 1985.

Blundell, T, G Dodson, D Hodgkin, and D Mercola. Insulin: The structure in the crystal and its reflecion in chemistry and biology. *Adv Protein Chem* 26:279–402, 1972.

Czech, MP. Insulin action. *Am J Med* 70:142–150, 1981.

Czech, MP. Insulin action and the regulation of hexose transport. *Diabetes* 29:399–409, 1981.

Dayhoff, MO. *Atlas of Protein Sequence and Structure*, Vol 5, Suppl 2, National Biomedical Research Foundation, Silver Spring, Maryland, 1976.

Deutsch, PJ, CF Wan, OM Rosen, and CS Rubin. Latent insulin receptors and possible precursors in 3T3-L1 adipocytes. *Proc Natl Acad Sci USA* 80:133–136, 1983.

Dick, APK, SI Harik, A Klip, and DM Walker. Identification and characterization of the glucose transporter of the blood–brain barrier by cytochalasin B binding and immunological activity. *Proc Natl Acad Sci USA* 81:7233–7237, 1984.

Eisenbarth, GS. Type I diabetes mellitus: A chronic autoimmune disease. *N Engl J Med* 314:1360–1368, 1986.

Faber, OK and C Binder. C-Peptide: An index of insulin secretion. *Diabetes Metab Rev* 2:331–345, 1986.

Fajans, SS. Heterogeneity of insulin secretion in type II diabetes. *Diabetes Metab Rev* 2:347–361, 1986.

Fujita-Yamaguchi, Y and S Kathuria. The monomeric $\alpha\beta$ form of the insulin receptor exhibits much higher insulin-dependent tyrosine-specific protein kinase activity than the intact $\alpha_2\beta_2$ form of the receptor. *Proc Natl Acad Sci (USA)* 82:6095–6099, 1985.

Gammeltoft, S and E van Obberghen. Protein kinase activity of the insulin receptor. *Biochem J* 235:1–11, 1986.

Gottschalk, WK and L Jarett. Intracelluar mechanisms of insulin action. *Diabetes Metab Rev* 1:229–259, 1985.

Greep, RO and EB Astwood (eds). *Handbook of Physiology*, Sect 7: *Endocrinology*: Vol 1, *Endocrine Pancreas*. Am Physiol Soc, 1972, 721 pp.

Gupta, S (ed). *Immunology of Clinical and Experimental Diabetes.* Plenum Medical Book, New York, 1984, 426 pp.

Hellman, B. Calcium transport in pancreatic β-cells: Implications for glucose regulation of insulin release. *Diabetes Metab Rev* 2:214–241, 1986.

Jacobs, S, and P Cuatrecasas. Insulin receptor: structure and function. *Endocrinol Rev* 2:251-263, 1981.

Jeanrenaud, B, S Halimi, and G van de Werve. Neuroendocrine disorders seen as triggers of the triad: Obesity—insulin resistance—abnormal glucose tolerance. *Diabetes Metab Rev* 1:261–291, 1985.

Kahn, BB and SW Cushman. Subcellular translocation of glucose trans-porters: Role in insulin action and its perturbation in altered metabolic states. *Diabetes Metab Rev 1*:203–227, 1985.

Kahn, CR, KL Baird, JS Flier, C Grunfeld, JT Harmon, FA Karlsson, M Kasuga, GL King, UC Lang, JM Podskalny, and E van Obberghen. Insulin receptors, receptor antibodies and the mechanism of insulin action. *Recent Prog Horm Res 37*:477–533, 1981.

Kasuga, M, Y Zick, DL Blith, FA Karlsson, HU Haring, and CR Kahn. Insulin stimulation of phosphorylation of the beta-subunit of the in-sulin receptor. *J Biol Chem 257*:9891–9894, 1982.

Larner, JL, K Cheng, C Schwartz, K Kikuchi, S Tamura, S Creacy, R Dubler, G Galasko, C Pullin, and M Katz. Insulin mediators and the control of metabolism through protein phosphorylation. *Recent Prog Horm Res 38*:511–522, 1982.

Levine, R. Insulin: The effects and mode of action of the hormone. *Vitam Horm 39*:145–173, 1982.

Malaisse, WJ. Stimulus-secretion coupling in the pancreatic B-cell: The cholinergic pathway for insulin release. *Diabetes Metab Rev 2*:243–259, 1986.

Meglasson, MD and FM Matschinsky. Pancreatic islet glucose metabol-ism and regulation of insulin secretion. *Diabetes Metab Rev 2*:164–214, 1986.

Morgan, HE and JR Neely. Insulin and membrane transport, In *Hand-book of Physiology*, (RD Greep and EB Astwood, eds). Sect 7, Vol 1, Am Physiol Soc, 1972, pp 323–330.

Noe, BD. Inhibition of islet prohormone to hormone conversion by incorporation of arginine and lysine analogs. *J Biol Chem 256*:4940–4946, 1981.

Orci, L. The insulin cell: Its cellular environment and how it pro-cesses (pro)insulin. *Diabetes Metab Rev 2*:71–106, 1986.

Polonsky, KS and AH Rubenstein. Current approaches to measurement of insulin secretion. *Diabetes Metab Rev 2*:315–329, 1986.

Robbins, DC, MD Tager, and AH Rubenstein. Biologic and clinical importance of proinsulin. *N Engl J Med 310*:1165–1175, 1984.

Robertson, RP. Arachidonic acid metabolite regulation of insulin secretion. *Diabetes Metab Rev 2*:261–296, 1986.

Sasaki, K, TP Cripe, SR Koch, TL Andreone, DD Petersen, EG Beale, and DK Granner. Multihormonal regulation of phospho*enol*pyruvate car-boxykinase gene transcription: The dominant role of insulin, *J Biol Chem 259*:15242–15251, 1984.

Shoelson, S, M Fickova, M Haneda, A Nahum, G Musso, ET Kaiser, AH Rubenstein, and H Tager. Identification of a mutant human insulin predicted to contain a serine-for-phenylalanine substitution. *Proc Natl Acad Sci USA 80*:7390–7394, 1983.

Tabarini, D, J Heinrich, and OM Rosen. Activation of S6 kinase activity in 3T3-L1 cells by insulin and phorbol ester. *Proc Natl Acad Sci USA 82*:4369–4373, 1985.

Ullrich, A, JR Bell, EY Chen, R Herrera, LM Petruzzelli, TJ Dull, A Gray, L Coussens, YC Liao, M Tsubokawa, A Mason, PH Seeburg, C Grunfield, OM Rosen, and J Ramachandran. Human insulin receptor and its relationship to the tyrosine kinase family of oncogenes. *Nature 313*:756–761, 1985.

Uyeda, K, E Furuya, and LJ Luby. The effect of natural and synthetic D-fructose-2,6-biphosphate on the regulatory kinetic properties of liver and muscle phosphofructokinase, *J Biol Chem 256*:8394–8399, 1981.

Ward, WK, JC Beard, and D Porte, Jr. Clinical aspects of islet B-cell function in non-insulin-independent diabetes mellitus. *Diabetes Metab Rev 2*:297–313, 1986.

Weir, GC, JL Leahy, and S Bonner-Weir. Experimental reduction of B-cell mass for the pathogenesis of diabetes. *Diabetes Metab Rev 2*:125–161, 1986.

White, MF, R Maron, and CR Kahn. Insulin rapidly stimulates tyrosine phosphorylation of a M_r-185,000 protein in intact cells. *Nature 318*:183–186, 1985.

Glucagon

Patzelt, C, HS Trager, RJ Carroll, and DF Steiner, Identification and processing of proglucagon in pancreatic islets. *Nature 282*:260–266, 1979.

Pilkis, SJ, CR Park, and TH Claus. Hormonal control of hepatic gluconeogenesis, *Vitam Horm 36*:383–460, 1978.

Richards, CS and K Uyeda. Changes in the concentration of activation factor for phosphofructokinase in hepatocytes in response to glucose and glucagon. *Biochem Biophys Res Comm 97*:1535–1540, 1980.

Ungar, RH and L Orci. Physiology and pathophysiology of glucagon. *Physiol Rev 56*:778–826, 1976.

Cortisol and Its Regulation

Brodish, A. Control of ACTH secretion by corticotropin-releasing factor(s). *Vitam Horm 37*:111–152, 1979.

Crapo, L. Cushing's syndrome: A review of diagnostic tests. *Metabolism 28*:955–976, 1979.

Eipper, BA and RE Mains. Structure and biosynthesis of pro-adrenocorticotropin/endorphin and related peptides. *Endocr Rev 1*:1–27, 1980.

Furutani, Y et al. Cloning and sequence analysis of cDNA for ovine corticotropin-releasing factor precursor. *Nature 301*:537–553, 1983.

Gold, EM. The Cushing syndromes: Changing views of diagnosis and treatment. *Ann Intern Med 90*:829–844, 1979.

Hollenberg, SM, C Weinberger, ES Ong, G Cerelli, A Oro, R Lebo, EB Thompson, MG Rosenfield, and RM Evans. Primary structure and expression of a functional human glucocorticoid receptor cDNA. *Nature 318*:635–641, 1985.

Keller-Wood, ME and MF Dallman. Corticosteroid inhibition of ACTH secretion. *Endocr Rev 5*:1–24, 1984.

Krieger, DT, AS Liotta, MJ Brownstein, and EA Zimmerman. ACTH, β-lipotropin and related peptides in brain, pituitary and blood. *Recent Prog Horm Res 37*:277–336, 1981.

Mininberg, DT, L Slevine, and MI New. Current concepts in CAH. *Invest Urol 17*:169–175, 1979.

Munck, A, PM Guyre, and NJ Holbrook. Physiological functions of glucocorticoids in stress and their relation to pharmacological actions. *Endocr Rev 5*:25–44, 1984.

Nakanishi, S, A Inoue, T Kita, M Nakamura, ACY CHang, SN Cohen, and S Numa. Nucleotide sequence of cloned cDNA for bovine corticotropin-β-lipotropin precursor. *Nature 278*:423–427, 1979.

Patthy, M, J Horvath, M Mason-Garcia, B Szoke, DH Schlesinger, and AV Schally. Isolation and amino acid sequence of corticotropin-releasing factor from pig hypothalami. *Proc Natl Acad Sci USA 82*:8762–8766, 1985.

Pedersen, RC. Polypeptide activators of cholesterol side-chain cleavage. Endocr Res 10:533–561, 1985.

Pedersen, RC and AC Brownie. Cholesterol side-chain cleavage in the rat adrenal cortex: Isolation of a cycloheximide-sensitive activator–peptide. Proc Natl Acad Sci USA 77:2239–2243, 1980.

Roberts, JL, C-CL Chen, JH Eberwine, MJQ Evinger, C Gee, E Herbert, and BS Schachter. Glucocorticoid regulation of proopiomelanocortin gene expression in rodent pituitary. *Recent Prog Horm Res 38*:227–250, 1982.

Seidah, NG, J Rochemont, J Hamelin, M Lis, and M Chretien. Primary structure of the major human pituitary pro-opiomelanocortin NH_2-terminal glycopeptide. *J Biol Chem 256*:7977–7984, 1981.

Shibahara, S, Y Morimoto, Y Furutani, M Notake, H Takahashi, S Shimizu, S Horikawa, and S Numa. Isolation and sequence analysis of the human corticotropin-releasing factor precursor gene. *EMBO J* 2:775–779, 1983.

Udelsman, R, JP Harwood, MA Millan, GP Chrousos, DS Goldstein, R Zimlichman, KJ Catt, and G Aguilera. Functional corticotropin releasing factor receptors in the primate peripheral sympathetic nervous system. *Nature 319*:147–150, 1986.

Vale, W, J Spiess, and C Rivier, and J Rivier. Characterization of a 41-residue ovine hypothalamic peptide that stimulates secretion of corticotropin and β-endorphin. *Science 213*:1394–1397, 1981.

Whitnall, MH, E Mezey, and H Gainer. Co-localization of corticotropin-releasing factor and vasopressin in median eminence neurosecretory vesicles. *Nature 317*:248–250, 1985.

Yasuda, N, MA Greer, and T Aizawa. Corticotropin-releasing factor. *Endocr Rev 3*:123–140, 1982.

Catecholamines

Dixon RAF, BK Kobilka, DJ Strader, JL Benovic, HG Dohlman, T Frielle, MA Bolanowski, CD Bennett, E Rands, RE Diehl, RA Mumford, EE Slater, IS Sigal, MG Caron, RJ Lefkowitz, and CD Strader. Cloning of the gene and cDNA for mammalian β-adrenergic receptor and homology with rhodopsin. *Nature 321*:75–79, 1986.

Exton, JH. Mechanisms involved in β-adrenergic effects of catecholamines. In *Adrenal Receptors and Catetholamine Action* (G Kunos, ed). John Wiley & Sons, New York, 1981, Ch 4.

Kopin, IJ. Catecholamines, adrenal hormones and stress. In *Neuroendocrinology* (DT Krieger and JC Hughes, eds). Sinauer Associates, Sunderland, Mass, 1980, Chap 17.

Leeb-Lundberg, LMF, S Cotecchia, JW Lomasney, JF DeBernadis, RJ Lefkowitz, and MG Caron. Phorbol esters promote α_1-adrenergic receptor phosphorylation and receptor uncoupling from inositol phospholipid metabolism. *Proc Natl Acad Sci USA 82*:5651–5655, 1985.

Shreeve, SM, CM Fraser, and JC Venter. Molecular comparison of α_1- and α_2-adrenergic receptors suggests that these proteins are structurally related "isoreceptors." *Proc Natl Acad Sci USA 82*:4842–4846. 1985.

Venter, JC and CM Fraser. β-Adrenergic receptor isolation and characterization with immobilized drugs and monoclonal antibodies. *Fed Proc 42*:273–278, 1983.

Integration

Cahill, GF, Jr. Starvation in man. *Clin Endocrinol Metab 5*:397–415, 1976.

Gerich, J, J Davis, M Lorenzi, R Rizza, N Bohannon, J Karam, S Lewis, R Kaplan, T Schultz, and P Cryer. Hormonal mechanisms of recovery from insulin-induced hypoglycemia in man. *Am J Physiol* *236*:E380–E385, 1979.

Press, M, WV Tamborlane, and RS Sherwin. Importance of raised growth hormone levels in mediating the metabolic derangements of diabetes. *N Engl J Med 310*:810–815, 1984.

Rizza, RA, PE Cryer, and JE Gerich. Role of glucagon, catecholamines and growth hormone in human glucose counterregulation. *J Clin Invest 64*:62–71, 1979.

Spence, JT and HC Pitot. Induction of lipogenic enzymes in primary cultures of rat hepatocytes. *Eur J Biochem 128*:15–20, 1982.

Unger, RH, RE Dobbs, and L Orci. Insulin, glucagon and somatostatin secretion in the regulation of metabolism. *Annu Rev Physiol 40*:307–343, 1978.

APPENDIX A Glossary of Abbreviations

a^a	avian
ACTH	corticotropin
ADH	antidiuretic hormone (vasopressin)
ADP	adenosine diphosphate
AIP	aldosterone-induced protein
AMP	adenosine monophosphate
ATP	adenosine triphosphate
b	bovine
cAMP	cyclic adenosine monophosphate
CCK	cholecystokinin (pancreozymin)
CLIP	corticotropinlike intermediate lobe polypeptide
CRH	corticotropin-releasing hormone
CS	chorionic somatomammotropin
DHEA	dehydroepiandrosterone
DHT	dihydrotestosterone
DIT	3,5-diiodotyrosine
E_2	estradiol
FSH	folliculotropin (follicle-stimulating hormone)
GH	somatotropin (growth hormone)
GIP	gastric inhibitory peptide
GnRH	gonadoliberin
GRF	see SRF
GRIH	see SRIH
h	human
LH	luteotropin (luteinizing hormone)
LPH	lipotropin
m	murine (mouse)
MIT	3-iodotyrosine
MSH	melanocyte-stimulating hormone
NP	neurophysin
o	ovine
$(OH)_2CC$	1,25-dihydroxycholecalciferol

[a]The source of a polypeptide hormone is designated by a lower-case letter attached
to the letter symbol of the hormone as a prefix.

OT	oxytocin
p	porcine
Pg	progesterone
POMC	proopiomelanocortin
PRA	plasma renin activity
PRF(H)	prolactoliberin [prolactin-releasing factor(hormone)]
PRL	prolactin
PTH	parathyroid hormone
r	rat
RIA	radioimmunoassay
rT_3	reverse T_3 (3,3',5'-triiodothyronine)
SM	somatomedin
SRF	somatocrinin (somatotropin-releasing factor)
SRIH	somatostatin (somatotropin release-inhibiting hormone)
STH	somatotropin (growth hormone)
T	testosterone
T_2	3,3'-diiodothyronine
T_3	3,3',5-triiodothyronine
T_4	thyroxine (3,3',5,5'-tetraiodothyronine)
VIP	vasoactive intestinal peptide
VP	vasopressin (ADH)

APPENDIX B   Units of Measurement

Abbreviation	Meaning	Fraction of a unit
m	milli	10^{-3}
μ	micro	10^{-6}
n	nano	10^{-9}
p	pico	10^{-12}
f	femto	10^{-15}

APPENDIX C   Amino Acid Codes

One-letter	Three-letter	Name
A	Ala	Alanine
C	Cys	Cysteine
D	Asp	Aspartic acid
E	Glu	Glutamic acid
F	Phe	Phenylalanine
G	Gly	Glycine
H	His	Histidine
I	Ile	Isoleucine
K	Lys	Lysine
L	Leu	Leucine
M	Met	Methionine
N	Asn	Asparagine
P	Pro	Proline
Q	Gln	Glutamine
R	Arg	Arginine
S	Ser	Serine
T	Thr	Threonine
V	Val	Valine
W	Trp	Tryptophan
Y	Tyr	Tyrosine

APPENDIX D   The Sequence of 18 Insulins

<——— B-CHAIN ———>   <——— A-CHAIN ———>

Position markers (B-chain): 1 · 8 9 · Zn · 10 11 · 20 25 · 30 33
Position markers (A-chain): 37 38 · 40 43 45 · 50 54 55

```
                    1                                                           20
                    -YVSQRLCG  SQLVDTLYSV  CRHRGF-YRP  ND-GIVDQCC  TNICSRNQLM  SYCND
Coypu               -YVSQRLCG  SQLVDTLYSV  CRHRGF-YRP  ND-GIVDQCC  TNICSRNQLM  SYCND
Guinea pig          -F   RH    N E         QDD F I  K            GT  T H Q      -

Mouse               -FVKQHLCG  PHLVEALYLV  CGERGFFYTP  KS-GIVDQCC  TSICSLYQLE  NYCN-
Spiny mouse          B          S
Rabbit               N          S
Human                N          S                       T           E
Elephant             N          S                       T           E           GV
Sheep                N          S                       A           E           AGV
Sperm whale          N          S                       A           E           AST

Chicken/Tky         -AANQHLCG  SHLVEALYLV  CGERGFFYSP  KA-GIVEQCC  HNTCSLYQLE  NYCN-
Duck                 P R                    F I          T           E P
Rattlesnake          P R                    F I  Y       RS          E T
Toadfish            MAPPOHLCG  SHLVDALYLV  CGDRGFFYNS  --GIVEQCC  HRPCDKFDLQ  SYCN-
```

398

	LCG	LV	L	C	GF	Y	MG	I	CC	C	L	YCN
Cod	V A					P	K--D		D		I	N
Angler fish	V P					P	K--G		E		NI	N
Tuna	- ANP					P	K--G		E		NI	N
Bonito	- RTTG	KD	E			QP	K--G		HZZ	K	BI	Z B
Atlantic hagfish			IA	V		DP	TKMG		VEQ	KR	SIYN	Q N
Common	LCG	LV	L	C	GF	Y	MG	I	CC	C	L	YCN
Alternatives	-FVNQH	SH	EA	YLV	GER	F	TP	KS	VEQ	TSP	SLYQ	E N –
	MAPPRR	PN	DT	FSI	QDD	-	NS	NT	HDZ	HNI	DIFD	Q S D
	VYASP	KQ	IA	RH	Y		S	RA		AGT	NRNN	M
	RTKG	D	N	V		I	TD			ERV	TKH	
	A				R		K			KR		
	T				Q							
					D							

Disulfide bonds link cysteines at positions 8 and 39 and 20 and 52 between the B and A chains and 38 and 43 in the A chain. An insulin hexamer has two zinc atoms, each coordinated to histidine-11 in three insulin monomers. Asterisks indicate residues thought to be involved in binding to the insulin receptor. Those insulins that are identical with any sequence shown and some for which the connecting peptide has been determined are shown in Appendix E. Differences are summarized in Figure 9.1.

Source: modified from the *Atlas of Protein Sequence and Structure*, 1976, p 128.

APPENDIX E   The Sequence of Nine Proinsulins

```
            |——————————————— B-CHAIN ———————————————>              <——————— C-PEPTIDE ———|
                                           8 5
             7 2                            |  |
             |                              |  |
             1  7                           2  3                    4
             0                              0  0                    0

Rat 2       FVKQHLCGS  HLVEALYLVC  GERGFFYTPM  SRREVEDPQV  AQLELGGGPG
Rat 1               P                       K                       P   E
Guinea pig  SR        S   N    T  S  QDD   I K  D//L        E T     M LG
Human       NQ        S H A    L     GER   T K  TRR  A  L   G V     G PG

Dog         FVNQHLCGS  HLVEALYLVC  GERGFFYTPK  A           DVELAGAPG
Horse                                          EAEDPQV  GE  G   G
Pig                                         RR  N    A      G  GL-
Bovine                                      RR  V  G  V   GAL  A  GPG
Duck        A A                    S        T//DV Q LV NGP-  H  EVG

Common         HLCG   LVE LY VC    GFFY P    RR  E       L

Alternatives FVNQ    S H A    L     GER   T K A  EV DPQV  GQVE GGGPG
             AAKR    P N T    S     QDD   I M T  DA NLLA  PAL- AMALE
             S                S           S   L G     EET  H EV-
                              D               Q      ADP
                                                     NG
```

```
├── C-PEPTIDE ──→          ├────────── A-CHAIN ──────────→

          5      6   6                 7 6 7   7 1           8     1 9
          0      0   5                 7 0 7   7 6           0     8 6
                                       0   1

              AGDLQTLALE  VARQKRGIVD  QCCTSICSLY  QLENYCN
Rat 2
Rat 1
Guinea pig    G  P --Q G L //          GT TRH      QS
Human         S  P ALE GSL KR  E       SI SLY      EN

              EGGLQPLALE  GALQ//GIVE  QCCTSICSLY  QLENYCN
Dog           L  A     PQ //           G
Horse         -  A  E  PP KR           S
Pig           A  ----E PP KR           ASV
Bovine        E-- PFQHEE --Y //        ENP
Duck

Common            L        QKRGIV      QCC  C     QL  YCN

Alternatives  AGG QPLALE  GAL    E     TSI SLY    EN
              E-D -T--Q   VPR    D     AGT TRH    QS
              L S PAQHEA  -SP          ENV
              - - -Q                   P
              - F                      Y
```

Disulfide bonds link cysteines at positions 7 and 72, 19 and 85, and 71 and 76.
Sources: modified from the *Atlas of Protein Sequence and Structure*, 1976, p 127.

APPENDIX F The Sequence of Human Somatotropin and Prolactin

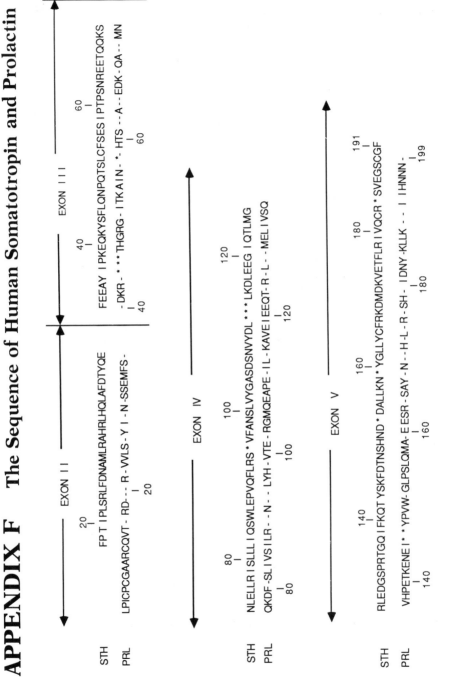

	EXON II
STH	FP T I PLSRLFDNAMLRAHRLHQLAFDTYQE
PRL	LPICPCGAARCQVT- RD--- R- VVLS- Y I -N -SSEMFS-

20

	EXON III
STH	FEEAY I PKEQKYSFLQNPQTSLCFSES I PTPSNREETQQKS
PRL	-DKR- * * *THGRG- I TKA I N- *- HTS - -A- - EDK- QA- - MN

40   60

40   60

EXON IV

STH	NLELLR I SLLL I QSWLEPVQFLRS * VFANSLVYGASDSNVYDL * * * LKDLEEG I QTLMG
PRL	QKDF-SL I VS I LR- - N- - LYH- VTE- RGMQEAPE - IL - KAVE I EEQT- R- L- - MEL I VSQ

80   100   120

80   100   120

EXON V

STH	RLEDGSPRTGQ I FKQT YSKFDTNSHND * DALLKN * YGLLYCFRKDMDKVETFLR I VQCR * SVEGSCGF
PRL	VHPETKENE I * * YPVW- GLPSLQMA- E ESR- SAY- N- -H- L- R- SH- - I DNY-KLLK- - - I I HNNN-

140   160   180   191

140   160   180   199

* The sequences are adjusted to maximize homologies; -, the residue in PRL is identical to that in STH.   Modified from Nicoll et al. Endocr Rev 7:173, 1986.

Index[a]

A

Ablation-replacement (technique), 27,28T
Acetylcholine, 58T
N-Acetylserotonin, 255,256F
Acromegaly, 121
Acrosome, bindin of, 259
ACTH (*see* Corticotropin)
Addison's disease, 171,380
Adenohypophysis (anterior pituitary), 54F,55F,57F,60
  cytology of, 61
  portal supply, 57F,60
Adenylate cyclase, 171
  in ACTH action, 177,230
  in α- and β-adrenergic response, 354
  in calcitonin action, 173T,174T, 212F
  in calcitonin secretion, 210
  coupling to receptors, 17
  in epinephrine/norepinephrine action, 353
  in FSH action, 227,243
  in glucagon action, 173T,174T, 336
  inhibition by ANH, 168,174
  in insulin secretion, 326
  in isoproterenol action, 173T, 174T
  in LH action, 227,230
  in potassium action, 177
  in PTH action, 173T,174T,212F
  in PTH secretion, 207,211

[Adenylate cyclase (con't.)]
  in STH secretion, 106
  in TSH thyrogenesis, 132
  in vasopressin action, 173T,174T
ADH (*see* Vasopressin)
Adrenal, fetal, 266
  steroid synthesis in, 267,268F
Adrenal androgen-stimulating h. (postulated), 283,284F
Adrenal gland, 26
Adrenal insufficiency, 162
Adrenal medulla
  laboratory tests, 380,381F
  pheochromocytoma, 382
Adrenaline (*see* Epinephrine)
Adrenarche, 283,284F
α-Adrenergic receptors
  characteristics of, 357
  comparison with β-adrenergic receptors, 355T
  subdivisions of, 354
  mechanisms of action of, 354
β-Adrenergic receptors
  characteristics of, 356T
  comparison with α-adrenergic receptors, 355T
  gene for β_2-receptor, 356
  homology with opsin, 356
  subdivisions of, 354
α-Adrenergic inhibition
  of insulin secretion, 323T,355T
  of PTH secretion, 207
β-Adrenergic stimulation
  of insulin secretion, 323T,355T
  of PTH secretion, 207

---

[a]T, table; F, figure; h, hormone; f, factor; X, appendix.

Adrenocorticotropic h (*see* Corticotropin)
Adrenocorticotropic hormone-
releasing h (see Corticoliberin)
Adrenogenital syndrome (*see* Congenital adrenal hyperplasia)
Adrenopathies
clinical tests for
ACTH stimulation, 374
dexamethasone suppression,
375
insulin stress, 374
metyrapone, 371,372F
dysfunction (*see* Congenital
adrenal hyperplasia)
hyperfunction (*see* Cushing's
syndrome)
hypofunction (*see* Addison's
disease)
laboratory tests for
plasma cortisol, 370,373
urinary free cortisol, 370
urinary 17-hydroxycortico-
steroids, 370,372
urinary 17-ketogenic steroids,
370,372F
Albumin, binding of T3 and T4 to,
142T
Aldosterone, 51T,156
actions of, 181,182T
biosynthesis of, 164F,165
mechanism of action of, 182-184
receptors for, 179,180T
regulation of synthesis/secretion
of, 56F,163,177
Aldosterone-stimulating factor
(ASF), 165
Ameloblasts, 201
Amenorrhea
from anatomical defects, 293
from androgen insensitivity,
295,296T
classification of, 294T

[Amenorrhea (con't.)]
from familial incomplete male
pseudohermaphroditism, 297
from male pseudohermaphroditism, 294
from ovarian failure, 298
from pituitary or hypothalamic
failure, 298
Amino acid codes, 397X
Amino acid sequences (see specific
substances by name)
γ-Aminobutyric acid (GABA), 58T,
257
Amnion, 259
Androgens (see also specific substances by name)
adrenal, 236
biological actions of, 238T
effect on plasma prealbumin
levels by, 141
effect on plasma TBG levels by,
141
in follicular fluid, 248
Leydig cell synthesis of, 254
LH secretion feedback suppression by, 255
during ontogeny, 270,271,273
in puberty, 283,284F
4-Androsten-3-one, 17β-hydroxy
(*see* Testosterone)
5-Androsten-17-one, 3β-hydroxy
(*see* Dehydroepiandrosterone)
ANF (*see* Atrial natriuretic factor)
Angiotensin, 52T,56F,156
amino acid sequence of, 163F
biosynthesis of, 162,163F
functions of, 163,169
mechanisms of action of, 177,229
receptors for, 178,179
Angiotensinogen
homology to CRH, 340
regulation of, 162
Anterior pituitary gland (*see*
Adenohypophysis)

Antibodies, monoclonal, 30
Antidiuretic h (ADH) (*see* both
  Vasopressin entries)
Antimullerian duct h, 270,272
  monoclonal antibody to, 31
APUD, 67
Arachidonic acid, 21,27,277,278
Arcuate nucleus, 240,242,274F
Arginine
  in STH stimulation, 107
  in insulin stimulation, 323
Arginine vasopressin (*see* Vasopressin, arginine)
ASF (*see* Aldosterone-stimulating
  factor)
Atrial natriuretic factor (ANF),
  52T,156
  adenylate cyclase inhibition by,
  168
  amino acid sequence of, 167F
  binding of, 174
  guanylate cyclase stimulation
  by, 168
  preproANH sequence of, 167F
  receptors for, 171,184
  source of, 165
  structure/activity of, 166

B

Baroreceptors, 168,175,176
Basal body temperature during
  menstrual cycle, 252,253F
Basal metabolic rate, 53T,129,143
Bindin, 259
  receptors for, 259
Binding proteins, 8
Biological rhythms/timing
  ACTH and, 10
  glucocorticoids and, 349
  hormonal, 10
  light-dark cycling, 255-257
  in sleep, 10,107,257
Blastocyst, 259

Blood-brain barrier, circumven-
  tion of, 169
Blood pressure/volume, 168,169,
  175,176,187F
Body temperature, 129
Bombesin, 52T
Bone
  compact, 197
  cortical, 197
  endochondral, 197
  perilacunar, 198

C

Calcitonin, 51T,56F
  amino acid sequence of, 209F
  bioactivity of, 210
  function of, 212
  gene for, 210
  in Paget's disease, 217
  receptors for, 171,173T,174T
  regulation of secretion of, 210
  sources of, 209
Calcium, 56F,177,196T
  crystalline, 197
  ionic, 207
  pools, 196
Calcium homeostasis
  effect of age on, 213
  hormones influencing, 205T
  nonhormonal factors, 204T
  RDA for, 219
  sex differences in, 213
Calcium transport protein, 211
Calmodulin, 14,15T,177,226
Cancer
  estradiol 16α-hydroxylation, 303
  GnRH superagonist, 304
Capacitation, 255
Catecholamines (see also specific
  types)
  adrenal synthesis of, 351
  in glucose counterregulation,
  357

[Catecholamines (con't.)]
  permissive action of thyroid hormones on, 144
  receptors for, 171,173T,174T
CCK (*see* Cholecystokinin)
Celiac disease, 93
Cementoblasts, 198
Central nervous system (CNS), 49, 54F,55F,170F
  angiotensin action on, 169,170F
  biological timekeeping by, 10
  definition of, 49
  endocrine system responses to, 54F
  neurotransmitters in, 58T
  water drinking and, 186F
Cerebrospinal fluid, melatonin in, 256
Children
  STH deficiency in, 121
  somatomedin deficiency in, 121
Cholecystokinin (CCK), 52T,69T
  amino acid sequence of, 72F
  as a calcitonin secretagogue, 210
  chemistry of, 74
  functions of, 76,76T
  regulation of, 74
Cholesterol, 24
  relationship to steroid hormones, 25F,26F
  side-chain cleavage of, 229,230F, 231F
Chorion, 259
Chorionic somatomammotropin (*see* Somatomammotropin, chorionic)
Chromosome, 6,24
Chymodenin, 52T
Circadian rhythms (*see also* Biological rhythms/timing), 10
Circumventricular organs, 169
Colchicine, as microtubular function inhibitor, 212
Collagen, type I, 198

Competitive protein-binding assay, 29
Congenital adrenal hyperplasia
  clinical features of, 378
  non-salt-losing form, 378
    virilization in, 378,379F
  salt-losing form, 377
Converting enzyme, 163,163F
Corpus luteum
  cellular changes in, 250
  life of, 249
  luteolytic agents of, 250,251
  luteotropic agents of, 250,251T
  progesterone synthesis by, 249
Corticoliberin, 50T
  amino acid sequence of, 339F
  homologues of, 340
  mechanism of action of, 339
  structure/function, 339
  synergism with vasopressin, 340
Corticosteroids
  (*see also* Glucocorticoids and specific steroids)
  circadian rhythms in, 10,349, 376
  in Cushing's syndrome, 376
  metabolism of, 344,346F,371F
  in stress response, 346,349
  synthesis of, 344,345F
Corticosterone, 51T,54F
  release of, 230
  secretion ratio to cortisol, 339
Corticotrope cells, 61T
Corticotropin (ACTH), 54F,177
  amino acid sequence of, 341F
  in proopiomelanocortin, 340, 341F
  in side-chain cleavage reaction, 229,230,231F
Corticotropin, placental, 266
Corticotropin-releasing h (CRH) (*see* Corticoliberin)
Corticotropinlike intermediate lobe polypeptide (CLIP), 340

Cortisol (hydrocortisone), 51T, 54F,339
  Cushing's syndrome levels of, 376
  in glucose counterregulation, 357
  in initiation of parturition, 277
  metabolism of, 344,346F,371F
  measurement in plasma, 370, 373
  measurement in urine, 370
  synthesis of, 344,345F
  transport of, 344
  TSH inhibition by, 132
Cretinism, 149
CRH (see Corticoliberin)
Cushing's syndrome
  ACTH plasma levels in, 376
  clinical features of, 375
  cortisol secretion in, 376
  diagnosis of, 377F
  types of, 375,377F
Cyclic AMP (cAMP) (see also Adenylate cyclase), 12,230
  cAMP-dependent protein kinases, 13
  interactions between Ca²⁺ and cAMP messenger systems, 21T
Cyclic center, hypothalamus, 252

D

Dehydration, 186F
Dehydroepiandrosterone (DHEA), 51T
  in adrenarche, 283,284F
  biological actions of, 238T
  biosynthesis of, 232F,344,345F
  values of, 237T
Dehydroepiandrosterone sulfate
  biosynthesis of, 232F
  as precursors of placental estrogen, 267
  values of, 237T

Dexamethasone
  as ACTH suppressor, 377
  in Cushing's syndrome diagnosis, 377
DHEA (see Dehydroepiandrosterone)
Diabetes insipidus (hypovasopressinemia), 186F
  drugs affecting, 184,185
  etiology for, 184
  types of, 184
Diabetes mellitus, 364-369
  classification of, 365T
  clinical aspects of, 364
  etiology of, 368
  and fetal development, 122
  insulin-dependent DM (type I), 366
  insulin-independent DM (type II), 367
  in neonates, 122
  STH and, 368
  tests for, 364,366F
Diabetogenic action
  of peptides contaminating STH, 102
  of STH, 102
Dihydrotestosterone (DHT), 7, 236,238FT
1α,25-Dihydroxycholecalciferol [(OH)₂CC], 52T,195
  biosynthesis of, 207,208F
  function, 211
Dihydroxyvitamin D (see Dihydroxycholecalciferol)
Diurnal rhythms (see Biological rhythms/timing)
L-Dopa
  in catecholamine synthesis, 352F
  STH response to, 107
Dopamine, 50T
  biosynthesis of, 352F
  as a PTH secretagogue, 207

[Dopamine (con't.)]
  in prolactin secretion inhibition, 58,257
  STH activation by, 58
  TSH secretion inhibition by, 130,131
Dopamine-beta-hydroxylase, 353
Drinking (see Water intake/drinking)
Dwarfism
  characteristics and diagnosis of, 121
  as STH deficiency, 121
  hypothalamic hypopituitarism in Laron, 121

E

EGF (see Epidermal growth factor)
Endorphin, 340,341F
  in response to calcitonin, 217
Enkephalin, 58T
Enteroglucagon, 69T
  chemistry of, 82
  regulation of, 83
Epidermal growth factor (EGF)
  biological effects of, 114
  chemistry of, 114
  receptor for, 114,117,248
  sources, 114
Epinephrine, 51T
  in adrenergic receptor stimulation, 354
  biosynthesis of, 351,352F
  effects of, 353
  as neurotransmitter, 353
  release of, 353
  as a stimulant of PTH secretion, 207
  stress activation of, 353
Erythropoietin, 52T

Estradiol, 52T
  antidopaminergic activity, 257
  biological properties of, 240T
  biosynthesis of, 232F
  critical concn for LH surge, 249,252
  follicular secretion of, 247
  menstrual cycle pattern, 253F
  negative feedback by, 241,255
  positive feedback by, 239,241
  receptor binding, 236
  sex difference in levels of, 236
  thyrotrope sensitization to TRH by, 132
  values of, 237T
1,3,5(10)-Estratriene-3,17β-diol
  (see Estradiol)
Estriol, 267
Estrogens (see also Estradiol and Ethinylestradiol)
  androgen coversion to, 232F, 236,239F
  angiotensinogen stimulation by, 162
  biological actions of, 239,240T
  effect on plasma TBG levels, 141
  effect on plasma prealbumin levels, 141
  in follicular fluid, 248
  melatonin suppression by, 257
  in therapy for osteoporosis, 215
  receptor monoclonal antibody of, 30
Estrus cycle regulation in the rat, 252
Ethanol in ADH inhibition, 175T
Ethinylestradiol, 122
Exercise and STH release, 107

F

Fallopian tubes, 258

Feedback, negative
  of endogenous glucocorticoids
    on CRH secretion, 346
  of synthetic glucocorticoids on
    ACTH secretion, 347
  of gonadal hormones on LH
    secretion, 238T,240T
  of folliculostatin on FSH secre-
    tion, 248
  of T4 on TSH secretion, 131
Feedback, positive, 239,241
Female
  brain sexuality, 274F
  gonadotropin secretion patterns
    in, 253F
  masculinization of, 273
  sex differentiation, 267,269F
α-Fetoprotein, 273
Fetus
  gonadotropin activation of, 270
  steroid biosynthesis in, 268F
FGF (see Fibroblast growth factor)
Fibroblast growth factor (FGF)
  amino acid sequence of, 120F
  biological properties of, 119
  chemistry of, 119
  fibronectin cell recognition site,
    119,120F
  ovarian action of, 248
  thyrotrope sensitization to TRH
    by, 132
Follicle-stimulating h (see
    Folliculotropin)
Follicle-stimulating hormone-
    releasing h (see Gonado-
    liberin)
Folliculogenesis
  in monotocous species, 243-248
  in polytocous species, 249
Folliculostatin, 51T
  chemistry of, 248
  inhibition of FSH secretion by,
    248

Folliculotropin (FSH), 50T
  amino acid sequence of FSHβ,
    264
  and aromatase activity, 236,
    239F
  biphasic action of estradiol on,
    241,242F
  effect of age on response to
    GnRH, 286F
  episodic release of, 251
  in folliculogenesis, 243
  folliculostatin inhibition of,
    248
  functions of, 227
  GnRH stimulation of, 240
  menstrual cycle pattern of,
    253F
  in precocious puberty, 301
  and spermatogenesis, 254
FSH (Follicle-stimulating hor-
    mone) (see Folliculotropin)
FSHRH (see Gonadoliberin)

G

G, guanine-binding protein (see
    Nucleotide-binding protein)
Gametotropin (see Folliculotropin)
Gastric acid, 73
Gastric inhibitory peptide (GIP),
    52T
  amino acid sequence of, 77F
  chemistry of, 79
  function of, 69T,79,80F,81T
  regulation of secretion of, 79
Gastrin-releasing peptide (GRP)
  amino acid sequence of, 84
  chemistry of, 83
  functions of, 69T,83
Gastrins
  amino acid sequences of, 72
  chemistry of, 71
  function of, 69T,73,73T
  regulation of secretion of, 73

Gastrointestinal tract
  anatomy of, 68F
  hormone-producing cells of, 69T
Genitalia, external, ontogeny of, 271,272F
Genetics, major histocompatibility complex, 33,34F
Genital tract differentiation, 267
GH (*see* Somatotropin)
GIP (*see* Gastric inhibitory peptide)
Glicentin, 82,334
Glossary of abbreviations, 395X
Glucagon, 52T,56F
  amino acid sequence of, 77F
  as a calcitonin secretagogue, 210
  chemistry of, 334
  function of, 69T, 334-337,338F
  in glucose counterregulation, 357
  in pancreatic islet α-cells, 318
  and permissive action of thyroid h, 144
  proglucagon, 334,335F
  regulation of secretion of, 83, 334
Glucocorticoids (*see also* Corticosterone, Cortisol, and Dexamethasone)
  decrease of plasma TBG levels by, 141
  effects of, 337,349,350T
  increase of plasma prealbumin level by, 141
  inhibition of ACTH secretion, 339
  inhibition of cartilage synthesis, 214
  production of secondary hyperparathyroidism, 214
Glucose-dependent insulinotropic peptide (*see* Gastric inhibitory peptide)

Glucose counterregulation, 357
GnRH (*see* Gonadoliberin)
Gonadal dysgenesis, 294T,296T, 298,301,302T
Gonadal function disorders, 293-303
Gonadarche, 283
Gonadoliberin (GnRH), 50T
  amino acid sequence of, 224
  analogues of, 227
  biphasic effect of, 226
  chemistry of, 224
  episodic release of, 240
  extrahypothalamic, 227
  gonadotropin response to, 240
  neuronal function of, 60
  preproGnRH, 224
  receptors for, 225
  second messenger for, 225
Gonadotrope cells, 61T
Gonadotropin, chorionic, human (hCG)
  amino acid sequence of hCGα, 261,263F
  amino acid sequence of hCGβ, 264F
  biosynthesis of, 261
  carbohydrate sequences of, 264, 265F
  in fetal testosterone synthesis, 270
  as a pregnancy test, 265
  and steroid hormone synthesis, 27
Gonadotropins (*see also* Folliculotropin and Luteotropin)
  biphasic effect of estradiol on, 241,242F
  effect of age on response to GnRH, 286F
  episodic secretion of, 24,251,283
  feedback inhibition of secretion of, 248,255

[Gonadotropins (con't.)]
supersensitivity of prepubes-
cents, 283
GnRH stimulation of, 240,251
menstrual cycle pattern of,
253F
in precocious puberty, 301
Gonadotropin-releasing h. (*see*
Gonadoliberin)
Granulosa cells, 226-228,236,239F,
240T
Graves disease, 150
GRF (*see* Somatocrinin)
GRH (*see* Somatocrinin)
GRIH (*see* Somatostatin)
Growth, childhood failure of,
121-123
Growth factors (GF) (see also
specific growth factors), 109T
Growth hormone (*see* Somato-
tropin)
Growth hormone release-inhibit-
ing h (*see* Somatostatin)
Growth hormone releasing h (*see*
Somatocrinin)
Guanine-binding protein (*see*
Nucleotide-binding protein)

H

Histamine
in gastric acid production, 73
synergism with gastrin, 73
Homeostasis, 9
Hormones (see also specific h.)
definition of, 2
properties of, 3,6
secretion of, 7
Howship's lacunae, 197
Hunter-Bolton reagent, 74,75F
Hydrocortisone (*see* Cortisol)
Hydroxyapatite, 197
Hydroxyindole-O-methyl trans-
ferase, 255

5-Hydroxytryptophan (*see*
Serotonin)
Hypercalcemia, 217T
Hypercortisolism (*see* Cushing's
syndrome)
Hyperepinephrinemia, 382
Hyperfunction (see also specific
organs and endocrinopathies),
31,36
Hyperparathyroidism, 217
Hyperpituitarism, 63
Hyperprolactinemia
etiology of, 228
infertility produced by, 228
Hypertension, 186
renin-angiotensin form of, 187F
Hyperthyroidism, 149
Hypervasopressinemia, 185
Hypocalcemia, 218T
Hypocortisolism (*see* Addison's
disease)
Hypofunction (see also specific
organs and endocrinopathies),
31,37
Hypoglycemia
catecholamine response to, 353
glucagon response to, 334
glucocorticoid response to, 346,
374
STH response to, 107
Hypogonadism, 298,300
Hypogonadotropic hypogonadism,
298,301
GnRH therapy in, 298
Hypoparathyroidism, 219
Hypophosphatemia, 217
Hypopituitarism (see also specific
endocrinopathies), 62
hypothalamic involvement in,
62
Hypothalamic releasing factors
(see specific h.)
Hypothalamus, 57F,59F
anatomy, 53

[Hypothalamus (con't.)]
arcuate nucleus and GnRH secretion, 240,242,274F
biological rhythms affecting, 10
neuroendocrine regulation by, 54F,55F
osmoreceptors in lateral pre-optic area, 168
paraventricular nucleus, 130,156
preoptic area in gonadotropin cycling, 252,273
supraoptic nucleus, 156
water intake and stimulation of, 168
Hypothyroidism
cretinism, 149
myxedema, 149
Hypoxia
angiotensinogen stimulation by, 162
suppression of iodide uptake by, 134

I

IGF (see Insulin-like growth factors)
Implantation, 259
Inhibin (see Folliculostatin)
Inositol, phospate esters of, 13F, 15,177,226,356
Insulin, 52T,56F
in ACTH activation, 373
amino acid sequence of, 398X
chemistry of, 316-318
crystoalographic structure of, 316
differences in sequences of, 317F
functions of, 69T
as a growth promoter, 108, 122
mechanism of secretion control of, 325
preproinsulin, 4,318
proinsulin, 4,318

[Insulin (con't.)]
amino acid sequences of, 400X
differences in sequences of, 319F
receptor for, 331-334
chemistry of, 331
on granulosa cells, 248
homology to GF receptors, 333
in Leprechaunism, 123
monoclonal antibody of, 31
phosphorylation of, 333
proreceptor, 331,332F
regulation of metabolism by, 326-330,329T
amino acid transport, 327
enzymatic activity, 328,329T
enzyme synthesis, 329,330T
glucose transport, 326,328
second messenger, 330
regulation of secretion of, 318-326
secretagogues of, 323T
amino acids, 323
glucose, 320,321F,322
hormones, 324
neural factors, 324
secretion phases of, 319
in STH activation, 108
Insulin-like growth factors (IGF-I and -II)
amino acid sequence of, 110F
carrier proteins of, 108
chemistry of, 108
comparison with insulin, 108
ovarian action of, 248
receptors for, 108,111T,117
Iodide, 134
Iodide pump, 134
Isoproterenol, 58
as a calcitonin secretagogue, 210
as a PTH secretagogue, 207

J, K

Juxtaglomerular cells, 169
Kallikrein, 6
Kininase II (*see* Converting enzyme), 163,163F

L

Lactation
  and conservation of calcium, 213
  hormone requirements for, 280
Lactose synthethase, regulation of B-subunit synthesis 281
LDL (*see* Low density lipoprotein)
Lactogen (*see* Prolactin and Somatomammotropin)
Lactotrope cells, 61T
Laron dwarfism, 121
Leu-enkephalin, 51T
Leydig cells, 226,254,269
LH (*see* Luteotropin)
LHRH (*see* Gonadoliberin)
Libido, 238T
Light-dark cycles
  and melatonin synthesis, 255
  pineal body response to, 256
Lipotropin, 340,341F,342
Low density lipoprotein
  apoB of, 26
  apoE of, 26
  as cholesterol carrier, 26,266
Luteinizing hormone (LH) (*see* Luteotropin)
Luteinizing hormone-releasing hormone (*see* Gonadoliberin)
Luteotropin (LH), 54F,56T
  amino acid sequence in LHβ, 264
  biphasic action of estradiol on, 241, 242F
  different negative feedback action of estradiol and testosterone, 255

[Luteotropin (LH) (con't.)]
  effect of age on response to GnRH, 286F
  episodic release of, 251
  in estrogen synthesis, 236,239F
  functions of, 227
  GnRH activation of, 240,242
  menstrual cycle pattern of, 253F
  in precocious puberty, 301
  prolactin secretion reciprocity with, 224
  in side-chain cleavage reaction, 229,230
  and steroid hormone synthesis, 27
  testosterone feedback on, 254
  in testosterone synthesis, 254
Lysine-8 vasopressin, amino acid sequence of, 157

M

Macula densa, 176
Masculinization, hormonal, in rats, 274
Median eminence, 57F,169
  vascular network of, 57F
Melanocyte-stimulating hormone (MSH), 340,341F,342
  γ_3-MSH in cholesterol esterase activity, 230,342
  pro-γ-MSH amino acid sequence, 343F
Melanocyte-stimulating hormone-releasing factor (*see* Melanoliberin)
Melanocyte-stimulating hormone release-inhibiting factor (*see* Melanostatin)
Melanoliberin, 50T
Melanostatin, 50T
Melatonin
  biosynthesis of, 255,256F
  in cerebrospinal fluid, 256
  sources of, 255

[Melatonin (con't.)]
  suppression of gonadal function by, 257
Menstrual cycle
  disorders of (see Amenorrhea)
  hormone patterns during, 253F
  lactation inhibition of, 248
  ovulation during, 249
  periodicity of, 251
  pregnancy inhibition of, 248
  regulation of, 240-243, 242F
Mental retardation in cretinism, 149
Metabolism
  coordinate control of, 357
  key enzymes in, 358,359T
  nutritional status in, 358-363, 360F-362F,363T
  regulation of, 53T
Met-enkephalin, 51T,340
Metyrapone, in Cushing's syndrome diagnosis, 371,372F
Milk letdown h (see Oxytocin)
Mineralization
  evidence for, 202,203T
  hypotheses for, 201
Monoamine neurotransmitters
  (see also specific type), 58T
  effects on pituitary h secretion, 58T
Morula, 259
Motilin, 52T,69T
  actions of, 91
  amino acid sequence of, 86F
  regulation of, 91
MRF (see Melanoliberin)
MRIF (see Melanostatin)
MSA (see Multiplication-stimulating activity)
MSH (see Melanocyte-stimulating hormone)
Mullerian duct system, 270F
Multiple endocrine neoplasia syndromes, 218

Multiplication-stimulating activity (MSA), 108
Myxedema, 149

N

N (see Nucleotide-binding protein)
Negative feedback, 8
Nerve growth factor (NGF)
  biologic properties of, 118
  chemistry of, 117
  receptor for, 118
Neurocrine hormones, 23
Neuroendocrine system, 49,60
Neurohypophyseal hormones
  oxytocin, 156,157F,279,281
  vasopressin, 156,157F,171-175
Neurohypophysis (posterior pituitary), 49,57F,60
  diabetes insipidus and, 184
  hormonal production (see Oxytocin)
  hypothalamic neural linkage, 60
Neurophysins
  amino acid sequences of, 157F, 158F
  biosynthesis of, 156
  chemistry of, 156,158,159
  hormone binding by, 158,159
Neurotensin
  actions of, 92
  amino acid sequence of, 86F
  function of, 69T
Neurotransmitters (see also
  Acetylcholine; Catecholamines; Norepinephrine; Serotonin)
  agonists/antagonists of, 53,58T
  STH secretion mediation by, 107
  in thyroliberin (TRH) release, 130
NGF (see Nerve growth factor)
Nonsuppressible insulinlike activity (NSILA),108

Noradrenaline (*see* Norepinephrine)
Norepinephrine (*see also* Catecholamines; Neurotransmitters), 51T
in adrenergic receptor stimulation, 354
biosynthesis of, 351,352F
effects of, 353
release of, 353
in somatotropin activity, 107
stress activation of, 353
thyroliberin activation by, 130
NSILA (see Nonsuppressible insulinlike activity)
Nucleotide-binding protein, 17

O

Obesity
cortisol and, in Cushing's syndrome, 375
hyperinsulinemia and, 366F,368
(OH)₂CC (*see* Dihydroxycholecalciferol)
Odontoblasts, 198
Oocyte meiosis inhibitor, 248
Oocyte meiosis stimulator, 248
Ontogeny, 267
Osmoreceptors, 168,171,174
Osmotic pressure, 155,156,184
extracellular, intracellular, 168,
169F
in vasopressin release, 174
water intake and, 168,170F
Osteitis fibrosa, 197
Osteoblasts, 198,214
Osteocalcin, 198,202
amino acid sequence of, 198,
199F
concentration of, 198
structure/function, 199
Osteochondral complex, 198
Osteoclast-activating f, monoclonal
antibody to, 31

Osteoclasts, 198,200,214
Osteocytes, 198,200
Osteomalacia, 216
causes of, 216
Osteonectin, 200,202
Osteoid, 198
Osteon, 198
Osteoporosis, 214
factors in, 215T
Osteoprogenitor cells, 198
Ovary (see also gonads) 26
asymmetrical function of, 243
corpus luteum formation of,
246F
dominant follicle of, 247
follicular recruitment in, 243
follicular selection in, 243
folliculogenesis in, 244F-246F
glomerulosa cells in, 236,239F,
243
as menstrual cycle Zeitgeber,
240,241
theca interna cells in, 236,239F
Ovulation
estradiol in activation of, 249
LH in activation of, 249
preoptic hypothalamus in, 252
reflex, 252
Oxytocin, 51T
action of, 281
amino acid sequence of, 157F
as hypothalamic hormone, 156
in induction of labor, 279
neurophysin and, 156
suckling stimulus for release of,
281

P

Paget's disease, 217
Pancreatic agenesis, 122
Pancreatic polypeptide (PP)
amino acid sequence of, 86F
biological properties of, 69T,86

[Pancreatic polypeptide (con't.)]
  chemistry of, 85
Pancreozymin (see Cholecystokinin)
Paracrine hormones, 23
Parathyroid h (PTH), 51T,56F,195
  amino acid sequence of, 206F
  function of, 211
  gene for, 206
  monoclonal antibody of, 31
  preproPTH, 4,5T,206
  proPTH, 4,5T,206
  receptors for, 171,173T,174T,211,
    212F
  regulation of secretion of, 206
  source of, 205
  structure/function, 206
Paraventricular nucleus, 57F,59F,
  156
Parturition, 273,277
  role of estrogen in, 279
  role of glucocorticoid in, 277
  role of oxytocin in, 279
  role of progesterone in, 277,279
  role of prostaglandins in, 276,
    279
  role of relaxin in, 275,279
PDGF (see Platelet-derived growth
  factor)
Pentagastrin, 71
  as a calcitonin secretagogue,
    210
Periosteum, 198
Phentolamine, 58T
Phenylethanolamine-N-methyl-
  transferase in catecholamine
  synthesis, 351
Pheromones, 252
Phosphatases, phosphoprotein, 17
Phosphoinositides (see Inositol)
Phospholipase C, 13
Phosphorylation, regulation of
  hormonal activity by,
    336-338F,357,359T

Pineal gland
  biological timing functions of,
    257
  hormone secretions of, 255
  light-dark responses by, 255
  photoreceptivity of, in lower
    vertebrates, 256
  receptors for sex steroids and
    PRL, 257
Pituitary (see also Adenohypo-
    physis and Neurohypophysis)
  in acromegaly, 121
  anatomy of, 60
  cell types of, 61,61T
  in Cushing's syndrome, 375,
    377F
Pituitary gland
  anatomy of, 60
  anterior (see Adenohypophysis)
  hormones released by (see
    Pituitary hormones)
  hypothalamic regulation of, 60
  posterior (see Neurohypophysis)
Pituitary hormones (see also spe-
    cific hormone), 54F,55F
Placenta, 26
Placental synthesis of
  ACTH, 266
  estrogen, 266
  hCS, 265
  hCG, 259-265
  progesterone, 266
Placental lactogen (see Somato-
    mammotropin)
Platelet-derived growth factor
    (PDGF)
  biology of, 115
  chemistry of, 109T,115
  receptor for, 111T,117
  viral homology of, 116,117
Portal system, pituitary-hypo-
    thalamic, 57F,60
Posterior pituitary gland (see
    Neurohypophysis)

Potassium ions
in aldosterone synthesis, 177
as a calcitonin secretagogue,
210
Precocious puberty
GnRH and gonadotropins in,
301
and growth, 122
Pregnancy (see also Parturition)
chorionic gonadotropin and,
259-265
chorionic somatomammotropin
and, 265
hormone production rates in,
265,266
progesterone action during,
266,280,281
4-Pregnen-18-al, 11β,21-dihy-
droxy-3,20-dioxo (see Aldosterone)
4-Pregnene-3,20-dione (see Progesterone)
4-Pregnene-3,20-dione, 11β,21-di-
hydroxy (see Corticosterone)
4-Pregnene-3,20-dione, 11β,17,21-
trihydroxy (see Cortisol)
Pregnenolone, biosynthesis of,
164F,229-231,342
Preoptic area, hypothalamus
in gonadotropin cycling, 252,273
as testosterone/estradiol target
tissue, 273
Preprohormones, 4
PRF (see Prolactin releasing
factor)
PRL (see Prolactin)
Proenkephalin, 5
Progesterone, 51T,54F
anesthesia of uterine endometrium, 266
biological actions of, 240T
fetoplacental synthesis, 266
inhibition of melatonin synthesis
and release, 257

[Progesterone (con't.)]
in menstrual cycle secretion,
253F
suppression of lactation, 266
transport of, 344
values of, 237T
Proglucagon, 6
Prohormones, 4
Prolactin, 50T
chemistry of, 228
dopamine inhibition of, 257
functions of, 228,257
genes of, 100
hypothalamic control of, 257
lactation and, 258,280
preprolactin, 4
receptors for, 258
release of, 48
secretion dysfunctions, 228
serotonin activation of, 257
sleep and secretion patterns, 10,
257
TRH stimulation of, 257
VIP stimulation of, 257
Prolactin release-inhibiting hormone (see Dopamine)
Prolactin releasing factor (see
Prolactoliberin)
Prolactoliberin, 50T
Proopiomelanocortin, 6,266,340,
341F
homology with calcitonin, 342
Propanolol, 58T
Propressophysin, 6
Prostaglandin E as a PTH
secretagogue, 207
Prostaglandin F$_{2\alpha}$ as a PTH secretion inhibitor, 207
Prostaglandins, 21
biological effects of, 277
biosynthesis of, 277,278F
induction of parturition by, 279
ovarian action of, 248
stimulation of somatocrinin
release, 106

Protein kinases
  cAMP-dependent protein
  kinases, 13,132
  calcium-calmodulin-dependent
  protein kinases, 14
  calcium-phospolipid-dependent
  protein kinases, 15,177,226
Pseudohypoparathyroidism, 219
Puberty
  adrenal androgen activity and,
  283
  CNS-neuroendocrine activation
  of, 285
  FSH response to GnRH in, 286F
  LH secretion patterns and,
  283,286F
  onset and development of, 282
  precocious (see Precocious
  puberty)
  supersensitive negative feedback in, 283

R

Radioimmunoassay, 29
Radioreceptor assay, 30
Receptors (see also specific hormones)
  downregulation, 226,227,334
  intracellular, 22,285
    activation-inactivation, 287
    transformation, 288,289F
    translocation, 291
    nuclear binding, 292
  of plasma membrane, 11
    chemical nature of, 12
    coupling to adenylate cyclase,
    17,18F,19F
    physical properties of, 111,
    332
  upregulation, 226,280
Relaxin, 51T
  amino acid sequence of, 110F
  biological activity of, 275

[Relaxin (con't.)]
  preprorelaxin, 275
  prorelaxin, 276F
  sources of, 275
Releasing hormones/factors (see
  specific substances)
Renin, 56F
  amino acid sequence of, 160,
  161F
  chemistry of, 159
  prorenin, 159
    activation of, 160,162F
    nucleotide sequence of, 161F
  release of, 176T
  sources of, 160
Reproductive tract, differentiation, 267
RIA (see Radioimmunoassay)
RRA (see Radioceptor assay)
Rickets
  vitamin D-dependent, 217
  vitamin D-resistant, 216

S

Saliva, salt intake and, 171
Salt (NaCl)
  depletion of and appetite for,
  171
  metabolism of, 53T
Saralasin, 169,188
Saturation analysis, 27
Sauvagine, 340
Second messengers
  calcium, 12,177,225,356
  cyclic AMP, 12,106,132,227,230,
  336
  diacylglycerol, 12,177
  inositol trisphosphate, 12,177
Secretin, 48,52T
  amino acid sequence of, 77F
  biological activities of, 69T,78,
  78T
  chemistry of, 76

[Secretin (con't.)]
  as a PTH secretagogue, 207
  regulation of, 78
Serotonin, 58T
  in somatotropin activity, 107
Sertoli cells
  folliculostatin production of, 254
  spermatogenesis and, 254
Setpoint, 9
Sex hormones (see specific type)
Sexual differences/differentiation
  anti-Mullerian duct hormone
    and, 270
  in brain development, 273,274F
  dihydrotestosterone in, 271
  of external genitalia, 271,272F
  α-fetoprotein in, 273
  gonadal steriod hormone pro-
    duction and, 237T
  HY antigen and gonadal dif-
    ferentiation, 267
  of internal reproductive organs,
    269,270F
  Jost model of, 269F
  multifactorial process of, 271
  in puberty, 282
  in secondary sex development,
    238T,240T
  temporal relationships in, 267,
    269F
  testosterone in, 270,271
Sexual precocity (see Precocious
    puberty)
Sleep
  ACTH secretion during, 349
  gonadotropin release during,
    283
  prolactin secretion and, 257
  serotonin in somatotropin re-
    sponse to, 107
  somatotropin secretion and, 10,
    107
Sodium, stimulation of plasma
    ANF by, 165

Somatocrinin, 50T
  amino acid sequence of, 104F
  and cAMP, 106
  chemistry of, 103
  glucocorticoid increases
    response to, 107
  preprosomatocrinin, 103,105F
  and somatostatin, 107
  and somatotropin, 106
  thyroid increases response to,
    107
Somatomammotropin, chorionic,
    human (hCS)
  growth-promoting properties of,
    113
  as a placental function test, 265
  role in pregnancy, 265
  presomatomammotropin, 4
Somatomedins
  amino acid sequence of, 110F,
    111T
  androgen noninvolvement with,
    113
  biological properties of, 112T
  in dwarfism diagnosis, 121
  glucocorticoid suppression of,
    113
  insulin compared with, 111T
  insulin-like growth factors and,
    108
  protein-calorie malnutrition
    and, 113
  somatomedin-C, 108
  somatotropin mediation of, 49
  as sulfation factor, 107
Somatostatin (somatotropin
    release-inhibiting hormone),
    50T,52T
  amino acid sequences of, 87,
    88F
  biological properties of, 48,87,
    91T
  chemistry of, 87
  distribution of, 87,318,320F

[Somatostatin (con't.)]
   function of, 69T,106,319
   inhibition of TSH secretion by,
      132
   regulation of, 90T
Somatotrope cells, 61T
Somatotropin, 50T
   in acromegaly, 121
   adrenergic response and, 107
   in carbohydrate metabolism, 357
   chemistry of, 100,102
   childhood deficiency of, 121
   diabetogenic action of, 102
   genes of, 100
   in gigantism, 121
   glucocorticoid suppression of,
      113
   hypersomatotropinemia, 121
   hyposomatotropinemia, 121
   monoclonal antibody of, 31
   neurotransmitter mediation of,
      58T
   presomatotropin, 4
   and promotion of osteoblastic
      function, 214
   secretagogues, 48,106
   serotonin response to, 107
   sleep-related activity of, 10
   somatocrinin and, 106
   somatomedins and, 107
   somatostatin and, 107
   species specificity of, 101
   structure-function relationships
      of, 101
Spermatogenesis
   hormonal factors in, 254
   light-dark modulation, 257
SRF (see Somatocrinin)
SRIH (see Somatostatin)
STH (see Somatotropin)
Stress
   catecholamine responses to, 353
   hypothalamoadenohypophyseal-
      adrenocortical responses to, 346

[Stress (con't.)]
   menstrual cycle response to, 243
   somatotropin response to, 107
Subfornical organ, in blood-brain
      barrier circumvention, 169,
      170F
Substance P
   function of, 52T,69T,85
   monoclonal antibody of, 31
Suckling, effect on menstrual
      cycle, 243
Sulfation factor (see Somato-
      medins)
Supraoptic nucleus, 156,174

T

T3 (see 3,3′,5-Triiodothyronine)
T3 resin uptake, 145,146F
rT3 (see 3,3′,5′-Triiodothyronine)
T4 (see Thyroxine)
Teprotide, 188
Testes (see also gonads), 26,254
Testicular disorders, 300
Testicular feminizing syndrome
      (see Amenorrhea, from andro-
      gen insensitivity)
Testosterone (see also gonadal
      hormones), 7,51T
   biological effects of, 238T
   biosynthesis of, 232F
   Leydig cell synthesis of, 254
   LH stimulation of, 254
   menstrual cycle pattern of, 253F
   negative feedback on LH by,
      255
   as a prohormone, 236,238F
   sex difference in, 236,237T
   in sex differentiation, 270
   in sperm production, 254
3,3′,5,5′-Tetraiodothyronine (see
      Thyroxine)
Theca interna cells, in LH syn-
      thesis of androgen, 236,239F

Thiourea compounds as inhibitors of
  iodothyronine synthesis, 137
  peripheral deiodination, 137
Thirst (*see also* Water intake/drinking)
  angiotensin levels and, 169
  renin-angiotensin system and, 163
Thyrocalcitonin (*see* Calcitonin)
Thyroglobulin
  cDNA of, 135
  chemistry of, 135
  iodination of, 136,138F
  iodothyronine synthesis on, 137, 139F
  storage of, 140
  usage of, 140
Thyroid gland
  C cells and calcitonin synthesis, 209,210
  hyperfunction of, 149
  hypofunction of, 148
  thyroid hormone production rates, 148T
  TSH action on, 132
Thyroid-stimulating hormone (TSH) (*see* Thyrotropin)
Thyroid uptake test, 145,147T
Thyroliberin (TRH), 50T
  amino acid sequence of, 130
  biosynthesis of, 129
  receptors for, 131
  stimulation of prolactin release by, 48,257
  stimulation of TSH synthesis/release by, 48,131
Thyroid-stimulating hormone-releasing h (*see* Thyroliberin)
Thyrotrope cells, 61T
Thyrotropin (TSH), 50T,54F
  biosynthesis of, 131
  chemistry of, 130

[Thyrotropin (TSH) (con't.)]
  dopamine inhibition of secretion of, 131
  effect of temperature on secretion of, 129,130
  feedback of T4, 131
  function of, 132
  monoamine transmitters and secretion of, 130
  receptor monoclonal antibody of, 30
  somatostatin inhibition of, 132
  TRH stimulation of, 131
Thyroxine (T4), 7,51T,54F
  amphibian metamorphosis by, 142
  binding to plasma proteins of, 140,142T,143T
  biosynthesis of, 132,134,141F
  blood transport of, 140
  in brain myelinization, 142
  negative feedback by, 131
  in osteoclastic activity, 214
  peripheral deiodination of, 141,145,148T
  permissive action of, 144
  plasma parameters of, 143T
  as a prohormone, 132
  receptors of, nuclear, 144
  regulation of basal metabolic rate, 143
  synthesis of α-glycerophosphateDHGase by, 143
Thyroxine-binding globulin (TBG), 140
Thyroxine-binding prealbumin, 140
TRH (*see* Thyroliberin)
Triiodothyronine (3,3',5-triiodothyronine; T3), 7,51T,54F
  binding to plasma proteins of, 140,142T,143T
  biosynthesis of, 132,134,141F
  blood transport of, 140

[Triiodothyronine (con't.)]
  kinetics of, 148T
  plasma parameters of, 143T
  production rate of, 141
  structure, 133F
Triiodothyronine (3,3′,5′-triiodo-
    thyronine; rT3)
  effects of, 142
  kinetics of, 148T
  occurrence of, 134
  potency of, 133
  structure of, 133F
Trophoblasts, 259
Tropical malabsorption, 93
TSH (see Thyrotropin)
Turner's syndrome, 122
Tyrosine hydroxylase, 351
Tyrosine kinase, 111T,117

U

Units, 397X
Urine, volume and osmolality, in
    diabetes insipidus, 184,186F
Urogastrone (see Epidermal
    growth factor)

V

Vasoactive intestinal peptide
    (VIP), 52T
  amino acid sequence of, 77F
  function of, 69T,82
  regulation of, 81
Vasopressin, arginine, 51T
  amino acid sequence of, 156,
    157F

[Vasopressin, arginine (con't.)]
  biosynthesis of, in hypothal-
    amus, 156
  in body fluid balance, 173
  as a corticotropin-releasing
    factor, 340
  in diabetes insipidus, 184,186F
  neurophysins and, 157F,158
  in portal blood, 340
  receptors for, 171,173T,174T
  release of, factors affecting,
    174,175T
  somatotropin secretion and, 107
  therapeutic administration of,
    184
Vasopressin, lysine-8, 157F
Vasotocin, 156,157F
Ventromedial nucleus, 57F,
    59F
Vinblastine, as a microtubular
    function inhibitor, 212
VIP (see Vasoactive intestinal
    peptide)

W, Z

Water intake/drinking, 168
  angiotensin levels and, 169
  ECF volume decrease and
    activation of, 168
  factors affecting, 169F
Water retention disorders, 184-188
Water excretion regulation,
    171-174
Wolffian duct system, 270F
Zollinger-Ellison syndrome, 92

About the Author

W. ROY SLAUNWHITE, Jr., is Professor Emeritus of Biochemistry at the State University of New York at Buffalo, where he taught from 1964 to 1987. He also served at SUNY-Buffalo as associate research professor of pediatrics and adjunct associate professor of medical technology. Formerly he conducted biochemical and cancer research at the University of Buffalo and at Roswell Park Memorial Institute in Buffalo. From 1967 to 1969 he was research director of the Medical Foundation of Buffalo and in 1969–1973 he was director of the Endocrine Laboratories at Children's Hospital of Buffalo. The author or coauthor of more than 110 articles and book chapters, he was an editor of the journal *Steroids*, and he previously edited the *Journal of Clinical Endocrinology and Metabolism* and *Journal of Immunoassay* (Marcel Dekker, Inc.). He is a member of the American Society of Biological Chemists and The Endocrine Society. Dr. Slaunwhite received the B.S. (1941), M.S. (1942), and Ph.D. (1948) degrees from the Massachusetts Institute of Technology in Cambridge, and he was a postdoctoral fellow (1952–1953) at the University of Utah Medical School in Salt Lake City.